T0230612

# AIRWAY WALL REMODELLING
# *in* ASTHMA

**Pharmacology and Toxicology: Basic and Clinical Aspects**

Mannfred A. Hollinger, Series Editor
University of California, Davis

**Forthcoming Titles**

*Antibody Therapeutics*, William J. Harris and John R. Adair
*Anabolic Treatment for Osteoporosis*, James F. Whitfield and Paul Morley
*Antisense Oligodeoxynucleotides as Novel Pharmacological
   Therapeutic Agents*, Benjamin Weiss
*Basis to Toxicity Testing, Second Edition*, Donald J. Ecobichon
*CNS Injuries: Cellular Responses and Pharmacological Strategies*, Martin Berry
   and Ann Logan
*Lead and Public Health: Integrated Risk Assessment*, Paul Mushak
*Molecular Bases of Anesthesia*, Eric Moody and Phil Skolnick
*Muscarinic Receptor Subtypes in Smooth Muscle*, Richard M. Eglen
*Receptor Characterization and Regulation*, Devendra K. Agrawal

**Published Titles**

*Inflammatory Cells and Mediators in Bronchial Asthma*, 1990,
   Devendra K. Agrawal and Robert G. Townley
*Pharmacology of the Skin*, 1991, Hasan Mukhtar
In Vitro *Methods of Toxicology*, 1992, Ronald R. Watson
*Basis of Toxicity Testing*, 1992, Donald J. Ecobichon
*Human Drug Metabolism from Molecular Biology to Man*, 1992, Elizabeth Jeffreys
*Platelet Activating Factor Receptor: Signal Mechanisms and Molecular Biology*,
   1992, Shivendra D. Shukla
*Biopharmaceutics of Ocular Drug Delivery*, 1992, Peter Edman
*Beneficial and Toxic Effects of Aspirin*, 1993, Susan E. Feinman
*Preclinical and Clinical Modulation of Anticancer Drugs*, 1993, Kenneth D. Tew,
   Peter Houghton, and Janet Houghton
*Peroxisome Proliferators: Unique Inducers of Drug-Metabolizing Enzymes*, 1994,
David E. Moody
*Angiotensin II Receptors, Volume I: Molecular Biology, Biochemistry,
   Pharmacology, and Clinical Perspectives*, 1994, Robert R. Ruffolo, Jr.
*Angiotensin II Receptors, Volume II: Medicinal Chemistry*, 1994,
   Robert R. Ruffolo, Jr.
*Chemical and Structural Approaches to Rational Drug Design*, 1994,
   David B. Weiner and William V. Williams
*Biological Approaches to Rational Drug Design*, 1994, David B. Weiner and
   William V. Williams

# Pharmacology and Toxicology: Basic and Clinical Aspects

## Published Titles Continued

# AIRWAY WALL REMODELLING
# *in* ASTHMA

*Edited by*

## *Alastair G. Stewart, Ph.D.*

*Chief Scientist, NH&MRC Research Fellow*
*Bernard O'Brien Institute of Microsurgery*
*St. Vincent's Hospital*
*Melbourne, Australia*

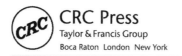

CRC Press
Taylor & Francis Group
Boca Raton  London  New York

CRC Press is an imprint of the
Taylor & Francis Group, an **informa** business

CRC Press
Taylor & Francis Group
6000 Broken Sound Parkway NW, Suite 300
Boca Raton, FL 33487-2742

© 1997 by Taylor & Francis Group, LLC
CRC Press is an imprint of Taylor & Francis Group, an Informa business

**Visit the Taylor & Francis Web site at**
**http://www.taylorandfrancis.com**

**and the CRC Press Web site at**
**http://www.crcpress.com**

*Dedicated to my sons*
*Michael,*
*Iain, and Timothy*

# PREFACE

Asthma is a prevalent disease in which the morbidity and mortality remain unacceptably high, despite apparently effective drug treatment regimens and increasing awareness of the need for better disease management. Hitherto regarded as a disorder of smooth muscle function, asthma is now widely recognised as a chronic inflammatory disease. Nevertheless, the involvement of smooth muscle in the manifestations of the disease should not be overlooked in the enthusiasm to embrace the concept that inflammation is the key feature of pathogenesis. In common with other chronic inflammatory diseases such as rheumatoid arthritis and atherosclerosis, there is a well-documented tissue remodelling process, the functional significance of which is only now emerging.

This book attempts to synthesize recent data and concepts that have been developed to determine the relationship between airway wall remodelling and the pathogenesis of asthma. The consequences of airway wall remodelling for airway hyperresponsiveness is the major focus of this volume. The first chapter reviews evidence for structural changes in asthmatic airways and elucidates the geometrical relationship between airway wall thickening and hyperresponsiveness. The following three chapters describe the relationship between cytokine production in the airways and tissue remodelling associated with inflammation. The significance of epithelial changes and the extracellular matrix are reviewed in the next two chapters. *In vivo* and *in vitro* experimental approaches to the assessment of remodelling are then described. The final two chapters detail the pharmacological and biochemical mechanisms which control smooth muscle cell proliferation.

I thank Mr. Paul Petralia and Mrs. Cindy Carelli of CRC Press for their patience and expert assistance in the preparation of this volume. I also thank Mrs. Joy Rogers for her secretarial assistance. I am deeply indebted to the authors for taking time out of their busy schedules to contribute to this book, which I believe will serve as an interim account of the recent advances in this area of research and catalyse further basic and clinical studies of airway wall remodelling.

Alastair G. Stewart

# THE EDITOR

**Alastair Stewart, Ph.D.,** is a National Health and Medical Research Council (Australia) Research Fellow, Chief Scientist at the Bernard O'Brien Institute of Microsurgery, St. Vincent's Hospital, Melbourne, and a Senior Associate in the Departments of Physiology, Pharmacology, and Surgery at the University of Melbourne.

Dr. Stewart completed his undergraduate and postgraduate training in the Department of Pharmacology, University of Melbourne, receiving his Ph.D. in 1984. After a two-year postdoctoral appointment at the Royal College of Surgeons of England, he returned to the Department of Physiology, University of Melbourne, as a C.R. Roper Research Fellow and in 1990 as a Research Fellow of the NH&MRC (Australia) before taking up his present position in 1992.

Dr. Stewart is a member of the Australasian Society of Clinical and Experimental Pharmacologists and Toxicologists, the British Pharmacological Society, the Australian Physiological and Pharmacological Society, the Australian and New Zealand Microcirculation Society, and the Society for Free Radical Research (Australia). He has presented over 20 lectures at national and international meetings, has given approximately 40 guest lectures at universities and institutes, and has published more than 60 research papers. His current research interests focus on pharmacological modulation of tissue remodelling in chronic inflammation.

# CONTRIBUTORS

**Tony R. Bai, M.D.**
University of British Columbia
  Pulmonary Research Laboratory
St. Paul's Hospital
Vancouver, British Columbia
Canada

**Peter Bradding, D.M.**
University Medicine
Southampton General Hospital
Southampton
United Kingdom

**Roy G. Goldie, Ph.D.**
Department of Pharmacology
University of Western Australia
Perth
Australia

**Stephen T. Holgate, B.Sc, M.D., D.Sc, FRACP**
University Medicine
Southampton General Hospital
Southampton
United Kingdom

**Stuart J. Hirst, Ph.D.**
Respiratory Research Laboratories
UMDS Department of Allergy and
  Respiratory Medicine
St. Thomas' Hospital
London
United Kingdom

**Alan L. James, MBBS, FRACP**
Department of Pulmonary Physiology
Sir Charles Gairdner Hospital
Perth
Australia

**Stephen A. Kilfeather, Ph.D.**
Sackler Institute of Pulmonary
  Pharmacology
Department of Thoracic Medicine
King's College School of Medicine
  and Dentistry
London
United Kingdom

**Xun Li, MBBS, M.D.**
Department of Medicine
Monash Medical School
Alfred Hospital
Prahran
Australia

**James G. Martin, M.D.**
Meakins-Christie Laboratories
McGill University
Montreal, Quebec
Canada

**John C. Marriott, B.Sc.**
Department of Physiology
University of Western Australia
Perth
Australia

**Howard W. Mitchell, Ph.D.**
Department of Physiology
University of Western Australia
Perth
Australia

**Peter K. McFawn, Ph.D.**
Department of Physiology
University of Western Australia
Perth
Australia

**Clive Page, Ph.D.**
Department of Pharmacology
King's College
University of London
London
United Kingdom

**Reynold A. Panettieri, Jr., M.D.**
Pulmonary and Critical Care Division
University of Pennsylvania Medical
  Center
Philadelphia, Pennsylvania

**Janet M. H. Preuss, Ph.D.**
Department of Pharmacology
King's College
University of London
London
United Kingdom

**Anthony E. Redington, D.M.**
University Medicine
Southampton General Hospital
Southampton
United Kingdom

**Leslie Schahte, M.Sc.**
Bernard O'Brien Institute of
  Microsurgery
St. Vincent's Hospital
Victoria
Australia

**Alastair G. Stewart, Ph.D.**
Bernard O'Brien Institute of
  Microsurgery
St. Vincent's Hospital
Victoria
Australia

**Malcolm P. Sparrow, Ph.D.**
Department of Physiology
University of Western Australia
Perth
Australia

**Paul R. Tomlinson, B.Sc.Hons.**
Bernard O'Brien Institute of
  Microsurgery
St. Vincent's Hospital
Victoria
Australia

**John W. Wilson, MBBS, Ph.D.,
FRACP, FCCP**
Department of Medicine
Monash Medical School
Alfred Hospital
Prahran
Australia

# TABLE OF CONTENTS

Chapter 1

# RELATIONSHIP BETWEEN AIRWAY WALL THICKNESS AND AIRWAY HYPERRESPONSIVENESS

Alan L. James

## CONTENTS

0-8493-7813-3/97/$0.00+$.50
© 1997 by CRC Press, Inc.

# I. INTRODUCTION

## A. CLINICAL FINDINGS IN ASTHMA

Patients with asthma report symptoms of variable wheeze, chest tightness, shortness of breath, cough, and sputum production. These symptoms occur either spontaneously or in response to a wide variety of trigger factors, such as allergens, cold or dry air, sulphur dioxide, cigarette smoke, exercise, laughing, coughing, grain dust, isocyanates, and smooth muscle agonists such as methacholine and histamine. Symptoms may occur at night resulting in disturbed sleep and are often at their worst first thing in the morning. Asthma persists over many years while varying in severity, and it can result in chronic airflow obstruction[1] and death.[2] Symptoms are relieved by agents that relax smooth muscle, and treatment with corticosteroids reduces the frequency and severity of symptoms.[3]

## B. PHYSIOLOGY OF ASTHMA

Asthma symptoms are accompanied (usually preceded) by a reduction in airway calibre, most often characterised by physiological measurements, such as the forced expired volume in 1 s ($FEV_1$), peak expiratory flow (PEF), or airway resistance (Raw). During acute exacerbations, lung volumes can increase markedly;[4,5] however, lung parenchymal recoil is usually normal.[6-8] Changes in airway calibre are associated with uneven distribution of ventilation throughout the lungs, resulting in reduced gas exchange and hypoxia.[9-11]

Compared with nonasthmatic subjects, patients with asthma have exaggerated airway responses to inhaled smooth muscle agonists such as methacholine and histamine. This has been characterised most often as increased *sensitivity* of the airways — same response at a lower dose[12,13] — but also as increased *reactivity* — greater increment of response per increment of dose.[14,15] With the recognition that airway narrowing is limited in nonasthmatic subjects and is excessive in asthmatic subjects,[16,17] it became clear that *increased maximal airway narrowing* (Figure 1) is the physiologically important abnormality in asthma, although in population studies maximal airway narrowing correlates with both sensitivity and reactivity.[18]

It seems likely, although remains to be proved, that the presence of chronic airway inflammation in asthma results in a change in airway wall structure, and possibly mechanical properties, leading to the development of excessive airway narrowing, symptoms, increased airway responsiveness, chronic airflow obstruction, and, in some cases, death.

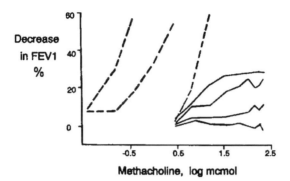

**FIGURE 1** Change in $FEV_1$, as a percent of baseline, in response to increasing doses of inhaled methacholine in selected subjects from a general population. Subjects who did not report asthma symptoms (solid lines) show limited maximal airway narrowing with flat dose–response curves shifted to the right. Subjects reporting asthma symptoms (dashed lines) have steep dose–response curves shifted to the left and do not reach a plateau within the constraints of the test. (From James, A. L. et al., *Am. Rev. Respir. Dis.*, 146, 895, 1992. With permission.)

## C. PATHOLOGY OF ASTHMA

Fatal asthma has long been characterised pathologically by airway wall inflammation with the infiltration of eosinophils, lymphocytes, mast cells, and plasma cells, increased amount of airway smooth muscle, plugging of airways with mucus, epithelial desquamation, "basement membrane" thickening, enlargement of mucous glands, and thickening of the airway wall.[19-35] Studies of airways from patients with asthma who have died of other causes or who have undergone lung resection have shown similar, although usually less severe, pathological changes.[23,24,36] The use of bronchial wall biopsy has shown that even in mild cases of asthma there is infiltration with eosinophils, lymphocytes, plasma cells, and mast cells,[37-50] thickening of the sub-basement membrane connective tissue,[25,45,51,52] possible epithelial disruption,[25,29,42,45,53,54] and goblet cell hyperplasia.[24,55] Bronchial biopsy and bronchoalveolar lavage studies have demonstrated that eosinophils and lymphocytes are recruited into the airway wall, where they are activated, releasing cytokines and other cell products which amplify the inflammatory response[39,46,56-58] and result in tissue damage.[59] Exposure to allergen[47,60-62] or occupational agents[63-67] will induce airway inflammation, and treatment with corticosteroids reduces the number of inflammatory cells in the airway wall.[68-73] What initiates the generally sustained, yet variable, airway inflammation in any individual and how this might be prevented or turned off remain to be determined.

## II. THEORETICAL CONSIDERATIONS

In 1971 Folkow[74] discussed the mechanical implications of adaptive structural changes in blood vessels in relation to systemic hypertension. A year later Freedman[75] used a similar theoretical approach to suggest that airway wall thickening in the presence of modest degrees of airway smooth muscle contraction could account for the wheezing and airway hyperresponsiveness that is observed in asthma. In 1985 Macklem[76] drew attention to the apparent paradox that, while airway narrowing is limited in nonasthmatic subjects *in vivo*,[16,17] *in vitro*, maximally stimulated airway smooth muscle has the ability to shorten by as much as 80% of its optimal relaxed length.[77] This degree of shortening of smooth muscle around the circumference of an airway should invariably cause airway closure. He suggested that powerful factors must act *in vivo* to limit airway narrowing in the nonasthmatic subject and that loss or alteration of these factors may result in excessive airway narrowing. He proposed that uncoupling of the contracting forces of stimulated smooth muscle from the surrounding distending forces of the parenchyma may be an important mechanism which could result in excessive airway narrowing.

Moreno et al.[78] described a multitude of factors which could modulate the change in airway resistance that occurs in response to an inhaled smooth muscle agonist. These factors include (1) those that might modulate the degree to which an inhaled agent is able to reach and activate smooth muscle, (2) those that modulate the amount that smooth muscle can shorten once it has been stimulated, (3) those that alter the amount of luminal narrowing that occurs as smooth muscle shortens, and (4) those that determine the change in pulmonary resistance that occurs as a result of the series and parallel changes in resistance of the elements of the bronchial tree and parenchyma (Table 1).

## TABLE 1
### Factors Affecting the Increase in Airway Resistance after Inhalation of a Bronchoconstricting Agent

Stimulus inhaled
↓      Deposition, mucociliary clearance, airway permeability, bronchial circulation, tissue enzymes, agonist-receptor interactions

Muscle stimulation
↓      Muscle contractility, length-tension characteristics, muscle bulk, tissue deformability, surface tension forces, lung parenchymal recoil, mucosal folding, cartilage stiffness

Muscle shortening
↓      Muscle orientation, surface liquid, wall thickness, mucus deposition

Lumen narrowing
↓      Flow regime, distribution of narrowed airways, parenchymal resistance

Increased pulmonary resistance

A vast amount of work has been undertaken to test the many hypotheses that were raised by Macklem[76] and Moreno et al.[78] in relation to factors affecting airway function in asthma and COPD. In this chapter, discussion will

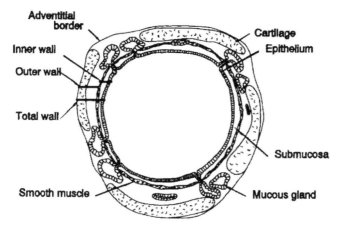

**FIGURE 2**  Airway structures and compartments (see Reference 79). In this chapter the *submucosa* will refer to the area of tissue between the basement membrane and the smooth muscle.

be related predominantly to factors affecting the thickness of the airway wall or the area of its structural components and the likely mechanical consequences. The compartments of the airway wall (Figure 2) will be those previously described.[79] The inner wall area includes the surface liquid, the epithelium, the basement membrane, the lamina propria, the submucosa, and, in this review, the airway smooth muscle. The outer wall area includes the airway wall from the outer border of the smooth muscle to the adventitial surface of the airway. It includes the mucous glands and the cartilage in the larger airways.

# III. QUANTITATIVE STUDIES OF AIRWAY WALL STRUCTURE

There have been a number of studies[19,23,26,28,30,31,34-36,80,81] undertaken which quantitatively compare airway structure in asthmatic and nonasthmatic subjects and allow the estimation of likely effects on airway function. These are summarised in Table 2. The methodology in these studies varies with respect to subject characteristics, the definition of disease, fixation of tissue, sampling of airways, staining and measurement of airway structures, analysis of data, and expression of results.

## A. COMPARISON OF QUANTITATIVE STUDIES — METHODOLOGY

Since airway dimensions will vary with airway size, it is important to ensure that airways are matched by size when comparing results from different subjects and from different studies. First, a reliable measure of airway size is needed. Markers of size, such as area of cartilage[26] or airway diameters,[30] are confounded by variability in the first instance or by artefact due to varying

## TABLE 2
## Quantitative Studies of Airway Wall Thickness and Area
## of Airway Wall Components

| Subjects | Airways | Measurements | Ref. |
|---|---|---|---|
| 6 fatal asthma; 7 controls | Central and peripheral; matched by outer diameter | Total wall thickness; mucous gland, eptihelial and subepithelial thickness | 30 |
| 12 fatal asthma; 11 controls | Segmental; matched by cartilage area | Percent of wall muscle, mucous gland, connective tissue | 26 |
| 4 "asthmatic bronchitis" with nonasthma deaths; 3 fatal asthma; control — historic | Left and right main bronchi and lobar bronchi | Percent of wall muscle, connective tissue, mucous gland; Reid index | 35 |
| 5 fatal asthma; 5 controls | LLL[a] bronchus, LLL posterior segment bronchus | Muscle area; number of muscle nuclei | 28 |
| 6 nonfatal asthma; 7 controls | Lobar bronchi, 10 parenchymal sections | Basement membrane thickness; percent of mucous gland, muscle | 36 |
| 18 asthma — 15 fatal asthma, 3 nonfatal asthma; 23 controls | Peripheral and central; matched by perimeter at epithelium | Inner wall area; areas of epithelium, muscle and submucosa | 31 |
| 16 fatal asthma; 13 COPD; 20 controls | Peripheral and central; matched by perimeter at basement membrane | Average thickness of muscle | 80 |
| 6 fatal asthma; 6 controls | Peripheral; matched by perimeter at epithelium | Total wall thickness; percent muscle; percent occlusion of lumen with mucus | 34 |
| 8 fatal asthma — 3 sudden, 5 slow and progressive; 4 controls | Peripheral and central; matched by perimeter at basement membrane | Percent of lumen occupied by mucus; percent mucous gland and goblet cells; thickness of epithelium | 19 |
| 11 fatal asthma; 13 nonfatal asthma; 11 controls | Peripheral and central; matched by perimeter at basement membrane | Wall areas — total, inner and outer; areas of cartilage, mucous gland and muscle; percent epithelial damage | 23 |
| 8 fatal asthma; 7 nonfatal asthma; 15 controls | Peripheral; matched by perimeter at basement membrane | Wall areas — outer and inner; areas of muscle and submucosa | 81 |

[a]  LLL, left lower lobe.

lung inflation or smooth muscle shortening in the latter. The use of the epithelial (internal perimeter — Pi) or basement membrane perimeter (Pbm) on transverse sections of airways has been validated as a marker of airway size that is independent of lung volume and smooth muscle shortening.[82-84]

Second, it is important to have a representative number of small and large airways to compare between subjects. Ideally, one should sample the same number of airways of the same size from each subject. This is rarely possible; however, where whole lungs are available, a standard sampling technique can be used to obtain similar numbers of large and small airways.[23] In studies where whole lungs are not available and where sampling is less than complete, the distribution of airway sizes from each subject may be very different. Where uniform sampling is not possible, a variety of analyses[85] can be used, depending upon the spread of the data obtained. These include crude pooling of the data, calculating the mean value of the means of each subject, and plotting airway dimensions against airway size for each case to obtain a slope and intercept of the fitted regression line. Using the latter approach, the data can then be combined to obtain the most representative regression equation to describe the relationship between airway size and airway dimensions for a group of asthmatic (fatal or nonfatal) or control subjects. This results in the mean data for a group of subjects being described in terms of mean slopes and intercepts.[81]

To summarise the data from the studies in Table 2, airways have been separated into four size groups defined by internal perimeter:[31] <2 mm — small membranous bronchioles; 2–4 mm — large membranous bronchioles; 4–10 mm — small cartilaginous bronchi; >10 mm — large cartilaginous bronchi. The median values of the internal perimeters for these size groups (1.5, 2.8, 7.3, 15 mm) were used to derive average values for airway dimensions in each size group.

Given that optimal sampling or statistical techniques have not been used in all of these studies, the crudely grouped data or interpolation of the linearised data has been used to calculate average airway dimensions for the airway size groups above. Lastly, in order to examine the qualitative trends of airway dimensions in asthma relative to control cases, airway dimensions of subjects with asthma have been expressed as the average percentage changes with reference to the control cases in each study.

## B.  INNER WALL AREA

Three studies[23,31,81] have measured the inner wall area in asthma (Table 3). Two of these studies included cases of nonfatal asthma,[23,81] and the study of Kuwano et al.[81] included only membranous airways. The epithelium was not included in the measurement of inner wall area in the study of Kuwano et al.[81] because of its variable loss from the basement membrane. In the other two studies, if more than 25% of the basement membrane was covered by epithelium, the internal perimeter was measured by extrapolating the epithelial surface between intact areas of epithelium. This was shown to be highly reproducible. The exclusion or inclusion of the thickness of the epithelium will result in variations in wall thickness which will be relatively greater in the peripheral airways, where the epithelium makes up a larger proportion of the airway wall (see below). However, the qualitative differences between asthmatic and nonasthmatic cases are likely to be the same.

## TABLE 3
### Inner Wall Area in Cases of Asthma
### (Percent Change from Control Cases)

|          | Membranous | | Cartilaginous | |
|----------|------------|-----------|------------|-----------|
|          | Small      | Large     | Small      | Large     |
| Fatal    | 64[a]      | 146       | 280        | 80        |
|          | (55–95)    | (133–162) | (258–302)  | (41–119)  |
| Nonfatal | 48         | 38        | 120        | 20        |
|          | (33–64)    | (24–52)   | —          | —         |

[a]  Mean (range).

## C. OUTER WALL AREA

Only two studies[23,81] have compared the wall area from the smooth muscle to the adventitial surface in asthmatic and nonasthmatic cases, and the data are shown separately in Table 4. The study of Carroll et al.[23] included large airways.

## TABLE 4
### Outer Wall Area in Cases of Asthma
### (Percent Change from Control Cases)

|          | Membranous | | Cartilaginous | |
|----------|------------|----------|------------|----------|
|          | Small      | Large    | Small      | Large    |
| Fatal    | 85, 91     | 93, 156  | 105        | 41       |
| Nonfatal | −11, 51    | 21, 60   | 38         | 7        |

## D. TOTAL WALL AREA

Four studies[23,30,34,81] have examined the entire wall area in asthmatic and nonasthmatic subjects (Table 5), although only two included large airways.[23,30]

## TABLE 5
### Total Wall Area in Cases of Asthma
### (Percent Change from Control Cases)

|          | Membranous | | Cartilaginous | |
|----------|------------|-----------|------------|----------|
|          | Small      | Large     | Small      | Large    |
| Fatal    | 72         | 108       | 80, 157    | 44, 57   |
|          | (45–100)   | (46–231)  | —          | —        |
| Nonfatal | 95         | 17        | 68         | 2        |
|          | (−7–102)   | (2–32)    | —          | —        |

## E. EPITHELIUM

The area of epithelium has been compared between asthmatic and nonasthmatic cases in transverse sections of large and small airways in only one study.[31] Compared with control cases, the area of epithelium in cases of asthma was increased in all airway sizes: small membranous bronchioles 67%, large membranous bronchioles 126%, small cartilaginous airways 156%, and large cartilaginous airways 57%. There have also been a number of quantitative studies of airway epithelial integrity and damage in asthmatic and nonasthmatic cases. Bronchial biopsy studies have shown increased epithelial damage in asthma,[86] although this was not seen in all studies.[45,54] Using a semiquantitative method in cases seen at autopsy, no differences were found in epithelial damage or desquamation between nonasthmatic cases and cases of fatal and nonfatal asthma.[23] Omari et al.[87] showed a correlation between epithelial damage and *in vitro* responsiveness in human bronchial segments, suggesting that the epithelium acts as a barrier to limit access to the smooth muscle of stimulants applied via the airway lumen. Epithelial damage measured by bronchial biopsy has been related to *in vivo* airway responsiveness in some studies,[45] but not in others.[86]

## F. SMOOTH MUSCLE

There have been nine studies[23,26,28,30,31,35,36,81,88] which have quantitatively compared the areas of smooth muscle in asthmatic and nonasthmatic cases (Table 6), mostly in fatal cases, but some studies have included nonfatal cases.[23,31,36,81]

### TABLE 6
### Smooth Muscle Area in Cases of Asthma
### (Percent Change from Control Cases)

|  | Membranous | | Cartilaginous | |
|---|---|---|---|---|
|  | Small | Large | Small | Large |
| Fatal | 48 | 152 | 230 | 185 |
|  | (7–123) | (62–269) | (140–378) | (108–267) |
| Nonfatal | 25 | 162 | 43 | 50 |
|  | (14–36) | (83–108) | — | (44–55) |

In the study of Ebina et al.[88] membranous and cartilaginous airways were examined in control cases and cases of fatal asthma. They observed that in some of their cases of asthma the area of smooth muscle was increased in both the large and small airways and that in others the increase in area of smooth muscle was confined to the central airways.

## G. MUCOUS GLANDS

Five studies[19,23,26,35,36] of mucous gland area in asthma have been undertaken. In cases of fatal asthma the average increase in mucous gland area compared with controls was 151% (61–285%) and in nonfatal cases was 25%

(22–27%). Extraparenchymal cartilaginous airways were predominantly examined, although in some studies any airway containing cartilage or glands was included. This could result in bias if mucous glands are present in a greater number of distal (smaller) airways in patients with asthma than in control cases. This would result in an underestimation of the average area of mucous glands in central airways for cases of asthma. It is unknown if the distribution of mucous glands down the bronchial tree changes in asthma.

## H. CARTILAGE

The area of cartilage in the airway wall of patients with asthma has been measured in only a few studies,[23,26,35] and there are few data regarding the distribution of cartilage down the bronchial tree in asthma. The data derived from each study are presented separately in Table 7 since there is a wide range of results. Only the study of Carroll et al.[23] showed an increase in the area of cartilage in asthma.

### TABLE 7
#### Cartilage Gland Area in Cases of Asthma
#### (Percent Change from Control Cases)

|          | Cartilaginous | |
|----------|-------|-------|
|          | Small | Large |
| Fatal    | 283   | −3    |
|          | —     | (−14–27) |
| Nonfatal | 53    | 10    |

## I. SUB-BASEMENT MEMBRANE CONNECTIVE TISSUE

Early studies noted that thickening of the basement membrane was a characteristic feature of asthma,[26,29,30] although not confined to this disease.[89] It was later confirmed that, in fact, the basement membrane, or lamina reticularis, is not thicker in cases of asthma but that there is substantial deposition of collagen types II and V and fibronectin beneath the basement membrane giving rise to the thickened appearance on light microscopy.[51] A number of studies have measured the thickness of the connective tissue below the basement membrane in cases of nonfatal, generally mild asthma.[25,45,51,52,69] These show an increased thickness of 60 and 90% compared with control cases. The increased thickness of the basement membrane in cases of fatal asthma has been invariably commented on, but infrequently measured. In the study of Huber and Koessler[30] the thickness of the basement membrane in cases of fatal asthma was similar to that seen in the cases of nonfatal asthma.

## J. BLOOD VESSELS

There are few published quantitative studies of blood vessels within the airway walls of asthmatic and nonasthmatic subjects. Using bronchial biopsy,

Beasley et al.[47] found similar numbers of submucosal blood vessels in asthmatic (mean 142, range 108–171 vessels/mm$^2$) and nonasthmatic (123, 106–135) subjects. Saetta et al.[34] examined the muscular arteries adjacent to membranous bronchioles in cases of fatal asthma. They found them to be of similar thickness to those in control cases, despite infiltration of inflammatory cells, predominantly into the vessel wall adjacent to the airway wall. Kuwano et al.[81] measured the number and areas of blood vessels in the adventitia and submucosa of membranous bronchioles in cases of asthma (fatal and nonfatal) and compared them with control cases. They found that although numbers per area of tissue were similar, the area (as a percent of tissue area, mean ± SD) was increased in asthma, both in the adventitia (12 ± 8% vs. 8 ± 4%) and in the submucosa (3 ± 1% vs. 1 ± 1%). These findings suggest that congestion of blood vessels is present in cases of asthma. These data are supported by recent preliminary findings from other laboratories.[90,91]

## K. DISCUSSION

In the studies examined above there were differences between cases with respect to cause of death, treatments, atopy, age, smoking habits, and severity and duration of disease. However, some consistencies appear among the studies. By definition, the cases of fatal asthma were severe and, in most cases, other contributing causes of death, such as heart disease and infection, had been excluded. In nearly all fatal cases there was a long history of persistent severe symptoms and requirement for regular treatment with inhaled and oral corticosteroids. The qualitative pathological findings were consistent with regard to mucus plugging, sub-basement membrane thickening, and infiltration of the airway wall with lymphocytes and eosinophils. The cases of nonfatal asthma tended to vary more in duration and frequency of symptoms and treatments administered, but in general they could be regarded as cases of mild to moderate asthma requiring treatment usually with inhaled β-agonists, occasionally with inhaled corticosteroids, but rarely with oral corticosteroids.

The differences in airway dimensions between case groups were consistent among studies except for areas of cartilage. Compared with nonasthmatic subjects, wall areas (inner, outer, and total) were increased from 50 to 300% in cases of fatal asthma and from 10 to 100% in cases of nonfatal asthma. In cases of fatal asthma, the thickening of the airway walls was most marked in the small cartilaginous airways and large membranous airways corresponding to internal diameters ranging from approximately 1–3 mm; however, significant differences were seen in all airway sizes. In cases of nonfatal asthma, the thickening of the airway walls was most marked in the small membranous airways (diameter <0.6 mm) and midsized airways (diameter 1–3 mm) and was much less marked in the central airways, in contrast to the fatal cases. These findings show that the increase in inner and outer airway wall thickness in asthma is related to severity and suggest that the increase in severity is associated with increased thickening of the midsized airways (1–3 mm diameter) and involvement of the large central airways.

The studies of airway wall components showed a consistent increase in the area of smooth muscle area ranging from 50 to 230% of control values in cases of fatal asthma and from 25 to 150% in cases of nonfatal asthma. The changes were most marked in central airways in cases of fatal asthma and in the large membranous bronchioles in cases of nonfatal asthma. The differences between the nonfatal and fatal cases with regard to smooth muscle were greatest in the cartilaginous airways. The area of mucous gland was increased in asthma, particularly in the fatal cases. In cases of asthma, epithelial damage was variable and subject to artefact due to post-mortem change or biopsy trauma; however, the area of the epithelium was increased. The data regarding the area of cartilage in cases of asthma are less consistent than for other airway wall structures.

In summary, the quantitative studies show that the increase in airway wall thickness that is present in asthma involves the inner wall *and* the outer wall and that all the components of the airway wall (with the possible exception of the cartilage) are involved. The degree to which the thickness of the airway wall is increased and the site (central or peripheral) where most of these changes occur appear to be related to the severity of the asthma.

## II. MODELLING THE EFFECTS OF AIRWAY STRUCTURE ON FUNCTION

The potential effects of the structural changes observed in asthma on airway function have been examined, in degrees of increasing complexity, using mathematical models. These models incorporate morphological and physiological measurements made in asthmatic and nonasthmatic tissues and include a number of assumptions regarding variables (and their interactions) which cannot or have not been measured.

The usefulness of these models lies in their ability to examine the effect of changing variables in isolation to assess, semiquantitatively, the likely effects of altered structure. The complexity of the models increases markedly if multiple variables are included and if allowance is made for the magnitude of the variables to change within the computations of the model.

### A. AIRWAY WALL THICKNESS

Freedman[75] and Moreno et al.[78] showed theoretically that increased airway wall thickness inside the smooth muscle layer will result in excessive airway luminal narrowing as smooth muscle shortens. Moreno et al.[78] formulated the relationship between the changes in airway resistance ($\Delta R$), relative to an arbitrary baseline value, the proportion of muscle shortening (PMS), the proportion of muscle in the airway perimeter (PMP), and the wall thickness of an observed airway (PW) relative to the wall thickness in the normal state (PWn):

$$\Delta R = \left( \sqrt{\left( (1 - \text{PMP} \times \text{PMS})^2 - \text{PW} \right)} \Big/ \sqrt{(1 - \text{PWn})} \right)^{-4}$$

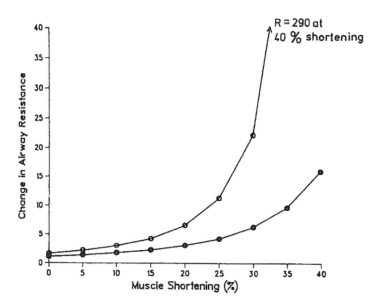

**FIGURE 3**  Calculated changes in airway resistance as airway smooth muscle shortens around an airway with an average inner wall area derived from control cases (closed circles) or from cases of fatal asthma (open symbols). (From James, A. L. et al., *Am. Rev. Respir. Dis.*, 139, 242, 1989. With permission.)

This formula allows simple calculations of the effects of increased inner wall thickness on resistance to flow through single airways, relative to control airways. Using data from nonasthmatic cases and from cases of predominantly fatal asthma, we showed that "usual" amounts of smooth muscle shortening (as much as 40% of fully relaxed, distended circumferential length) would result in a maximum 15-times increase in resistance in nonasthmatic airways and 290-times increase in resistance in asthmatic airways (Figure 3).[31] Interestingly, the 15-times increase in resistance is similar to the maximum increase in pulmonary resistance seen *in vivo* after challenge with methacholine.[92] It should also be noted that the increased inner wall area seen in subjects with asthma has a negligible effect on airway resistance in the absence of smooth muscle shortening — the baseline resistance. Therefore, the increased airway wall thickness (due to inflammation) will not be apparent functionally until airway smooth muscle shortening occurs. These calculations demonstrate that altered airway structure, occurring as a result of airway inflammation, may itself account for the excessive airway narrowing in asthma.

Wiggs et al.[93] developed a model based on that of Moreno et al.,[78] but which included morphometric measurements of normal airway diameters and lengths[94] and a dynamic component[95] so that the effects of various changes in airway structure on total pulmonary resistance could be assessed. Using data obtained from cases of asthma, the model showed that thickening of the inner airway wall resulted in excessive airway narrowing with smooth muscle shortening of as much as 40%, as noted above, and that the effects of increased wall thickness were greater if they were present in the peripheral airways.[96] In another study[97] using the same model, it was shown that increased inner airway wall area will also account for the increased bronchodilator response seen in patients with asthma. Increased thickness of the airway wall may have other effects, including altered permeability and altered mechanical properties which could decrease or increase the loads opposing muscle thickening (see below).

The model of Wiggs et al.[97] also showed that thickness of the increased outer wall could result in uncoupling of airway smooth muscle from the distending loads imposed by the elastic recoil of the lung parenchyma. This could occur in two ways. First, if the outer wall expanded as the smooth muscle contracted, then the expected increase in elastic load imparted by the surrounding lung parenchyma would be less. Second, if the parenchymal recoil forces are distributed over a greater airway adventitial surface area, the stress (force/area) transferred to the smooth muscle will be less. Both of these mechanisms will tend to allow more airway narrowing when the smooth muscle is stimulated. The reduction in total airway wall stress could account for the bronchoconstriction that occurs after a deep inspiration in some patients with asthma.[98-100] It will tend to exaggerate the reduction in loads opposing smooth muscle shortening that occurs as lung volume decreases after a deep inspiration. This will tend to reduce airway hysteresis, relative to parenchymal hysteresis, and result in bronchoconstriction.

## B. OTHER PROPERTIES OF THE AIRWAY WALL
## RELATED TO STRUCTURE

The discussion above and the effects of airway wall thickness derived from models are predominantly related to the space-occupying effect of increased airway wall thickness. However, a number of other factors need to be considered when trying to estimate the likely effects of increased airway wall thickness on luminal cross-sectional area as smooth muscle shortens.

### 1. Factors Affecting Stimulation and Contraction
### of Smooth Muscle

The factors that alter airway smooth muscle stimulation relate to delivery of the stimulus, its deposition in the bronchial tree, its access to airway smooth muscle, its half-life in the bronchial wall, and agonist–receptor interactions. These factors may be altered indirectly by changes in the airway wall thickness. The permeability of the airways is said to be increased in asthma in some studies,[101] but not in others.[102] These studies have difficulty in separating the permeability of the parenchyma and the airways. There are a number of animal studies that have shown increased penetration of macromolecules into the airway wall following tissue injury.[103,104] On the other hand, it has been shown that increased mucous secretions will reduce access of stimuli to the airway smooth muscle and result in reduced airway responsiveness to inhaled agonists.[105] Loss of, or damage to, the epithelium will reduce wall thickness on the one hand but may allow increased access of stimuli to airway smooth muscle on the other.[87] Little is known about the relative permeabilities of the epithelium and submucosa in asthma.

There are large capacitance blood vessels present in the nasal submucosa,[106] and these can cause significant obstruction in their own right. Although the morphometric data above suggest that submucosal vascular congestion occurs in asthma, capacitance vessels have not been reported. However, changes in the bronchial circulation may alter the strength and duration of an inhaled stimulus.[107] More data are required on the dynamic changes that occur in the submucosal bronchial wall vessels in asthma.

### 2. Inhomogeneity of the Bronchial Tree

Most models of the bronchial tree use a symmetrically dichotomous branching system as described by Weibel,[94] assigning mean values for airway dimensions (length, diameter) at each generation. This greatly simplifies the calculation required to examine the effects of disease at different levels of the bronchial tree on changes in airway resistance as smooth muscle shortens. However, the branching of the bronchial tree in humans is asymmetric as described by Horsfield and Cumming,[108] giving not only a range of airway dimensions at each generation (or order), but also a range of path lengths from central to peripheral airways. Assuming that the dimensions and properties of airway generations are uniform may be misleading, and a much greater range of values for airway resistances and airway responsiveness can be estimated if the inhomogeneities of the bronchial tree are taken into account.[109] The inhomogeneity of the bronchial tree will also be important when considering airway responses to, and the distribution of, externally applied stimuli.

The bronchial tree varies not only in terms of airway segments in parallel, but also in terms of airways in series. The changes in airway structure that occur as one moves from the central to peripheral airways include reduced absolute amount of tissue, such as cartilage, muscle, mucous gland, and connective tissue; increased thickness of the airway wall relative to total airway cross-sectional area; increased relative thickness of the epithelium and decreased relative thickness of the submucosa and adventitia; increased relative thickness of smooth muscle down to the respiratory bronchioles, after which the smooth muscle becomes increasingly sparse; and reduced numbers of submucosal and adventitial blood vessels. From these anatomic observations it is to be expected that in individual airways any increase in wall area will have a relatively greater effect in the peripheral airways compared with the central airways. This will include fluid or mucus on the airway surface. We have seen that in modelling studies,[96,97] if all airways in a generation of the bronchial tree are affected equally by changes in structure, the changes in function that result will be greater if those structural changes occur in the peripheral airways than if they occur in the central airways. However, the exponential increase in the number of airway segments, and therefore the cross-sectional area of the bronchial tree, as one moves towards the periphery of the lung means that a very large number of peripheral airways must have structural alterations before this is detected as a change in airway function measured at the mouth as $FEV_1$ or airway resistance. This has long been recognised with regard to the small airway disease in smokers.[110,111]

## 3. Loads Opposing Airway Smooth Muscle Shortening

When smooth muscle shortens in the airway wall it does not do so isotonically,[112] since the loads opposing shortening change during the process of smooth muscle shortening. Lambert et al.[113] showed that the tension (TN) that smooth muscle must develop to shorten is a resultant of a number of forces (Figure 4). The passive tension (Pp) within the tissues of the airway wall (including the smooth muscle) tends to narrow the airway, except at very small lung volumes. As the smooth muscle develops tension, it initially unloads the passive wall tension. As smooth muscle shortening increases and the airway wall becomes compressed, Pp becomes a tension that tends to dilate the airway and increases rapidly as the smooth muscle shortens. The static elastic recoil of the lung parenchyma $(P_L)$, which is critically related to lung volume, and the forces required to distort the lung parenchyma around the airway $(\Delta P)$ must be overcome to allow muscle shortening. Figure 4 shows that the importance of these three forces varies as smooth muscle shortens and that, between 40–60% muscle shortening, TN changes direction — that is, *less* tension is needed to shorten the muscle. This represents a potentially hazardous situation!

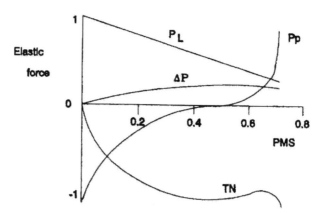

FIGURE 4  The changing elastic forces against which airway smooth muscle must develop tension as it shortens. Positive forces are those tending to open the airway and negative forces are those tending to narrow the airway. Pp is the force required to distort the airway wall tissue, $P_L$ is force opposing the passive elastic recoil of the lung parenchyma, $\Delta P$ is the force required to distort the lung parenchyma around the airway and TN is the total tension in the smooth muscle. PMS = proportion of muscle shortening. (From Lambert, R. K. et al., *J. Appl. Physiol.*, 74, 2771, 1993. With permission.)

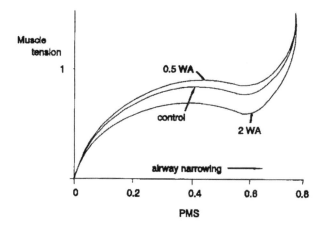

**FIGURE 5** Muscle tension in arbitrary units against proportion of muscle shortening (PMS). For any given PMS the tension that needs to be developed by the smooth muscle is less in an airway where the outer wall area (WAo) is increased. (From Lambert, R. K. et al., *J. Appl. Physiol.*, 74, 2771, 1993. With permission.)

The same model also showed that, for any degree of muscle shortening, the total tension in the smooth muscle was less in airways with increased outer wall thickness (Figure 5). Finally, the model showed that the increased thickness in the airway smooth muscle may be the most important determinant of maximal airway narrowing in asthma. However, the morphometric measurements of airway wall thickness used in this model did not include the epithelium, which makes up a greater proportion of the submucosa in peripheral vs. central airways. This may have led to an overestimation of the importance of smooth muscle thickness in determining maximal airway narrowing. In addition, the mechanical forces required to buckle the epithelium were not included, and this will similarly alter the results. As in other studies the model again shows that increased airway wall thickness results in increased maximal airway narrowing.

In the model described above, the mechanical properties of the airway wall tissues were inferred from studies of isolated, usually normal tissues.[114] There are a number of reasons why the mechanical properties of the airway wall might be different from those assumed. The increased deposition of collagen beneath the basement membrane that is seen in asthma[51] might increase the stiffness of airway wall tissue and oppose both narrowing and distension of the airway wall.[115] On the other hand, release of inflammatory products might decrease tissue elastance[116] and increase the ability of stimulated muscle to shorten.[117] Reduced stiffness will decrease the loads opposing smooth muscle shortening.[82,118] Increased cartilage area may add to airway wall thickness but may also add to airway wall stiffness and, therefore, reduce responsiveness.

It is clear that modelling studies are useful in examining the possible effects of elastic loads and altered airway structure on airway narrowing and point to areas of interest that can be tested in the laboratory. However, more studies of the effects of inflammation on airway tissue matrix and the mechanical properties of asthmatic and normal tissues are required.

### 4. Folding of the Airway Mucosa

In order for the airway lumen to narrow, the mucosa must buckle and fold. The forces required to achieve this are to some extent determined by tissue properties as discussed above and by the number of folds that occur in the mucosa around the airway perimeter.[119] Lambert calculated that a reduced number of folds would result in an increased narrowing response in a stimulated airway. Little is known about the factors that determine how many folds occur, how changes in airway wall thickness might affect folding, and whether or not the number of folds differs in asthmatic and nonasthmatic subjects. Preliminary work suggests that the number of folds is similar.[120] Further calculations have shown that the increased thickness of the folding mucosa in asthma may increase the stiffness of the airway wall to a greater extent than the decrease in stiffness that will occur because of a decrease in the number of folds.[121]

### 5. Effects of Fluid and Mucus on the Airway Surface

In most models of airway narrowing the effects of surface lining fluid and mucus have not been included. This is partly because trying to include their effects greatly adds to the complexity of the model and partly because there is little quantitative data regarding the thickness of the fluid and mucus in nonasthmatic and asthmatic subjects during life and how it behaves as airways narrow. The amount of mucus on the surface of the airway is difficult to measure because of problems of fixation and staining. Mucus also may move centrally or peripherally at the time of death or be pushed peripherally by fixative fluids instilled into the airway. Aikawa et al.[19] studied the amount of the lumen area (calculated relaxed dimensions) that was occupied by mucus in cases of asthma and control cases after lungs were fixed only by immersion. In central airways they found this to be 15% in cases dying shortly after coming to hospital, 5% in cases dying after some weeks in hospital, and <1% in control cases. Values were similar in peripheral airways. We recently calculated the maximum area that mucus might occupy in the airway lumen, assuming that the entire area of submucosal mucous gland could be transferred to the lumen.[122] This gave a figure of 6% occupation of the airway lumen in nonfatal asthma and 12% in fatal asthma, compared with 3% in control cases. This amount of mucus in the lumen will exaggerate airway narrowing as smooth muscle shortens and might greatly increase the contribution of the central airways to increased resistance to flow in asthma.

Liquid on the airway surface may have other functional effects. Yager et al.[123] demonstrated that by filling the interstices and folds of the airway, surface liquid will reduce the cross-sectional area of the lumen, amplifying the effect of smooth muscle shortening. They also showed that inflammatory products are likely to increase the surface tension of the air–liquid interface and add to the forces tending to narrow the airway. The magnitude of these effects *in vivo* in humans has not been studied.

## V. CLINICAL IMPLICATIONS

It can be seen from Figure 6 that changes in airway wall thickness may be used to explain how airway inflammation results in the clinical manifestations and the responses to treatment that are seen in asthma. Airway A represents a relaxed airway from a nonasthmatic subject with an arbitary resistance of 1. It can respond to a variety of bronchoconstricting stimuli, but since maximal airway smooth muscle shortening is usually limited (in this case to 40% of relaxed length) so that only a 14-times increase in resistance is possible (B), despite increasing doses of inhaled agonist, a plateau response is observed (see Figure 1). Therefore, symptoms of chest tightness, wheeze, and shortness of breath do not occur. In the presence of airway inflammation the airway becomes thickened as in C, although in the relaxed state there is little change in airway resistance — 1.4 times normal. However, if the airway smooth muscle shortens to the same extent as in B (40%) in response to a bronchoconstricting stimulus, excessive airway narrowing results with a nonphysiological 75-times increase in airway resistance (D). Increased thickness of the outer wall might also allow the smooth muscle to be uncoupled from the distending forces of the surrounding tissues. This may allow smooth muscle shortening of 40% to occur more readily, i.e., with less tension development, or may allow increased maximal smooth muscle shortening to occur. These events will give rise to wheeze, shortness of breath, and chest tightness, symptoms that can be relieved temporarily by a bronchodilator. The greater the thickening of the airway wall, the more likely that excessive airway narrowing will occur when smooth muscle is stimulated. That is, symptoms will be more readily produced, even by stimuli that may not usually cause symptoms. Therefore, the airways will appear to be "twitchy" and responsive to a greater range of stimuli.

Treatment of the airway inflammation with corticosteroids reduces airway inflammation and may, therefore, result in thinning of the airway walls, reduced airway responsiveness, and resolution of symptoms. The degree of reversibility of airway wall thickening will presumably be related to the structural changes. Cellular infiltration and oedema may be reversible within hours, whereas the accumulation of mucus, hypertrophy of smooth muscle, and deposition of collagen may take days, weeks, or months to reverse — or may be irreversible.

An alternative mechanism might also result in excessive airway narrowing. If airway smooth muscle shortening is usually limited because of submaximal stimulation of the smooth muscle via the airway, increased epithelial or submucosal permeability could allow greater smooth muscle stimulation and, therefore, greater shortening. Thus, markedly increased resistance could occur

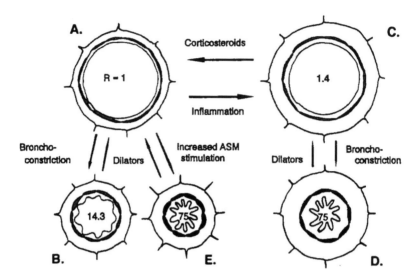

**FIGURE 6**  Schematic airways showing the effects of muscle shortening, wall thickness and increased smooth muscle stimulation on airway resistance and the effects of treatment. See text for details.

(as in E) despite the presence of normal tissue recoil forces. Given the epithelial damage that is observed in asthma and the increase in airway responsiveness that occurs following viral infections,[124,125] which are known to cause epithelial damage,[126] this mechanism deserves further study.

## VI. SUMMARY AND CONCLUSIONS

The qualitative results of morphometric studies of the airway wall in asthma and models of airway narrowing point towards the following conclusions:

1.  The thickness of the airway wall is increased in asthma and related to severity. The increase in thickness is due to increases in most tissue compartments, including smooth muscle, epithelium, submucosa, adventitia, and mucous glands. The number of blood vessels in the submucosa does not seem to be increased in asthma, although congestion is evident in preliminary studies.
2.  Increased wall thickness has little effect on airway resistance in the absence of smooth muscle shortening.
3.  Increased wall thickness will amplify the effects of smooth muscle shortening on airway narrowing, and the effect is in direct relation to the degree of increased thickness.
4.  The increased adventitial area may result in uncoupling of the distending, elastic recoil of the lung from the smooth muscle and, therefore, greater maximal smooth muscle shortening.

5. The magnitude of the functional effects predicted from the structural changes in asthma more than adequately accounts for the excessive airway narrowing, the occurrence of symptoms, and the responses to treatment that are observed in asthma.

The relative importance of the many possible mechanical effects of increased wall thickness, the mechanical properties of the tissue matrix, cartilage, and smooth muscle in nonasthmatic and asthmatic airways, the magnitude of the airway wall elastic loads during shortening, the distribution of structural changes throughout the bronchial tree in asthma, and the factors which limit the degree to which the airway smooth muscle can be stimulated require further study.

It seems likely that airway inflammation is the basis of the altered structure and function in asthma (although it is yet to be established that excessive airway narrowing, as observed in asthma, cannot occur in the absence of airway structural change). The factors that cause and sustain the inflammation and methods of treatment that can prevent the inflammation remain to be elucidated.

## ACKNOWLEDGMENTS

I would like to thank Neil Carroll for his helpful comments. This work is partly supported by a grant from the National Health and Medical Research Council.

## REFERENCES

1. Brown, P. J., Greville, H. W., and Finucane, K. E., Asthma and irreversible airflow obstruction, *Thorax*, 39, 131, 1984.
2. Benatar, S. R., Fatal asthma, *N. Engl. J. Med.*, 314, 423, 1986.
3. Jenkins, C. R. and Woolcock, A. J., Effect of prednisone and beclomethasone dipropionate on airway hyperresponsiveness in asthma: a comprehensive study, *Thorax*, 43, 378, 1988.
4. Freedman, S., Tattersfield, A. E., and Pride, N. B., Changes in lung mechanics during asthma induced by exercise, *J. Appl. Physiol.*, 38, 974, 1975.
5. Woolcock, A. J. and Read, J., Lung volumes in exacerbations of asthma, *Am. J. Med.*, 41, 259, 1966.
6. Woolcock, A. J. and Read, J., The static elastic properties of the lungs in asthma, *Am. Rev. Respir. Dis.*, 98, 788, 1968.
7. Finucane, K. E. and Colebatch, H. J. H., Elastic behaviour of the lung in patients with airway obstruction, *J. Appl. Physiol.*, 26, 330, 1969.
8. Colebatch, H. J. H., Finucane, K. E., and Smith, M. M., Pulmonary conductance and elastic recoil relationships in asthma and emphysema, *J. Appl. Physiol.*, 34, 143, 1973.
9. Bentivoglio, L. G., Beerel, F., Bryan, A. C., Stewart, P. B., Rose, B., Ball, W. C., and Bates, D. V., Regional pulmonary function with bronchial asthma, *J. Clin. Invest.*, 42, 1193, 1963.

10. Roca, J., Ramis, L. I., Rodriguez-Roisin, R., Ballester, E., Montserrat, J. M., and Wagner, P. D., Serial relationships between ventilation-perfusion inequality and spirometry in acute severe asthma requiring hospitalisation, *Am. Rev. Respir. Dis.*, 137, 1055, 1988.

11. Wagner, P. D., Dantzker, T. R., Iacovoni, V. E., Tomlin, W. C., and West, J. B., Ventilation-perfusion inequality in asymptomatic asthma, *Am. Rev. Respir. Dis.*, 118, 511, 1978.

12. Orehek, J., Gayrard, P., Smit, A. P., Grimaud, C., and Charpin, J., Airway response to carbachol in normal and asthmatic subjects. Distinction between bronchial reactivity and sensitivity, *Am. Rev. Respir. Dis.*, 115, 937, 1977.

13. Hargreave, F. E., Ryan, G. R., Thomson, N. C., O'Byrne, P. M., Latimer, K., Juniper, E. F., and Dolovich, J., Bronchial responsiveness to histamine or methacholine in asthma: measurement and clinical significance, *J. Allergy Clin. Immunol.*, 68, 347, 1981.

14. Malo, J.-L., Cartier, A., Pineau, L., Gagnon, G., and Martin, R., Slope of the dose-response curve to inhaled histamine and methacholine and PC20 in subjects with symptoms of hyperexcitability and in normal subjects, *Am. Rev. Respir. Dis.*, 132, 644, 1985.

15. Cockroft, D. W. and Berscheid, B. A., Slope of the dose-response curve: usefulness in assessing bronchial response to inhaled histamine, *Thorax*, 38, 55, 1983.

16. Sterk, P. J., Daniel, E. E., Zamel, N., and Hargreave, F. E., Limited bronchoconstriction to methacholine using partial flow-volume curves in nonasthmatics, *Am. Rev. Respir. Dis.*, 131, A289, 1985.

17. Woolcock, A. J., Salome, C. M., and Yan, K., The shape of the dose-response curve to histamine in asthmatic and normal subjects, *Am. Rev. Respir. Dis.*, 130, 71, 1984.

18. James, A. L., Lougheed, M. D., Pearce-Pinto, G., Ryan, G., and Musk, A. W., Maximal airway narrowing in a general population, *Am. Rev. Respir. Dis.*, 146, 895, 1992.

19. Aikawa, T., Shimura, S., Sasaki, H., Ebina, M., and Takashima, T., Marked goblet cell hyperplasia with mucus accumulation in the airways of patients who died of severe acute asthma attack, *Chest*, 101, 916, 1992.

20. Azzawi, M., Jeffrey, P. K., Frew, A. J., Johnston, P., and Kay, A. B., Activated eosinophils in bronchi obtained at postmortem from asthma deaths, *J. Clin. Exp. Allergy*, 19, 118, 1989.

21. Bullen, S. S., Correlation of clinical and autopsy findings in 176 cases of asthma, *J. Allergy*, 23, 193, 1952.

22. Cardell, B. S. and Pearson, R. S. B., Death in asthmatics, *Thorax*, 14, 341, 1959.

23. Carroll, N. G., Elliot, J., Morton, A. R., and James, A. L., The structure of large and small airways in nonfatal and fatal asthma, *Am. Rev. Respir. Dis.*, 147, 405, 1993.

24. Cutz, E., Levison, H., and Cooper, D. M., Ultrastructure of airways in children with asthma, *Thorax*, 8, 207, 1978.

25. Dunnill, M. S., The pathology of asthma with special reference to changes in the bronchial mucosa, *J. Clin. Pathol.*, 13, 27, 1960.

26. Dunnill, M. S., Massarella, G. R., and Anderson, J. A., A comparison of the quantitative anatomy of the bronchi in normal subjects, in status asthmaticus, in chronic bronchitis, and in emphysema, *Thorax*, 24, 176, 1969.

27. Earle, B. V., Fatal bronchial asthma. A series of fifteen cases and a review of the literature, *Thorax*, 8, 195, 1953.

28. Heard, B. E. and Hossain, S., Hyperplasia of bronchial muscle in asthma, *J. Pathol.*, 110, 319, 1971.

29. Houston, J. C., De Navasquez, S., and Trounce, J. R., A clinical and pathological study of fatal cases of status asthmaticus, *Histopathology*, 2, 407, 1953.

30. Huber, H. L. and Koessler, K. K., The pathology of bronchial asthma, *Arch. Intern. Med.*, 30, 689, 1922.

31. James, A. L., Pare, P. D., and Hogg, J. C., The mechanics of airway narrowing in asthma, *Am. Rev. Respir. Dis.*, 139, 242, 1989.

32. Messer, J. W., Peters, G. A., and Bennett, W. A., Causes of death and pathologic findings in 304 cases of bronchial asthma, *Dis. Chest*, 38, 616, 1960.

33. Richards, W. and Patrick, J. R., Death from asthma in children, *Am. J. Dis. Child*, 110, 6, 1965.

34. Saetta, M., Di Stefano, A. D., Rosina, C., Thiene, G., and Fabbri, L. M., Quantitative structural analysis of peripheral airways and arteries in sudden fatal asthma, *Am. Rev. Respir. Dis.*, 143, 138, 1991.
35. Takizawa, T. and Thurlbeck, W. M., Muscle and mucous gland size in the major bronchi of patients with chronic bronchitis, asthma, and asthmatic bronchitis, *Am. Rev. Respir. Dis.*, 104, 331, 1971.
36. Sobonya, R. E., Quantitative structural alterations in long-standing allergic asthma, *Am. Rev. Respir. Dis.*, 130, 289, 1984.
37. Azzawi, M., Johnston, P. W., Majumdar, S., Kay, A. B., and Jeffrey, P. K., T-lymphocytes and activated eosinophils in airway mucosa in fatal asthma and cystic fibrosis, *Am. Rev. Respir. Dis.*, 145, 1477, 1992.
38. Wardlaw, A. J., Dunnett, S., Gleich, G. J., Collins, J. V., and Kay, A. B., Eosinophils and mast cells in bronchoalveolar lavage in mild asthma: relationship to bronchial hyperreactivity, *Am. Rev. Respir. Dis.*, 137, 62, 1988.
39. Bousquet, J., Chanez, P., Lacoste, J. Y., Barneon, G., Ghavanian, N., Enander, I., Venge, P., Ahlstedt, S., Simony-Lafontaine, J., Godard, P., and Michel, F. B., Eosinophilic inflammation in asthma, *N. Engl. J. Med.*, 323, 1033, 1990.
40. Poston, R. N., Chanez, P., Lacoste, J. Y., Litchfield, T., Lee, T. H., and Bousquet, J., Immunohistochemical characterization of the cellular infiltration in asthmatic bronchi, *Am. Rev. Respir. Dis.*, 145, 918, 1992.
41. Djukanovic, R., Lai, C. K. W., Wilson, J. W., Britten, K. M., Wilson, S. J., Roche, W. R., Howarth, P. H., and Holgate, S. T., Bronchial mucosal manifestations of atopy: a comparison of markers of inflammation between atopic asthmatics, atopic nonasthmatics and healthy controls, *Eur. Respir. J.*, 5, 538, 1992.
42. Laitinen, L. A., Laitinen, A., and Haahtela, T., Airway mucosal inflammation even in patients with newly diagnosed asthma, *Am. Rev. Respir. Dis.*, 147, 697, 1993.
43. Pesci, A., Foresi, A., Bertorelli, A. C., and Oliveri, D., Histochemical characteristics and degranulation of mast cells in epithelium and lamina propria of bronchial biopsies from asthmatic and normal subjects, *Am. Rev. Respir. Dis.*, 147, 684, 1993.
44. Fournier, M., Lebargy, F., Ladurie, L., Lenormand, E., and Pariente, R., Intraepithelial T-lymphocyte subsets in the airways of normal subjects and of patients with chronic bronchitis, *Am. Rev. Respir. Dis.*, 140, 737, 1989.
45. Jeffery, P. K., Wardlaw, A. J., Nelson, F. C., Collins, J. V., and Kay, A. B., Bronchial biopsies in asthma: an ultrastructural, quantitative study and correlation with hyperreactivity, *Am. Rev. Respir. Dis.*, 140, 1745, 1989.
46. Bradley, B. L., Azzawi, M., Jacobson, M., Assoufi, B., Collins, J. V., Irani, A. A., Schwartz, L. B., Durham, S. R., Jeffery, P. K., and Kay, A. B., Eosinophils, T-lymphocytes, mast cells, neutrophils, and macrophages in bronchial biopsy specimens from atopic subjects with asthma: comparisons with biopsy specimens from atopic subjects without asthma and normal control subjects and relationship to bronchial hyperresponsiveness, *J. Allergy Clin. Immunol.*, 88, 661, 1991.
47. Beasley, R., Roche, W., Roberts, J. A., and Holgate, S. T., Cellular events in the bronchi in mild asthma and after bronchial provocation, *Am. Rev. Respir. Dis.*, 139, 806, 1987.
48. Foresi, A., Bertorelli, G., Pesci, A., Chetta, A., and Olivieri, D., Inflammatory markers in bronchoalveolar lavage and in bronchial biopsy in asthma during remission, *Chest*, 98, 528, 1990.
49. Djukanovic, R., Wilson, J. W., Britten, K. M., Wilson, S. J., Walls, A. F., Roche, W. R., Howarth, P. H., and Holgate, S. T., Quantitation of mast cells and eosinophils in the bronchial mucosa of symptomatic atopic asthmatics and healthy control subjects using immunohistochemistry, *Am. Rev. Respir. Dis.*, 142, 863, 1990.
50. Ollerenshaw, S. L. and Woolcock, A. J., Characteristics of the inflammation in biopsies from large airways of subjects with asthma and subjects with chronic airflow limitations, *Am. Rev. Respir. Dis.*, 145, 922, 1992.

51. Roche, W. R., Williams, J. H., Beasley, R., and Holgate, S. T., Subepithelial fibrosis in the bronchi of asthmatics, *Lancet*, 1, 520, 1989.
52. Brewster, C. E. P., Howarth, P. H., Djukanovich, R., Wilson, J., Holgate, S. T., and Roche, W. R., Myofibroblasts and subepithelial fibrosis in bronchial asthma, *Am. J. Respir. Cell Mol. Biol.*, 3, 507, 1990.
53. Naylor, B., The shedding of the mucosa of the bronchial tree in asthma, *Thorax*, 157, 69, 1962.
54. Lozewicz, S., Wells, C., Gomez, E., Ferguson, H., Richman, P., Devalia, J., and Davies, R. J., Morphological integrity of the bronchial epithelium in mild asthma, *Thorax*, 45, 12, 1990.
55. Glynn, A. A. and Michaels, L., Bronchial biopsy in chronic bronchitis and asthma, *Thorax*, 15, 142, 1960.
56. Mattoli, S., Mattoso, V. L., Soloperto, M., Allegra, L., and Fasoli, A., Cellular and biochemical characteristics of bronchoalveolar lavage fluid in symptomatic nonallergic asthma, *J. Allergy Clin. Immunol.*, 87, 794, 1991.
57. Corrigan, C. J. and Kay, A. B., CD4 T-lymphocyte activation in acute severe asthma. Relationship to disease severity and atopic status, *Am. Rev. Respir. Dis.*, 141, 970, 1990.
58. Ackerman, V., Marini, M., Vittori, E., Bellini, A., Vassali, G., and Mattoli, S., Detection of cytokines and their cell sources in bronchial biopsy specimens from asthmatic patients, *Chest*, 105, 687, 1994.
59. Frigas, E. and Gleich, G. J., The eosinophil and pathophysiology of asthma, *J. Allergy Clin. Immunol.*, 77, 527, 1986.
60. de Monchy, J. G. R., Kauffman, H. F., Venge, P., Koeter, G. H., Jansen, H. M., Sluiter, H. J., and De Vries, K., Bronchoalveolar eosinophilia during allergen-induced late asthmatic reactions, *Am. Rev. Respir. Dis.*, 131, 373, 1985.
61. Brusasco, V., Crimi, E., Gianiorio, P., Lantero, S., and Rossi, G. A., Allergen-induced increase in airway responsiveness and inflammation in mild asthma, *J. Appl. Physiol.*, 69, 2209, 1990.
62. Bentley, A. M., Menz, G., Robinson, D. S., Hamid, Q., Kay, A. B., and Durham, S. R., Increases in activated T lymphocytes, eosinophils, and cytokine mRNA expression for interleukin-5 and granulocyte/macrophage colony-stimulating factor in bronchial biopsies after allergen inhalation challenge in atopic asthmatics, *Am. J. Respir. Cell Mol. Biol.*, 8, 35, 1993.
63. Bentley, A. M., Maestrelli, P., Saetta, M., Fabbri, L. M., Robinson, D. S., Bradley, B. L., Jeffery, P. K., Durham, S. R. and Kay, A. B., Activated T-lymphocytes and eosinophils in the bronchial mucosa in isocyanate-induced asthma, *J. Allergy Clin. Immunol.*, 89, 821, 1992.
64. Fabbri, L. M., Boschetto, P., Zocca, E., Milani, G., Pivirotto, F., Plebani, M., Burlina, A., Licata, B., and Mapp, C. E., Bronchoalveolar neutrophilia during late asthmatic reactions induced by toluene diisocyanate, *Am. Rev. Respir. Dis.*, 136, 36, 1987.
65. Lam, S., LeRiche, J., Phillips, D., and Chan-Yeung, M., Cellular and protein changes in bronchial lavage fluid after late asthmatic reaction in patients with red cedar asthma, *J. Allergy Clin. Immunol.*, 80, 44, 1987.
66. Saetta, M., Maestrelli, P., Di Stefano, A., De Marzo, N., Milani, G. F., Pivirotto, F., Mapp, C. E., and Fabbri, L. M., Effect of cessation of exposure to toluene diisocyanate (TDI) on bronchial mucosa of subjects with TDI-induced asthma, *Am. Rev. Respir. Dis.*, 145, 169, 1992.
67. Paggiaro, P., Bacci, E., Paoletti, P., Bernard, P., Dente, F. L., Marchetti, G., Talini, D., Menconi, G. F., and Giuntini, C., Bronchoalveolar lavage and morphology of the airways after cessation of exposure in asthmatic subjects sensitized to toluene diisocyanate, *Chest*, 98, 536, 1990.
68. Djukanovic, R., Wilson, J. W., Britten, K. M., Wilson, S. J., Roche, W. R., Howarth, P., and Holgate, S. J., The effect of beclomethasone dipropionate treatment on clinical indices of asthma and inflammatory cells in the asthmatic airways, *Eur. Respir. J.*, 3, 237, 1990.

69. Jeffery, P. K., Godfrey, R. W., Adelroth, E., Nelson, F., Rogers, A., and Johansson, S. A., Effects of treatment on airway inflammation and thickening of basement membrane reticular collagen in asthma. A quantitative light and electron microscopic study, *Am. Rev. Respir. Dis.*, 145, 890, 1992.

70. Lundgren, R., Soderberg, M., Horstedt, P., and Stenling, R., Morphological studies of bronchial mucosal biopsies fr n asthmati s before and after ten years of treatment with inhaled steriods, *Eur. J. Respir. Dis* 1, 883, 1988.

71. Laitinen, L. A., Laitinen, ., and Haahtela, T., A comparative study of the effects of an inhaled corticosteroid, budesonid. , and a beta-2 agonist, terbutaline, on airway inflammation in newly diagnosed asthma: a randomized, double-blind, parallel-group controlled trial, *J. Allergy Clin. Immunol.*, 90, 32, 1992.

72. Laursen, L. C., Taudorf, E., Borgeskov, S., Kobayashi, T., Jensen, H., and Weeke, B., Fiberoptic bronchoscopy and bronchial mucosal biopsies in asthmatics undergoing long-term high-dose budesoni . aerosol treatment, *Allergy*, 43, 284, 1988.

73. Djukanovic, R., Wilson, J. W., Britten, K., Wilson, S. J., Walls, D. F., Roche, W. R., Howarth, P., and Holgate, S. T., Effect of an inhaled corticosteroid on airway inflammation and symptoms in asthma, *Am. Rev. Respir. Dis.*, 145, 669, 1992.

74. Folkow, B., The haemodynamic consequences of adaptive structural changes of the resistance vessels in hypertension, *Clin. Sci.*, 41, 1, 1971.

75. Freedman, R. J., The functional geometry of the bronchi. The relationship between changes in external diameter and calibre, and a consideration of the passive role played by the mucosa in bronchoconstriction, *Bull. Eur. Physiopathol. Respir.*, 8, 45, 1972.

76. Macklem, P. T., Bronchial hyporesponsiveness, *Chest*, 158s, 1985.

77. Stephens, N. L., Kroeger, E., and Metha, J. A., Force-velocity characteristics of respiratory airway smooth muscle, *J. Appl. Physiol.*, 26, 685, 1969.

78. Moreno, R. H., Hogg, J. C., and Pare, P. D., Mechanics of airway narrowing, *Am. Rev. Respir. Dis.*, 133, 1171, 1986.

79. Bai, A., Eidelman, D. H., Hogg, J. C., James, A. L., Lambert, R. K., Ludwig, M. S., Martin, J., McDonald, D. M., Mitzner, W. A., Okazawa, M., Pack, R. J., Pare, P. D., Schellenberg, R. R., Tiddens, H. A. W. M., Wagner, E. M., and Yager, D., Proposed nomenclature for quantifying subdivisions of the bronchial wall, *J. Appl. Physiol.*, 77, 1011, 1994.

80. Ebina, M., Yaegashi, H., Takahashi, T., Motomiya, M., and Tanemura, M., Distribution of smooth muscle along the bronchial tree: a morphometric study of ordinary autopsy lungs, *Am. Rev. Respir. Dis.*, 141, 1322, 1990.

81. Kuwano, K., Bosken, C. H., Pare, P. D., Bai, T. R., Wiggs, B. R., and Hogg, J. C., Small airways dimensions in asthma and in chronic obstructive pulmonary disease, *Am. Rev. Respir. Dis.*, 148, 1220, 1993.

82. James, A. L., Moreno, R., Pare, P. D., and Hogg, J. C., Quantitative measurement of smooth muscle shortening in the isolated pig trachea, *J. Appl. Physiol.*, 63, 1360, 1987.

83. James, A. L., Hogg, J. C., Dunn, L. A., and Pare, P. D., The use of the internal perimeter to compare airway size and to calculate smooth muscle shortening, *Am. Rev. Respir. Dis.*, 138, 235, 1988.

84. James, A. L., Pare, P. D., and Hogg, J. C., Effects of lung volume, bronchoconstriction, and cigarette smoke on morphometric airway dimensions, *J. Appl. Physiol.*, 64, 913, 1988.

85. Feldman, H. A., Families of lines: random effects in linear regression analysis, *J. Appl. Physiol.*, 64, 1721, 1988.

86. Laitenen, L. A., Heino, M., Laitenen, A., Kava, T., and Haahtela, T., Damage of the airway epithelium and bronchial reactivity in patients with asthma, *Am. Rev. Respir. Dis.*, 131, 599, 1985.

87. Omari, T. I., Sparrow, M. P., and Mitchell, H. W., Responsiveness of human isolated bronchial segments and its relationship to epithelial loss, *Br. J. Clin. Pharmacol.*, 35, 357, 1993.

88. Ebina, M., Yaegashi, H., Chiba, R., Takahashi, T., Motomiya, M., and Tanemura, M., Hyperreactive site in the airway tree of asthmatic patients revealed by thickening of the bronchial muscles. A morphometric study, *Am. Rev. Respir. Dis.*, 141, 1327, 1990.

89. Bohrod, M. G., Pathologic manifestations of allergic and related mechanisms in diseases of the lungs, *Int. Arch. Allergy,* 13, 39, 1958.

90. James, A. L., Kan, R., and Carroll, N. G., Bronchial blood vessel dimensions in asthma, *Am. Rev. Respir. Dis.,* 147, A455, 1993.

91. Wilson, J. W. and Li, X., Bronchial vessels in mild asthma are dilated, *Aust. N.Z. J. Med.,* 25, A414, 1995.

92. Ding, D. J., Martin, J. G., and Macklem, P. T., Effects of lung volume on maximal methacholine induced bronchoconstriction in normal humans, *J. Appl. Physiol.,* 62, 1324, 1987.

93. Wiggs, B., Moreno, R., James, A., Hogg, J. C., and Pare, P., in *A Model of the Mechanics of Airway Narrowing in Asthma,* Kaliner, M. A., Barnes, P. J., and Persson, C. G. A., Eds., Marcel Dekker, New York, 1991, 74.

94. Weibel, E. R., *Morphometry of the Human Lung,* Springer-Verlag, Berlin, 1963.

95. Pedley, T. J., Schroter, R. C., and Sudlow, M. F., in *Gas Flow and Mixing in the Airways,* West, J. B., Ed., Marcel Dekker, New York, 1977, 163.

96. Wiggs, B. R., Bosken, C., Pare, P. D., James, A. L., and Hogg, J. C., A model of airway narrowing in asthma and in chronic obstructive pulmonary disease, *Am. Rev. Respir. Dis.,* 145, 1251, 1992.

97. Pare, P. D., Wiggs, B. R., James, A. L., Hogg, J. C., and Bosken, C., The comparative mechanics and morphology of airways in asthma and in chronic obstructive pulmonary disease, *Am. Rev. Respir. Dis.,* 143, 1182, 1991.

98. Pliss, L. B., Ingenito, E. P., and Ingram, R. H., Responsiveness, inflammation, and effects of deep breaths on obstruction in mild asthma, *J. Appl. Physiol.,* 66, 2298, 1989.

99. Fish, J. E., Peterman, V., and Cudgell, D., Effect of deep inspiration on airway conductance in subjects with allergic rhinitis and allergic asthma, *J. Allergy Clin. Immunol.,* 60, 41, 1970.

100. Fairshter, R., Effect of deep inhalation on maximal expiratory flow in normals and patients with chronic obstructive pulmonary disease, *Bull. Eur. Physiopathol. Respir.,* 22, 119, 1986.

101. Ilowite, J. S., Bennett, W. D., Sheetz, M. S., Groth, M. L., and Nierman, D. M., Permeability of the bronchial mucosa to $^{99m}$Tc-DTPA in asthma, *Am. Rev. Respir. Dis.,* 139, 1139, 1989.

102. Elwood, R. K., Kennedy, S., Belzberg, A., Hogg, J. C., and Pare, P. D., Respiratory mucosal permeability in asthma, *Am. Rev. Respir. Dis.,* 128, 523, 1983.

103. Simani, A. S., Inoue, S., and Hogg, J. C., Penetration of the respiratory epithelium of guinea-pigs following exposure to cigarette smoke, *Lab. Invest.,* 31, 75, 1974.

104. Boucher, R. C., Pare, P. D., Gilmore, N. J., Moroz, L. A., and Hogg, J. C., Airway mucosal permability in the *Ascaris suum*-sensitive rhesus monkey, *J. Allergy Clin. Immunol.,* 60, 134, 1977.

105. Drazen, J. M., O'Cain, C. F., and Ingram, R. H., Experimental induction of chronic bronchitis in dogs, *Am. Rev. Respir. Dis.,* 126, 75, 1982.

106. Widdicombe, J. G., Comparison between the vascular beds of upper and lower airways, *Eur. Respir. J.,* 3 (Suppl. 12), 564, 1990.

107. Kelly, L., Kolbe, J., Mitzner, W., Spannhake, E. W., Bromberger-Barnea, B., and Menkes, H., Bronchial blood flow affects recovery from constriction in dog lung periphery, *J. Appl. Physiol.,* 60, 1954, 1986.

108. Horsfield, K. and Cumming, G., Morphology of the bronchial tree in man, *J. Appl. Physiol.,* 24, 373, 1968.

109. Bates, J. H. T., Stochastic model of the pulmonary airway tree and its implications for bronchial responsiveness, *J. Appl. Physiol.,* 75, 2493, 1993.

110. Hogg, J. C., Macklem, P. T., and Thurlbeck, W. M., Site and nature of airflow obstruction in chronic obstructive lung disease, *N. Engl. J. Med.,* 278, 1355, 1968.

111. Cosio, M., Ghezzo, H., Hogg, J. C., Corbin, R., Loveland, M., Dosman, J., and Macklem, P. T., The relations between structural changes in small airways and pulmonary-function tests, *N. Engl. J. Med.,* 298, 1277, 1977.

112. Ishida, K., Pare, P., Blogg, T., and Schellenberg, R. R., Effects of elastic loading on porcine trachealis muscle mechanics, *J. Appl. Physiol.*, 69(3), 1033, 1990.

113. Lambert, R. K., Wiggs, B. R., Kuwano, K., Hogg, J. C., and Pare, P. D., Functional significance of increased airway smooth muscle in asthma and COPD, *J. Appl. Physiol.*, 74, 2771, 1993.

114. Lambert, R. K., Wilson, T. A., Hyatt, R. E., and Rodarte, J. R., A computational model for expiratory flow, *J. Appl. Physiol.*, 52, 44, 1982.

115. Wilson, J. W., Li, X., and Pain, C. F., The lack of distensibility of asthmatic airways, *Am. Rev. Respir. Dis.*, 148, 806, 1993.

116. Bramley, A. M., Roberts, C. R., and Schellenberg, R. R., Increased contractility of human bronchial smooth muscle after collagenase treatment, *Am. Rev. Respir. Dis.*, 147, A844, 1993.

117. Bramley, A. M., Thomson, R. J., Roberts, C. R., and Schellenberg, R. R., Hypothesis: excessive bronchoconstriction in asthma is due to decreased airway elastance, *Eur. Respir. J.*, 7, 337, 1994.

118. Moreno, R. H., Lisboa, C., Hogg, J. C., and Pare, P. D., Limitation of airway smooth muscle shortening by cartilage stiffness and lung elastic recoil in rabbits, *J. Appl. Physiol.*, 75(2), 738, 1993.

119. Lambert, R. K., Role of bronchial basement membrane in airway collapse, *J. Appl. Physiol.*, 71, 666, 1991.

120. James, A. L. and Carroll, N. G., Mucosal folding in asthmatic and nonasthmatic airways, *Am. J. Respir. Crit. Care Med.*, 151, A133, 1995.

121. Lambert, R. K., Codd, S. L., Alley, M. R., and Pack, R. J., Physical determinants of bronchial mucosal folding, *J. Appl. Physiol.*, 77, 1206, 1994.

122. James, A. J. and Carroll, N. G., The theoretical effects of mucous gland discharge on airway resistance in asthma, *Chest*, 107, 110S, 1995.

123. Yager, D., Butler, J. P., Bastacky, J., Israel, E., Smith, G., and Drazen, J. M., Amplification of airway constriction due to liquid-filling of airway interstices, *J. Appl. Physiol.*, 66, 2873, 1989.

124. Empey, D. W., Laitinen, L. A., Jacobs, L., Gold, W. M., and Nadel, J. A., Mechanisms of bronchial hyperreactivity in normal subjects following upper respiratory tract infection, *Am. Rev. Respir. Dis.*, 113, 131, 1976.

125. Cheung, D., Dick, E. C., Timmers, M. C., De Klerk, E. P. A., Spaan, W. J. M., and Sterk, P. J., Rhinovirus inhalation causes prolonged excessive airway narrowing to methacholine in asthmatic subjects *in vivo*, *Am. J. Respir. Crit. Care Med.*, 149, A47, 1994.

126. Walsh, J. J., Dietlein, L. F., Low, F. N., Burch, G. E., and Mogabgab, W. J., Bronchotracheal response in human influenza, *Arch. Intern. Med.*, 108, 376, 1961.

127. Ebina, M., Takahashi, T., Chiba, T., and Motomiya, M., Cellular hypertrophy and hyperplasia of airway smooth muscle underlying bronchial asthma, *Am. Rev. Respir. Dis.*, 148, 720, 1993.

Chapter 2

# AIRWAY WALL REMODELLING IN THE PATHOGENESIS OF ASTHMA: CYTOKINE EXPRESSION IN THE AIRWAYS

Peter Bradding, Anthony E. Redington, and Stephen T. Holgate

## CONTENTS

## I. INTRODUCTION

Airway inflammation has become accepted as the pathological hallmark of asthma and is likely to account, at least in large part, for the pathophysiological manifestations of the disease. Studies using fibreoptic bronchoscopy to obtain specimens from the airways have allowed a detailed characterisation of this inflammatory response.[1-12] Typically, there is infiltration of the bronchial mucosa with activated eosinophils, activation of mast cells and T-lymphocytes within the airways, and, in some studies, infiltration with monocytes and plasma cells. These cellular changes are believed to be orchestrated by a complex network of cytokines which controls the nature of the response and determines whether there is continued inflammation or resolution with or

0-8493-7813-3/97/$0.00+$.50

without fibrosis. The major challenge in the last few years has been to understand the nature of this cytokine network, and although much still remains
unknown, enormous progress has been made.

In this chapter, we will first discuss some of the practical difficulties arising
when attempting to study cytokine expression and to interpret such studies.
We will then consider the theoretical background relating to some of the
cytokines which are believed to be of key importance in allergic asthma: those
involved in the regulation of IgE synthesis, in the control of eosinophil function, in the process of leukocyte recruitment into the airways, and in the
development of airway wall thickening. Finally, we will review the current
state of knowledge regarding the expression of these cytokines *in vivo* in
asthma.

## II. INVESTIGATION OF THE ROLE OF CYTOKINES IN ALLERGIC INFLAMMATION

In the last few years cytokine research has greatly improved our understanding of cell biology and highlighted important aspects of tissue inflammation, but the study of cytokine biology is fraught with difficulties. Many
studies have focussed on the biological properties of individual cytokines *in
vitro*. Although clearly important, these studies need to be interpreted with
caution. The complex cytokine–cytokine and cytokine–matrix interactions
existing *in vivo* mean that responses of isolated cells studied out of context *in
vitro* may be misleading. Furthermore, a cell removed from its normal tissue
milieu to a culture dish may undergo significant changes in its phenotype. For
example, the β-receptor for platelet-derived growth factor (PDGF) is expressed
by porcine smooth muscle cells and human skin fibroblasts in culture, but not
by these cells *in situ* .[13]

Many studies have approached the investigation of cytokine expression in
the airways by studying mRNA for the molecule of interest using such techniques as Northern blot analysis, *in situ* hybridisation, and most recently the
reverse transcriptase polymerase chain reaction (RT-PCR). However, when
interpreting such studies it must be remembered that the presence of mRNA
does not necessarily imply that there is translation into protein,[14] let alone
protein secretion. An alternative approach has been to investigate the expression of cytokine protein using immunohistochemistry. However, the presence
of immunoreactive cytokine protein within the airways may not provide an
accurate reflection of its release. It is probably too simplistic to assume that
quantification of numbers of cytokine-expressing cells in a tissue can provide
an accurate guide to cytokine activity in a disease setting.

A further level of complexity is added by the fact that, once released, many
cytokines do not remain in the soluble phase but bind in a specific fashion to
components of the extracellular matrix (ECM) and that these interactions can
profoundly alter the biologic properties of the cytokines. For example, heparan
sulphate proteoglycans (HSPGs) are ubiquitous components of the ECM which

are located predominantly in basement membranes and on the surfaces of many cells. These molecules are capable of binding many cytokines including the haematopoietic growth factors interleukin 3 (IL-3) and granulocyte/macrophage colony-stimulating factor (GM-CSF),[15,16] members of the chemokine family such as IL-8,[17] and the potent fibrogenic and angiogenic cytokine, basic fibroblast growth factor (bFGF).[18,19] In the case of IL-8 this interaction serves to increase the activity of the cytokine as a neutrophil activator,[17] presumably by facilitating its precise spatial orientation when presented to the target cell. On the other hand, in the case of bFGF its interaction with basement membrane HSPGs is believed to create an extracellular reservoir of cytokine which can be released in response to specific stimuli.[18,20,21] Presentation of cytokines as cell surface molecules is also important in the process of juxtacrine signalling,[22] whereas in the case of bFGF this cytokine must first bind to cell surface HSPGs in order to be presented to its high-affinity receptors.[23] The role that cytokine–matrix interactions play in cytokine biology has received relatively little attention, and their significance is likely to become increasingly evident with further research. The recognition of their importance also draws attention to the need to exert caution when interpreting measurement of quantities of "free" cytokine in a biologic fluid, as these may not provide a true reflection of its biologic activity. Ideally, when studying cytokine expression, evidence of mRNA and protein synthesis, together with cytokine release and biologic activity, should all be investigated.

# III. CYTOKINES IMPLICATED IN ALLERGIC INFLAMMATION

Although the list of known cytokines is continually expanding, a number stand out as being of particular significance when considering the processes of airway inflammation and remodelling in allergic asthma. These are those which (1) regulate IgE synthesis; (2) influence eosinophil function; (3) facilitate leukocyte recruitment through their ability to influence endothelial cell adhesion molecule expression; and (4) may be implicated in the development of chronic structural changes in the airway wall. The potential role of specific cytokines in these processes will be discussed briefly before describing the patterns of cytokine expression and cellular localisation in bronchial mucosal inflammation.

## A. REGULATION OF IgE SYNTHESIS

Atopy is dependent on the presence of mast cell–bound IgE directed against specific allergens and is intimately related to the development of cutaneous and mucosal allergic disease. *In vitro* studies first indicated the essential role played by IL-4 in the isotype switching and subsequent production of IgE by human B cells.[24,25] However, although IL-4 alone is sufficient to induce germline ε transcription,[26] additional costimulatory signals are required in order for IgE synthesis to occur. These signals depend on direct cell–cell contact and involve both cognate interactions, between B cell MHC class II antigen and the T cell receptor/CD3 complex,[27] and noncognate T cell–B cell interactions,[28] for example, between CD40 expressed on B cells and its complementary ligand expressed by activated T cells[29,30] and between the B7 and CD28 receptor families.[31] *In vitro*, the requirement for T cells can be replaced by stimulation with anti-CD40[32] or by infection of B cells with the Epstein–Barr virus (EBV).[33] An alternative signal may also be provided by hydrocortisone,[34,35] which may explain why, despite the negative effects of hydrocortisone on IL-4 gene expression and protein production *in vitro*,[36,37] long-term corticosteroid therapy fails to reduce serum IgE levels *in vivo*.[38]

In addition to acting as an isotype switch, IL-4 increases the expression of the low affinity IgE receptor (CD23/FcεRII) and MHC class II antigen by B cells, events which are also important during the process of IgE synthesis.[39-43] In contrast, IFNγ and IFNα inhibit both IL-4-induced MHC class II antigen and CD23 expression on B cells[39,44] and reduce the level of IL-4-induced IgE synthesis.[24,25]

The importance of IL-4 in the regulation of IgE synthesis has been confirmed *in vivo* in mice. Polyclonal IgE responses following infection with the parasite *Nippostrongylus brasiliensis* are completely inhibited by administration of a neutralising anti-IL-4 monoclonal antibody,[45] and mice homozygous for a mutation that inactivates the IL-4 gene in most cases have undetectable serum IgE levels.[46] In contrast, transgenic mice that overexpress the IL-4 gene develop high levels of circulating IgE, as well as a severe chronic conjunctivitis, characterised by mononuclear, mast cell, and eosinophil infiltration, changes similar to those observed in human allergic mucosal inflammation.[47]

Recently, a further cytokine, designated interleukin-13, has been identified which is able to support the synthesis of IgE by human[48] and murine B-lymphocytes *in vitro* independently of IL-4. This cytokine is encoded as part of the IL-4 gene cluster on chromosome 5 and shares approximately 30% homology at the amino acid level with IL-4 itself.[49] It also shares many properties with IL-4, including the ability to increase the expression of CD23 on resting B-lymphocytes and to stimulate B-lymphocyte proliferation,[48,50] but unlike IL-4 it has no known effects in relation to T cells. The actions of IL-13 are mediated through a discrete receptor which shares a signal-transducing component with the IL-4 receptor.[51] In mice, the failure of most IL-4 "knockout" animals to synthesise any IgE[46] suggests that IL-13 alone is insufficient to support this process *in vivo*, whereas in humans this remains to be established.

## B. CONTROL OF EOSINOPHIL FUNCTION

### 1. Eosinophil Production

Production of eosinophils from progenitor cells in human liquid and semi-solid bone marrow cultures can be stimulated by the cytokines IL-3, IL-5, and GM-CSF.[52-57] However, of these, only IL-5 is specific for eosinophils, as IL-3 and GM-CSF also promote the production of neutrophils, basophils, and macrophages. IL-5 appears to be a late-acting factor, in contrast to IL-3 and

GM-CSF which act at an earlier stage in development to increase the number of IL-5-responsive eosinophil colony-forming cells.

The role of these cytokines in eosinophil production *in vivo* has been studied extensively in murine systems. Administration of neutralizing anti-IL-5 antibody to mice infected with *N. brasiliensis*[58] or *Schistosoma mansoni*[59] completely inhibits the development of eosinophilia, revealing the essential role played by IL-5 in the eosinophilic responses to these infections. Conversely, lethally irradiated mice transplanted with bone marrow cells infected with a retrovirus carrying the IL-5 coding sequence develop a marked eosinophilia which persists for at least 12 months, in association with eosinophilic infiltration of bone marrow, spleen, liver, lung, and gastrointestinal tract.[60] Similarly, transgenic mice that overexpress the IL-5 gene develop a lifelong blood eosinophilia associated with marked eosinophilic infiltration of bone marrow and multiple organs.[61,62] However, in spite of the massive blood and tissue eosinophilia, these animals remain healthy, indicating that other factors are necessary to initiate eosinophil-mediated tissue damage. In contrast, mice that overexpress the genes for either IL-3[63] or GM-CSF[64,65] develop a fatal myeloproliferative syndrome, in which not only eosinophil numbers are substantially increased, but also those of many other haematopoietic cell lineages.

## 2. Eosinophil Chemotaxis

The three cytokines IL-3, IL-5, and GM-CSF which profoundly influence eosinophil development are also chemoattractants for eosinophils, but this property is only evident at relatively high concentrations.[66,67] At concentrations which are too low to induce chemotaxis, all three can prime eosinophils for an increased chemotactic response to small molecules, such as platelet-activating factor (PAF) and leukotriene (LT)B$_4$.[67-69]

Other cytokines have also been identified which are more potent as eosinophil chemotactic stimuli. Of these, several belong to the family of small cytokines known as chemokines. These can be subdivided into an α, or C-X-C subfamily, in which two cysteine residues in a conserved four-cysteine motif are separated by an intervening residue, and a β, or C-C family, in which they are adjacent.[70] IL-8 (NAP-1), a member of the α family, was originally identified as a potent neutrophil chemoattractant and activating agent.[71] However, when eosinophils from nonatopic donors are first primed by exposure to the cytokines IL-3, IL-5, or GM-CSF they also respond chemotactically to IL-8.[67,72] Eosinophils from atopic subjects respond directly to IL-8, suggesting they have already undergone a priming process *in vivo*.[73] Members of the β chemokine subfamily, including RANTES[74-78] and MIP-1α,[75,77] also exhibit chemotactic activity for eosinophils. In the case of RANTES, activity is increased if the cells are first primed with IL-5.[78]

## 3. Eosinophil Survival

The length of time that eosinophils can survive within tissues is unclear, but is thought to be on the order of several weeks or even months. IL-3, IL-5,

GM-CSF, and IFNγ all prolong the survival of eosinophils *in vitro,*[79-82] and in the case of IL-5 this effect is mediated by a delay in programmed cell death (apoptosis).[83,84] The ability of cytokines to prolong eosinophil survival is inhibited by corticosteroids,[85] which may explain in part how these drugs exert their beneficial effects in eosinophil-related diseases. Interestingly, higher concentrations of IL-5 are able to overcome the proapoptotic effect of corticosteroids, providing one possible mechanism for glucocorticoid resistance.[85]

### 4. Eosinophil Priming and Activation

The cytokines IL-3, IL-5, and GM-CSF all increase the functional capacity of eosinophils as assessed using various *in vitro* assays. For example, all three are able to enhance Ig-induced degranulation, with IL-5 being the most potent in this respect.[86] These cytokines are also able to increase $LTC_4$ release, reactive oxygen production, and cytotoxic potential in appropriate assays.[52,79,80] IFNγ also increases eosinophil cytotoxicity, but in contrast to the cytokines discussed above this effect is delayed, not being apparent until 24 h.[82] Finally, tumour necrosis factor-alpha (TNFα) enhances the toxicity of eosinophils towards *S. mansoni* larvae,[87] as well as priming them for increased superoxide[88] and $LTC_4$[89] generation. However, TNFα has no apparent effect on eosinophil degranulation.[88]

Once activated, eosinophils are capable of producing a large number of mediators which may be important for host defence in response to parasitic infection, but which may also be responsible for tissue damage in allergic responses. These include reactive oxygen intermediates, lipid mediators such as $LTC_4$ and PAF, and the four cationic granule proteins: major basic protein (MBP); eosinophil cationic protein (ECP); eosinophil-derived neurotoxin (EDN); and eosinophil peroxidase (EPO). The release of these mediators *in vivo* is likely to occur in response to contact with Ig- or complement-coated targets. The observation that tissue damage does not occur in IL-5 transgenic mice[61] demonstrates that priming with IL-5 alone is insufficient to mediate this response.

### C. LEUKOCYTE RECRUITMENT

The recruitment of circulating leukocytes to sites of allergic inflammation involves a series of stepwise processes (Figure 1). Initial contact with the vessel wall is likely to be largely a random event, although perhaps influenced by local alterations in blood flow. Under flow conditions, the leukocyte then first rolls along the vessel wall before subsequently flattening and firmly adhering to the endothelial cell surface. The leukocyte next crawls over the endothelial surface until it reaches an intercellular junction, where it is finally able to transmigrate between endothelial cells and continue its migration towards the site of inflammation. At each stage these processes depend upon interactions between complementary pairs of adhesion molecules on the surfaces of the two cells, and the expression of these molecules is regulated by cytokines (Table 1).

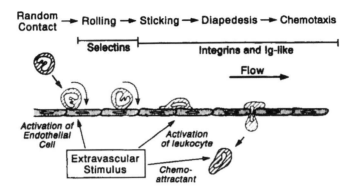

**FIGURE 1** Stages in the process of leukocyte recruitment. (From Carlos T.M. and Harlan J.M., *Blood*, 84, 2068, 1994. With permission.)

## TABLE 1
### Endothelial Adhesion Molecules, Their Leukocyte Ligands, and Inducing Stimuli Relevant to Allergic Inflammation

| Endothelial adhesion molecule | Leukocyte ligand(s) | Inducing stimuli |
|---|---|---|
| P-selectin | sLeˣ-containing glycoprotein | Histamine |
| E-selectin | sLeˣ-containing glycoprotein | IL-1, TNFα |
| ICAM-1 | LFA-1, Mac-1 | — |
| VCAM-1 | α4β1 (VLA-4), α4β7 (Act-1) | IL-1, TNFα, IL-4 |
| PECAM-1 | ? | ? |

*Note:* sLeˣ, sialyl Lewisˣ; IL, interleukin; TNFα, tumour necrosis factor-alpha; ICAM-1, intercellular adhesion molecule-1; LFA-1, lymphocyte function associated antigen-1; VCAM-1, vascular cell adhesion molecule-1; VLA-1, very late activation antigen-1; PECAM-1, platelet endothelial cell adhesion molecule-1.

The selectins form a family of adhesion proteins which possess in common a C-type $NH_2$-terminal lectin-like domain.[90] Two members of this family, P-selectin and E-selectin, are expressed on endothelial cells and have been extensively studied using preparations of human umbilical vein endothelial cells (HUVECs). P-selectin is stored intracellularly in Weibel–Palade bodies[91,92] and is rapidly translocated to the surface of the cell following endothelial activation with such mediators as histamine.[92,93] In contrast, expression of E-selectin by HUVECs requires *de novo* protein synthesis, with cell surface expression becoming detectable 1–2 h following activation, peaking at 4 h, and disappearing again by 16 h.[94,95] The third member of the selectin family, L-selectin, is expressed constitutively on the surface of most peripheral blood leukocytes. The counterstructures to which the selectins bind are still poorly defined. They are known to contain carbohydrate moieties, notably the oligosaccharide motif sialyl Lewis x which binds to all three,[96] but the nature of the protein backbone to which these are attached has proved elusive. However, the recent identification of heavily glycosylated protein ligands for P-selectin[97] and L-selectin[98,99] suggests the existence of a novel family of sialomucin adhesion molecules which present carbohydrates to the selectins.[100] Interactions involving all three selectins are important during the initial stages of the adhesion process; they mediate the loose form of attachment in which the leukocyte "rolls" along the endothelial cell surface under conditions of flow.[101-103]

After this initial stage of loose adhesion, leukocyte activation occurs with the shedding of L-selectin from the cell surface by proteolytic cleavage and the engagement of a second set of complementary pairs of adhesion molecules which mediate firm adhesion. These comprise the endothelial molecules intercellular adhesion molecule-1 (ICAM-1) and vascular cell adhesion molecule-1 (VCAM-1), which are members of the immunoglobulin supergene family, and their counterreceptors on leukocytes, the $\beta_2$-integrins lymphocyte function-associated antigen-1 (LFA-1) (CD11a/CD18) and Mac-1 (CD11b/CD18), and the $\beta_1$-integrin very late antigen-4 (VLA-4) (CD49d/CD29), respectively.[104-106] The leukocyte integrins on circulating cells are expressed in a low-affinity state in which they bind their endothelial ligands either weakly or not at all.[107] In order for firm adhesion to occur, the integrin receptors must first undergo an activation process, in which there is a change to a high-affinity conformation, and this step is likely to represent a major determinant of integrin-mediated leukocyte adhesion. E-selectin binding can itself induce integrin activation,[108] but more recently attention has focussed on the role of chemokines in this process. By using a vessel wall construct, it was shown that IL-8 is produced by cytokine-activated endothelial cells and that this chemokine is able to promote neutrophil adherence by inducing integrin activation and the shedding of L-selectin.[109] Similarly, MIP-1α bound to endothelial cell proteoglycans has been shown to facilitate VLA-4-dependent T-lymphocyte adhesion.[110] The binding of these chemokines to endothelial cell surface proteoglycans is likely to be representative of a more widespread mechanism for facilitating their presentation to leukocytes and, thus, an important means of conferring specificity to the process of leukocyte recruitment.[111]

Changes in the level of surface expression of endothelial adhesion molecules are likely to provide a further element of regulatory control, and such changes can also be induced by cytokines. In the case of HUVECs, E-selectin is not expressed by unstimulated cells but can be induced by exposure to the cytokines IL-1 and TNFα.[94,95,112] In contrast, ICAM-1 is expressed constitutively, but its expression is increased by IL-1, TNFα, and IFNγ,[112] as is that of VCAM-1 by IL-1, IL-4, and TNFα.[113-116] The induction of ICAM-1 and VCAM-1 is slower than that of E-selectin, with expression peaking at about 12 and 6 h, respectively, after exposure and persisting for at least 72 h. There are also complex interactions between these cytokines; for example, IL-4 synergises with IL-1 and TNFα in inducing the expression of VCAM-1, but partially antagonises the expression of E-selectin and ICAM-1 induced by these cytokines.[115] In the case of VCAM-1, initial expression is increased by TNFα while IL-4 stabilises mRNA and prolongs the period of time that the adhesion molecule is expressed on the endothelial surface. These interactions have been used to suggest a possible mechanism for the selective recruitment of eosinophils rather than neutrophils in allergic inflammation. Interactions between VLA-4 and VCAM-1 have been shown to be important in the adherence of eosinophils,[117-119] lymphocytes,[105,114,120,121] and monocytes[122,123] to cytokine-activated HUVECs, whereas neutrophils do not express VLA-4 and so cannot use this pathway.[119] Expression of IL-4 by T-lymphocytes and mast cells is increased in asthma, and as a consequence IL-4-induced upregulation of VCAM-1 may offer at least a partial explanation for the selective recruitment of eosinophils rather than neutrophils in this disease.

Interactions between CD11/CD18 and ICAM-1 are also important determinants of the transmigration of neutrophils across activated endothelium.[124-126] However, this particular pathway appears not to be essential for the transendothelial migration of eosinophils, lymphocytes, or monocytes, as illustrated by the appearance of these cells in inflammatory lesions in patients with leukocyte adhesion deficiency (LAD) type I, a disorder characterised by deficiency of $\beta_2$-leukocyte integrins.[127] In the case of eosinophils, a role for VLA-4 in endothelial transmigration has been clearly demonstrated using a vascular construct of HUVECs cultivated on ECM derived from human fibroblasts.[128] By using this system, IL-4 pretreatment induced not only eosinophil adherence, but also impressive layer penetration, while it had no effect on neutrophils. Eosinophils from atopic subjects were able to penetrate the IL-4-activated vascular constructs spontaneously, whereas those from nonatopic donors required priming with GM-CSF, IL-3, or IL-5, indicating that eosinophils in allergic subjects have undergone a priming process *in vivo*. Another adhesion protein that has been implicated in transendothelial migration is platelet-endothelial cell adhesion molecule-1 (PECAM-1), a further member of the immunoglobulin gene superfamily.[129,130] This molecule is constitutively expressed on the surfaces of endothelial cells, where it is localised to the region of intercellular junctions. The importance of PECAM-1 in leukocyte diapedesis has been demonstrated,[131,132] but its expression is not increased by exposure to the cytokines IL-1 or TNFα.[130]

## D. AIRWAY WALL REMODELLING

Early studies of post-mortem tissue obtained from asthma fatalities first drew attention to thickening of the airway wall in this condition.[133] More recently, morphometric studies have confirmed that the wall area is increased in both large and small airways of asthmatic subjects. Many elements contribute to this thickening, including an increase in airway smooth muscle and the presence in the submucosal tissue of oedema, inflammatory cell infiltration, glandular hypertrophy, and connective tissue deposition.[134,135] The changes in airway smooth muscle appear to result predominantly from hyperplasia rather than from hypertrophy.[136] These alterations are likely to have important physiological consequences as they reduce the calculated smooth muscle shortening required to cause airway closure.[134] Mathematical modelling of airway dysfunction in asthma[137] has shown that the magnitude of airway wall thickening is sufficient to contribute substantially to airway hyperresponsiveness, which is characteristic of asthma.

An additional feature noted in the early post-mortem studies was apparent thickening of the basement membrane.[133,138-140] Electron microscopy later demonstrated that this thickening is confined to the lamina reticularis, whereas the lamina rara and the lamina densa are unaltered.[141,142] Using specific monoclonal antibodies, we have shown that the subepithelial connective tissue which is deposited is composed predominantly of collagens types I, III, and V and fibronectin.[143] In contrast, collagen IV, which is classically epithelially derived, is not increased in amount. The significance of subepithelial fibrosis is at present unclear; no correlation has been demonstrated with any clinical index of disease expression, but its pathophysiological consequences are likely to be proportionately greater in small airways. Moreover, subepithelial fibrosis may serve as a marker for fibrosis more generally in the airway wall. The most likely origin for this collagen is a population of myofibroblasts which underlie the bronchial epithelium. These are present in normal airways, but they are increased in number in asthma, and furthermore these numbers correlate with the degree of collagen thickness[144] (Figure 2). They possess long, branching dendritic processes which are likely to form an interlacing network through which inflammatory cells, such as eosinophils, must pass in order to reach the epithelium.

The stimuli responsible for airway wall remodelling in asthma are not yet well defined. Several proinflammatory cytokines also have the capacity to induce a fibrogenic response. For example, in mice IL-4 stimulates fibroblast proliferation,[145] whereas in humans this cytokine is a potent chemoattractant for dermal fibroblasts[146] and also induces the synthesis of ECM components such as types I and III collagen and fibronectin.[147] TNFα is also a fibroblast mitogen[148] and chemoattractant,[149] but collagen synthesis is inhibited[150,151] while collagenase synthesis is increased.[152,153] A role for TNFα *in vivo* in tissue remodelling and fibrosis is supported by the observation that chronic subcutaneous infusion of TNFα results in a dense accumulation of fibroblasts accompanied by neovascularisation and epidermal hyperplasia.[154]

A number of other cytokines exist which are likely to influence airway fibrotic responses. Transforming growth factor-beta (TGFβ) denotes a family of three closely related molecules denoted TGFβ1, TGFβ2, and TGFβ3. TGFβ1 is an extremely potent modulator of the ECM. It enhances the synthesis by fibroblasts of very many components of the ECM, including collagen types I and III,[155-158] fibronectin,[155,157-160] tenascin,[161] and proteoglycans.[162] It also

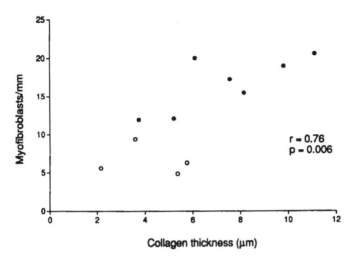

**FIGURE 2** Relationship between subepithelial collagen thickness and number of myofibro-blasts per millimetre basement membrane length. Open circles represent nonasthmatics, filled circles represent asthmatics. (Redrawn from Brewster, C.E.P. et al., *Am. J. Respir. Cell Mol. Biol.*, 3, 507, 1990. With permission.)

increases expression of cell surface receptors for several of these molecules,[160,163] so as to facilitate cell–matrix interactions. In addition, TGFβ decreases the synthesis of several enzymes which are involved in the degradation of ECM components, such as plasminogen activator,[164] type I collagenase, and metalloproteinases,[165] and conversely increases the synthesis of molecules which inhibit these enzymes, such as type I plasminogen activator inhibitor (PAI-I)[166] and tissue inhibitor of metalloendoproteinase (TIMP).[165] Most studies have reported that TGFβ1 exerts an inhibitory effect on fibroblast proliferation.[167]

Evidence for the *in vivo* ability of TGFβ1 to induce fibrotic responses derives from experiments showing that when injected subcutaneously in mice it results in the rapid development of fibroblast activation, collagen production, and angiogenesis.[156] In addition, a number of investigators have provided compelling evidence for the role of TGFβ1 in lung fibrosis, both that induced experimentally in rodents by bleomycin exposure[168,169] and naturally occurring pulmonary fibrosis in humans.[170,171]

A further molecule of interest in the context of airway wall remodelling is bFGF. This cytokine was originally identified on the basis of its mitogenicity for fibroblasts[172,173] but is also a potent mitogenic factor for endothelial cells.[174,175] When implanted in sponges in rats, bFGF induces the formation of highly vascularised granulation tissue.[176] It also leads to the formation of provisional matrix but, unlike TGFβ, is insufficient alone to cause collagen deposition,[177] suggesting that the additional actions of other mediators are required for the latter response *in vivo*. In the morphometric studies referred to above[135] proliferation of new vessels was reported in the submucosal tissue of asthmatic subjects, although not disproportionate to the overall increase in submucosal tissue, and thus bFGF is a candidate mediator for this response.

## IV. CYTOKINE EXPRESSION IN ASTHMA

Cytokines normally function at low concentration and in a local manner so that it is unsurprising that they are frequently not detectable in peripheral blood. Nevertheless, several investigators have reported measurable quantities of cytokines in serum in asthma in certain circumstances. In one study, IL-1β, TNFα, IFNγ, and GM-CSF were undetectable in the serum of mild asthmatic subjects, but there were measurable concentrations of GM-CSF in acute severe asthma.[178] Other studies have also shown increased serum concentrations of IL-5[179] and IFNγ[180] in subjects with acute exacerbations of asthma, and of IL-5 in a proportion of patients with chronic corticosteroid-dependent asthma.[181] Increased concentrations of IL-4 have been reported in subjects with mild-to-moderate asthma in comparison with normal subjects[182] although this observation remains to be confirmed.

The procedure of bronchoalveolar lavage (BAL) allows sampling of epithelial lining fluid, and several groups have measured cytokine concentrations in BAL fluid in asthma. There are a number of methodological difficulties with such studies, including variable dilution, variable recovery of BAL fluid, and the possibility of degradation of cytokines by BAL fluid proteases. Nevertheless, Walker et al.[183] reported increased concentrations of IL-4 and IL-5 in BAL fluid from allergic asthmatic subjects and increased concentrations of IL-2 and IL-5 in nonallergic asthmatic subjects compared with nonasthmatic control subjects. In this study, BAL fluid was concentrated up to 18–21 times, but, even so, cytokine concentrations were in the lower ranges of the assays employed. Using a similar approach, Broide et al.[184] compared symptomatic with asymptomatic atopic asthmatic subjects and reported elevated levels of IL-1β, IL-2, IL-6, TNFα, and GM-CSF in concentrated BAL fluid. IL-4, however, was not detectable in this study, probably because of the relatively high detection limit of the assay employed (200 pg/ml). In our own studies we have shown that levels of TNFα in concentrated BAL fluid are increased in mild atopic asthmatic subjects when compared with healthy control subjects.[185] However, neither IL-4 nor IFNγ were measurable in the control subjects, and these cytokines were only detectable in a small proportion of the asthmatic subjects.

The technique of *in situ* hybridisation has allowed the quantification of cytokine mRNA-expressing cells in BAL fluid and bronchial biopsies in asthma. In BAL fluid there are increased proportions of cells expressing mRNA for IL-2, IL-3, IL-4, IL-5, and GM-CSF, but not IFNγ, in subjects with mild atopic asthma compared with normal control subjects, suggesting the existence of a predominant Th2-like T cell population in the airways in asthma.[186,187] Similar studies have demonstrated an increased proportion of BAL cells expressing mRNA for TNFα in stable atopic asthma.[188] Following allergen challenge, it was possible to demonstrate an increase in the proportion of BAL cells expressing mRNA for IL-4, IL-5, and GM-CSF, but not IL-2, IL-3, or IFNγ.[189] In bronchial biopsies, a similar pattern of mRNA expression has been described. Thus, there is an increase in the numbers of cells expressing mRNA+ for IL-4 and IL-5 in mildly symptomatic asthmatic subjects compared with asymptomatic asthmatic and normal control subjects,[187] and 24 h after allergen inhalation challenge there is increased expression of mRNA for IL-5 and GM-CSF.[190]

Studies employing immunohistochemistry have identified the presence of immunoreactive IL-4, IL-5, IL-6, and TNFα in the bronchial mucosa of both normal subjects and those with atopic asthma.[191,192] We have demonstrated a disease-related increase in the numbers of cells expressing immunoreactivity for IL-4 and for TNFα in asthma, but no difference in the numbers of cells expressing IL-5 or IL-6 (Figure 3). These findings provide the first direct evidence for the increased expression of IL-4 and TNFα at the protein level in the airway mucosa in asthma and, in view of the known biologic activities of these two cytokines as discussed above, support the view that they may be central mediators in the pathogenesis of allergic mucosal inflammation.

When used in isolation, immunohistochemistry has a number of limitations. In particular, it gives no information about whether or not the protein identified is being actively synthesised and released, so that simple quantification of numbers of cells expressing immunoreactivity for a particular protein may be misleading. This is illustrated by the observation that numbers of tryptase-immunostaining mast cells are similar in bronchial biopsies from normal subjects and from patients with atopic asthma,[8,9] and yet there is clear evidence of mast cell activation in this disease when assessed by measurement of mediators in lavage fluid[1,193] or by the ultrastructural appearance of the cells as assessed by electron microscopy.[4,8] Thus, although we have been unable to demonstrate a difference between asthmatic and control subjects in the numbers of IL-5- and IL-6-immunoreactive cells in bronchial biopsies,[192] this does not exclude the possibilities of increased release and/or increased availability of these cytokines.

In addition to studying the expression of disease-related cytokines in terms of their quantity, it is clearly important to identify which cell types are responsible for their production. The application of immunohistochemistry to glycol methacrylate (GMA)-embedded bronchial biopsies sectioned at 2 μm thickness has greatly facilitated cell–cytokine colocalisation. Of great interest was the observation that immunoreactive IL-4, IL-6, and TNFα were localised predominantly to mast cells, while IL-5 was localised to both mast cells and eosinophils.[192] Ohkawara et al.[194] have also reported TNFα immunolocalisation to mast cells in human lung fragments, and, in skin biopsies from normal subjects and from patients with atopic dermatitis, it has recently been reported that mast cells are a major source of IL-4 immunoreactivity.[195]

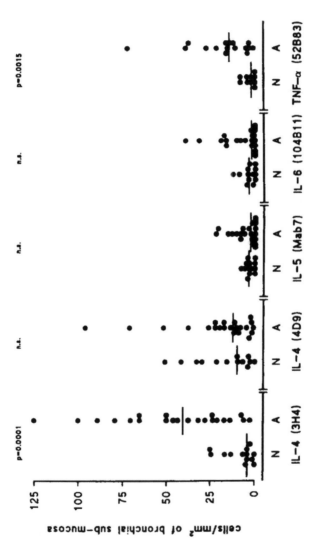

**FIGURE 3**  Comparison of cytokine-immunoreactive cells in bronchial biopsies from normal (N) and asthmatic (A) subjects. Monoclonal antibodies 3H4 and 4D9 recognise different epitopes of IL–4. (From Bradding, P. et al., *Am. J. Respir. Cell Mol. Biol.*, 10, 471, 1994. With permission.)

Several recent observations have confirmed that mast cells also express mRNA for these cytokines and release them in response to IgE-dependent activation. Using *in situ* hybridization and RT-PCR technology on isolated skin and lung mast cells, we have demonstrated expression of mRNA for IL-4, IL-5, and IL-6, although the signals for IL-5 and IL-6 were relatively weak in the skin mast cells.[196] We have also demonstrated that isolated human lung mast cells release IL-4 in response to IgE-dependent activation[191] (Figure 4), and others have reported similar findings in relation to IL-5.[197] The rapid time course of cytokine release in these studies suggests that they are stored in a preformed state within mast cell granules, as has previously been demonstrated using immunogold localisation in the case of TNFα in rodent mast cells.[198] The presence of immunoreactive IL-4, IL-5, IL-6, and TNFα in mast cells from nonasthmatic subjects might also suggest that these cytokines are stored in a preformed state. By using an approach combining immunohistochemistry and *in situ* hybridisation, expression of mRNA for IL-4 and IL-5 has also been demonstrated by approximately 17 and 25%, respectively, of mast cells in bronchial biopsies from atopic asthmatic subjects.[187] Taken together, these studies of mast cell cytokine synthesis and release *in vitro* and mRNA expression *in vivo* support the conclusions with regard to cellular localisation reached by immunohistochemical studies.

These observations have major implications for the role of the mast cell in asthma (Figure 5). Both the induction of *de novo* cytokine expression after cellular activation and the induction of adhesion molecule expression in response to cytokine exposure usually take several hours. Therefore, the rapid release of preformed cytokines from mast cell granules in response to allergen exposure could represent a crucial initiating stimulus in the chain of events leading to the recruitment of leukocytes from the circulation into the airways, a process which begins as early as 3 h.[199] The identification of TNFα release into nasal lavage fluid 2 min after allergen challenge supports this hypothesis,[200] as do the *in vitro* observations that IL-4, IL-5, and TNFα are released from purified human mast cells through an IgE-dependent mechanism.[191,194,197] Thus, mast cell–derived TNFα and IL-4 may be critical in inducing the endothelial expression of the adhesion molecules E-selectin, ICAM-1, and VCAM-1[112-116] which, as discussed above, are believed to be important in the recruitment of eosinophils. Within the airways, mast cell–derived IL-4, IL-5, and TNFα would then act to induce the chemoattraction, survival, and priming of eosinophils.[87,201,202] Indeed, evidence from animal studies suggests that overexpression of IL-4 alone is sufficient to induce pathological eosinophilic inflammation.[47,203,204] The question also arises of whether or not the mast cell might, under certain circumstances, provide the initial source of IL-4 required for the development of the Th2 subset of T-lymphocytes.[205,206] Mast cells have been shown to induce IgE synthesis by B-lymphocytes *in vitro* through an interaction with CD40.[207] In this study the mast cells were not activated through an IgE-dependent mechanism and exogenous IL-4 was also required, but it nevertheless indicates that mast cells may in principle influence IgE production.

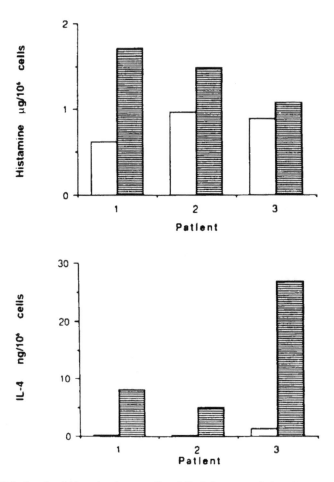

FIGURE 4   Levels of histamine (top panel) and IL-4 (lower panel) in culture supernatants following challenge of purified human lung mast cells with either anti-IgE (shaded bars) or saline control (open bars). (From Bradding, P. et al., *J. Exp. Med.*, 176, 1381, 1992. With permission of The Rockefeller University Press.)

In our studies of biopsies from asthmatic and normal subjects we have been unable to detect immunoreactivity for cytokines localised to T cells. Nevertheless, there is good evidence that T cells do synthesise cytokines in the human airway mucosa. For example, the majority of allergen-specific CD4+ T cell clones derived from bronchial biopsies obtained 48 h after inhalation challenge of atopic asthmatic subjects with relevant allergen have been reported to secrete a Th2-like cytokine profile (IL-4+ and IL-5+).[208] Robinson et al.[186] have demonstrated that 42 and 59% of T cells in BAL fluid from asthmatic subjects express mRNA for IL-4 and IL-5, respectively, with significantly greater numbers of cytokine mRNA-positive cells in asthmatic subjects compared with normal controls. Similarly, numbers of cells expressing

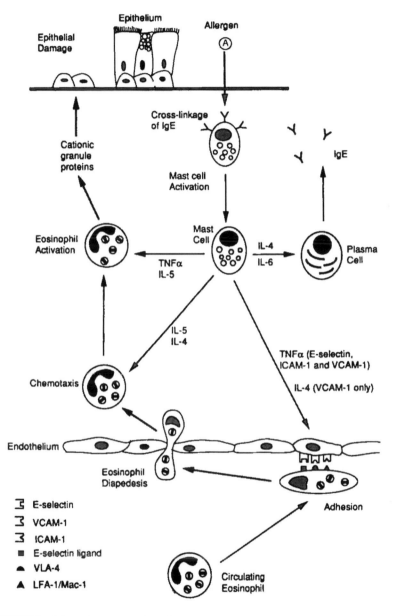

**FIGURE 5** Schematic representation of potential sites at which mast cell cytokines may be involved in the regulation of allergic inflammation. (From Redington, A.E. and Howarth, P.H., *Can. Respir. J.*, 1, 118, 1994. With permission.)

mRNA for IL-4 and IL-5 in BAL fluid from atopic asthmatic subjects increase following allergen challenge, with 45 and 59% of T cells expressing mRNA for IL-4 and IL-5, respectively, after provocation.[189] In bronchial biopsies from atopic asthmatic subjects it has been estimated that approximately 11 and 23% of T-lymphocytes express mRNA for IL-4 and IL-5, respectively.[187] However, the significance of these findings is uncertain in light of a recent report from the same group suggesting that only 1 in 300 to 1 in 5000 T cells in the airways of atopic subjects are allergen specific.[209] This would suggest that most of the Th2-like T-lymphocytes are not allergen specific.

The apparent discrepancy between the results from immunohistochemistry and *in situ* hybridisation is likely to result at least in part from the fact that T cells are unable to store cytokines. Instead, cytokine synthesis only occurs in response to cellular activation, and secretion takes place in a highly specific and localised manner,[210] making detection of intracellular protein difficult in biopsy material. This interpretation is further supported by observations from our own studies using flow cytometry. When activated with PMA and iono-mycin, T cells from an IL-4-producing clone stain poorly for cytokines. However, when export from the Golgi apparatus is blocked using monensin, cytokine immunoreactivity becomes much easier to detect. Using this method to block cytokine secretion, we have recently completed a study comparing the cytokine-producing potential of peripheral blood and BAL T cells from atopic asthmatic subjects in comparison with atopic and nonatopic nonasthmatic controls.[211] In contrast to the studies investigating the expression of cytokine mRNA, we have found increased numbers of IFNγ-producing T cells in BAL fluid of asthmatic subjects, whereas only a small proportion of BAL T cells (median <1%) produce IL-4. This latter observation is perhaps more in keeping with our findings in mucosal biopsies.

Eosinophils were also a source of cytokines in our studies. In approximately 25% of the biopsies of patients with allergic asthma, about 20% of eosinophils contained immunoreactive IL-5.[192] In addition, we found that a small proportion of eosinophils expressed immunoreactivity for IL-4.[192] These findings are compatible with the reports that the majority of eosinophils recovered by BAL 24 h after local allergen challenge express mRNA for IL-5[212] and that in bronchial biopsies from atopic asthmatic patients approximately 20 and 2% of eosinophils express mRNA for IL-5 and IL-4, respectively.[187] In addition, recent reports have confirmed the ability of eosinophils *in vitro* to release IL-5 in response to Ig-dependent activation.[213] Thus, eosinophils are likely to make a significant contribution to the total expression of both IL-4 and IL-5 within the airways. In the case of IL-5, this cytokine may act in an autocrine manner to amplify eosinophilic inflammation.

In the case of a number of other cytokines, the predominant site at which immunoreactivity is localised is not inflammatory cells but the bronchial epithelium. In the case of IL-8 we have demonstrated localisation of immu-noreactivity to the bronchial epithelium in biopsies from both asthmatic and control subjects with increased expression in the former[214] (Figure 6). Other groups have also shown similar findings in relation to GM-CSF[215,216] and two other chemokines, RANTES[217] and monocyte chemoattractant protein-1

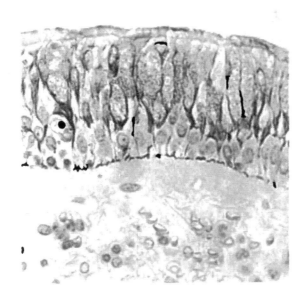

**FIGURE 6** Immunoreactivity for IL-8 in a bronchial biopsy specimen showing predominant localisation to bronchial epithelial cells and to the basement membrane region.

(MCP-1).[218] These findings are in keeping with *in vitro* studies using transformed or cultured human airway epithelial cells which can synthesise and release GM-CSF,[219-222] IL-8,[222] and RANTES,[223] particularly after stimulation with either IL-1 or TNFα. The production of cytokines such as these may provide a means for the directed recruitment of eosinophils into the epithelial compartment and their activation once there.

In the studies on cytokine production by cultured bronchial epithelial cells, two further cytokines were demonstrated, IL-6 and TNFα.[220,224] However, we have not been able to localise immunoreactivity for either of these cytokines to bronchial epithelial cells in biopsies from either asthmatic or control subjects.[214] The explanation for this apparent discrepancy is unclear. It may be that these cytokines are produced in quantities which are below the limit of detection using our methodology. Alternatively, they may be synthesised but very rapidly exported from the cells so that there is insufficient intracellular accumulation to allow detection using immunohistochemistry, as discussed above in relation to T cells. However, a third possibility is that this represents a significant difference between the metabolic behaviour of cultured cells and those *in situ* in tissues. Similar divergent profiles of cytokine production have been reported between freshly isolated and cultured upper airway epithelial cells,[225] and these findings draw further attention to the need to exert caution when extrapolating from *in vitro* studies to the *in vivo* situation.

In the case of IL-8 an additional feature which we observed in our immunohistochemical studies was the localisation of immunoreactivity to the interepithelial spaces and subepithelial basement membrane region. The basement membrane is a complex structure, but one component which may be of particular relevance is the proteoglycan HSPG. IL-8 can bind to HSPG and its activity as a neutrophil activator is increased by this interaction.[17] Furthermore, recent discussion has focussed on the possibility that, rather than acting in soluble form, many mediators involved in leukocyte recruitment do so when bound to the ECM, a process referred to as haptotaxis. Neutrophil migration *in vitro* in response to IL-8 has been shown to take place via such a haptotactic mechanism.[226] Thus, our demonstration of the basement membrane localisation of IL-8 in biopsies may reflect a mechanism whereby, once released from bronchial epithelial cells, this cytokine is maintained at a high concentration locally and so can subserve a role in leukocyte haptotaxis.

In the case of fibrogenic cytokines, interaction with components of the ECM are likely to be of even greater importance. Using a monoclonal antibody which recognises all three isoforms of TGFβ, we have shown that in addition to immunostaining of bronchial epithelial cells and inflammatory cells in the subepithelial tissues, a major site of immunoreactivity was the ECM. Here, staining was seen in an interstitial pattern and, comparing adjacent sections, was distributed in a fashion similar to immunoreactivity for the small proteoglycan decorin. Many components of the ECM have been reported to be capable of binding TGFβ, including collagen IV[227] and fibronectin.[228] However, the particular significance of decorin is that its interaction with TGFβ inhibits the biologic activity of this cytokine both *in vitro*[229] and *in vivo*.[230] Thus, the colocalisation of immunoreactivity which we have observed may reflect a mechanism to control the activity of this cytokine. Although the pattern of immunohistochemical staining was similar in asthmatic and control subjects, we have been able to detect increased quantities of TGFβ recoverable in BAL fluid in asthma.[231] In this study TGFβ was detected using an ELISA incorporating an acidification step so that total quantities of the cytokine were measured. However, it is probable that only a small proportion of the cytokine is present in an active form *in vivo*. As TGFβ is an extremely potent stimulus for ECM formation, its activation is likely to be tightly controlled by a number of mechanisms, including binding to ECM components such as decorin.

Interactions with components of the ECM are also likely to be of major importance in the case of bFGF. In bronchial biopsies from both normal and asthmatic subjects, we have shown that immunoreactivity for bFGF is predominantly localised extracellularly in association with basement membranes of the vascular endothelium and bronchial epithelium.[232] At these basement membrane sites there is colocalisation of immunoreactivity for bFGF and HSPG. As bFGF is known to bind to HSPG *in vitro*,[18,19] it seems likely that the staining pattern we have observed reflects the existence of such an interaction *in vivo*. When thus bound to HSPG, bFGF is protected from inactivation by proteases[18,233] and other stimuli such as heat and extremes of pH.[234] It has therefore been proposed that this mechanism acts to provide a reservoir of cytokine which can be released in response to specific stimuli.

To examine the release of bFGF within the airways *in vivo* in response to a physiologically relevant stimulus, we have performed segmental broncho-provocation with allergen and saline in a group of atopic asthmatic subjects. At a time point of 10 min after challenge, there was approximately a fivefold increase in the concentration of bFGF in BAL fluid recovered from allergen-challenged segments in comparison with control saline-challenged sites. The most likely explanation for this observation may be the rapid release of extra-cellular bFGF from basement membrane–binding sites. One possible mechanism by which this might be achieved is via the actions of mast cell degranulation products released in response to allergen exposure. Mast cell heparin also binds bFGF and is generally considered to have an affinity for the cytokine at least equal to that of any HSPG preparation. Thus, mast cell heparin might compete with HSPG for binding of bFGF and elute the cytokine from its matrix-bound state in a biologically active form. This explanation is supported by the demonstration that heparin can induce the rapid *in vitro* release of bFGF from ECM secreted by cultured bovine endothelial cells[21] and from preparations of bovine corneal Descemet's membrane.[20] Furthermore, administration of heparin to rabbits by intravenous infusion results in the rapid release of bFGF-like activity into the circulation.[235] Alternatively, mast cell–derived enzymes might be implicated in the release of bFGF. bFGF bound to ECM HSPGs can be released in a fully active form when these are degraded by the specific endoglycosidase heparanase,[21] and mast cell degranulation is known to result in the release of an endoglycosidase that can degrade heparan sulphate in subendothelial ECM.[236]

We have also reported increased concentrations of bFGF recoverable in BAL fluid from asthmatic subjects at baseline in comparison with normal subjects.[232] Theoretically, this might reflect differences in synthesis, release, degradation, or any combination of these. However, mast cell activation is evident in mild stable asthma, as indicated by increased levels of mast cell mediators in BAL fluid[1,193] and ultrastructural appearances of mast cell degranulation.[4,8] Thus, one possible explanation for the increased concentrations of bFGF in mild stable asthma may be ongoing mast cell degranulation with the release of heparin and/or enzymes which influence the distribution of bFGF between its matrix-bound and soluble states.

## V. CONCLUSIONS

The availability of fibreoptic bronchoscopy as a relatively noninvasive means to obtain biologic samples has resulted in an increasing number of studies being performed in the last few years to examine the expression of cytokines in the airways in asthma. Most of these studies have concentrated on those cytokines which are likely to be involved in the more acute aspects of the inflammatory response, but interest is now increasing in the chronic structural changes in the airway wall which are also characteristic of this condition.

However, it must be recognised that the majority of these studies have produced information which is of a largely descriptive or correlative nature. To prove unequivocally that the expression of a particular cytokine is functionally important, it will be necessary to examine the effect of specifically inhibiting its expression. Studies with experimental gene-knockout animals have provided some information in this respect, but their interpretation is complicated by the possibility of compensatory mechanisms developing during ontogeny. To date, no naturally occurring cytokine deficiencies in humans have been reported. Clinical studies using agents such as specific cytokine receptor antagonist and anticytokine antibodies are certain to be performed in the next few years and may well produce some surprises. Lessons need to be learned from experience with PAF. This lipid mediator has many biologic properties which are relevant to allergic inflammation, and throughout the 1980s it seemed highly likely that PAF would prove to be an important mediator in asthma.[237] However, a recent study using a potent and selective PAF antagonist failed to show any evidence of benefit in clinical asthma,[238] and it now seems very doubtful that PAF will prove to be a mediator of major importance.

# REFERENCES

1. Casale, T. B., Wood, D., Richerson, H. B., Trapp, S., Metzger, W. J., Zavala, D., and Hunninghake, G. W., Elevated bronchoalveolar lavage fluid histamine levels in allergic asthmatics are associated with methacholine bronchial hyperresponsiveness, *J. Clin. Invest.*, 79, 1197, 1987.
2. Wardlaw, A. J., Dunnette, S., Gleich, G. J., Collins, J. V., and Kay, A. B., Eosinophils and mast cells in bronchoalveolar lavage in subjects with mild asthma: relationship to bronchial reactivity, *Am. Rev. Respir. Dis.*, 137, 62, 1988.
3. Lozewicz, S., Gomez, E., Ferguson, H., and Davies, R. J., Inflammatory cells in the airways in mild asthma, *Br. Med. J.*, 297, 1515, 1988.
4. Beasley, R., Roche, W. R., Roberts, J. A., and Holgate, S. T., Cellular events in the bronchi in mild asthma and after bronchial provocation, *Am. Rev. Respir. Dis.*, 139, 806, 1989.
5. Jeffery, P. K., Wardlaw, A. J., Nelson, F. C., Collins, J. V., and Kay, A. B., Bronchial biopsies in asthma: an ultrastructural, quantitative study and correlation with hyperreactivity, *Am. Rev. Respir. Dis.*, 140, 1745, 1989.
6. Azzawi, M., Bradley, B., Jeffery, P. K., Frew, A. J., Wardlaw, A. J., Knowles, G., Assoufi, B., Collins, J. V., Durham, S., and Kay, A. B., Identification of activated T lymphocytes and eosinophils in bronchial biopsies in stable atopic asthma, *Am. Rev. Respir. Dis.*, 142, 1407, 1990.

7. Bousquet, J., Chanez, P., Lacoste, J. Y., Barneon, G., Ghavanian, N., Enander, I., Venge, P., Ahlstedt, S., Simony-Lafontaine, J., Godard, P., and Michel, F.-B., Eosinophilic inflammation in asthma, *N. Engl. J. Med.*, 323, 1033, 1990.

8. Djukanovic, R., Wilson, J. W., Britten, K. M., Wilson, S. J., Walls, A. F., Roche, W. R., Howarth, P. H., and Holgate, S. T., Quantitation of mast cells and eosinophils in the bronchial mucosa of symptomatic atopic asthmatics and healthy control subjects using immunohistochemistry, *Am. Rev. Respir. Dis.*, 142, 863, 1990.

9. Bradley, B. L., Azzawi, M., Jacobson, M., Assoufi, B., Collins, J. V., Irani, A. A., Schwartz, L. B., Durham, S. R., Jeffery, P. K., and Kay, A. B., Eosinophils, T-lymphocytes, mast cells, neutrophils, and macrophages in bronchial biopsy specimens from atopic subjects with asthma: comparison with biopsy specimens from atopic subjects without asthma and normal control subjects and relation to bronchial hyperresponsiveness, *J. Allergy Clin. Immunol.*, 88, 661, 1991.

10. Laitinen, L. A., Laitinen, A., and Haahtela, T., Eosinophilic airway inflammation during exacerbation of asthma and its treatment with inhaled corticosteroid, *Am. Rev. Respir. Dis.*, 143, 423, 1991.

11. Poston, R. N., Chanez, P., Lacoste, J. Y., Lichfield, T., Lee, T. H., and Bousquet, J., Immunohistochemical characterization of the cellular infiltration in asthmatic bronchi, *Am. Rev. Respir. Dis.*, 145, 918, 1992.

12. Laitinen, L. A., Laitinen, A., and Haahtela, T., Airway mucosal inflammation even in patients with newly diagnosed asthma, *Am. Rev. Respir. Dis.*, 147, 697, 1993.

13. Terracio, L., Rönnstrand, L., Tingström, A., Rubin, K., Claesson-Welsh, L., Funa, K., and Heldin, C.-H., Induction of platelet-derived growth factor receptor expression in smooth muscle cells and fibroblasts upon tissue culturing, *J. Cell Biol.*, 107, 1947, 1988.

14. Schall, T. J., O'Hehir, R. E., Goeddel, D. V., and Lamb, J. R., Uncoupling of cytokine mRNA expression and protein secretion during the induction phase of T cell anergy, *J. Immunol.*, 148, 381, 1992.

15. Gordon, J., Millsum, M. J., Guy, G. R., and Ledbetter, J. A., Compartmentalisation of a haematopoietic growth factor (GM-CSF) by glycosaminoglycans in the bone marrow microenvironment, *Nature*, 326, 403, 1987.

16. Roberts, R., Gallagher, J., Spooncer, E., Allen, T. D., Bloomfield, F., and Dealer, T. M., Heparan sulphate bound growth factors: a mechanism for stromal cell mediated haemopoiesis, *Nature*, 332, 376, 1988.

17. Webb, L. M. C., Ehrengruber, M. U., Clark-Lewis, I., Baggiolini, M., and Rot, A., Binding to heparan sulfate or heparin enhances neutrophil responses to interleukin 8, *Proc. Natl. Acad. Sci. U.S.A.*, 90, 7158, 1993.

18. Saksela, O., Moscatelli, D., Sommer, A., and Rifkin, D. B., Endothelial cell-derived heparan sulfate binds basic fibroblast growth factor and protects it from proteolytic degradation, *J. Cell Biol.*, 107, 743, 1988.

19. Vigny, M., Ollier-Hartmann, M. P., Lavigne, M., Fayein, N., Jeanny, J. C., Laurent, M., and Courtois, Y., Specific binding of basic fibroblast growth factor to basement membrane-like structures and to purified heparan sulfate proteoglycan of the EHS tumor, *J. Cell Physiol.*, 137, 321, 1988.

20. Folkman, J., Klagsbrun, M., Sasse, J., Wadzinski, M., Ingber, D., and Vlodavsky, I., A heparin-binding angiogenic protein — basic fibroblast growth factor — is stored within basement membranes, *Am. J. Pathol.*, 130, 393, 1988.

21. Bashkin, P., Doctrow, S., Klagsbrun, M., Svahn, C. M., Folkman, J., and Vlodavsky, I., Basic fibroblast growth factor binds to subendothelial extracellular matrix and is released by heparitinase and heparin-like molecules, *Biochemistry*, 28, 1737, 1989.

22. Zimmerman, G. A., Lorant, D. E., McIntyre, T. M., and Prescott, S. M., Juxtacrine intercellular signaling: another way to do it, *Am. J. Respir. Cell Mol. Biol.*, 9, 573, 1993.

23. Yayon, A., Klagsbrun, M., Esko, J. D., Leder, P., and Ornitz, D. M., Cell surface, heparin-like molecules are required for binding of basic fibroblast growth factor to its high affinity receptor, *Cell*, 64, 841, 1991.

24. Del Prete, G., Maggi, E., Parronchi, P., Chrétien, I., Tiri, A., Macchia, D., Ricci, M., Banchereau, J., de Vries, J., and Romagnani, S., IL-4 is an essential factor for the IgE synthesis induced *in vitro* by human T cell clones and their supernatants, *J. Immunol.*, 140, 4193, 1988.

25. Pène, J., Rousset, F., Brière, F., Chrétien, I., Bonnefoy, J. Y., Spits, H., Yokota, T., Arai, N., Arai, K. I., Banchereau, J., and de Vries, J. E., IgE production by normal human lymphocytes is induced by interleukin-4 and suppressed by interferons γ and α and prostaglandin E2, *Proc. Natl. Acad. Sci. U.S.A.*, 85, 6880, 1988.

26. Gauchat, J.-F., Lebman, D. A., Coffman, R. L., Gascan, H., and de Vries, J. E., Structure and expression of germline ε transcripts in human B cells induced by interleukin 4 to switch to IgE production, *J. Exp. Med.*, 172, 463, 1990.

27. Vercelli, D., Jabara, H. H., Arai, K., and Geha, R. S., Induction of human IgE synthesis requires IL-4 and T/B cell interactions involving the T cell receptor/CD3 complex and MHC class II antigens, *J. Exp. Med.*, 167, 1406, 1989.

28. Parronchi, P., Tiri, A., Macchia, D., De Carli, M., Biswas, P., Simonelli, C., Maggi, E., Del Prete, G., Ricci, M., and Romagnani, S., Noncognate contact-dependent B cell activation can promote IL-4-dependent *in vitro* human IgE synthesis, *J. Immunol.*, 144, 2102, 1990.

29. Spriggs, M. K., Armitage, R. J., Strockbine, L., Clifford, K. N., Macduff, B. M., Sato, T. A., Maliszewski, C. R., and Fanslow, W. C., Recombinant human CD40 ligand stimulates B cell proliferation and immunoglobulin E synthesis, *J. Exp. Med.*, 176, 1543, 1992.

30. Castle, B. E., Kishimoto, K., Stearns, C., Brown, M. L., and Kehry, M. R., Regulation of expression of the ligand for CD40 on T helper lymphocytes, *J. Immunol.*, 151, 1777, 1993.

31. June, C. H., Bluestone, J. A., Nadler, L. M., and Thompson, C. B., The B7 and CD28 receptor families, *Immunol. Today*, 15, 321, 1994.

32. Zhang, K., Clark, E. A., and Saxon, A., CD40 stimulation provides an IFN-γ-independent and IL-4-dependent differentiation signal directly to human B cells for IgE production, *J. Immunol.*, 146, 1836, 1991.

33. Thyphronitis, G., Tsokos, G. C., June, C. H., Levine, A. D., and Finkelman, F. D., IgE secretion by Epstein–Barr virus-infected purified human B lymphocytes is stimulated by interleukin 4 and suppressed by interferon γ, *Proc. Natl. Acad. Sci. U.S.A.*, 86, 5580, 1989.

34. Wu, C. Y., Sarfati, M., Heusser, C., Fournier, S., Rubio-Trujillo, M., Peleman, R., and Delespesse, G., Glucocorticoids increase the synthesis of immunoglobulin E by interleukin 4-stimulated human lymphocytes, *J. Clin. Invest.*, 87, 870, 1991.

35. Nüsslein, H. G., Träg, T., Winter, M., Dietz, A., and Kalden, J. R., The role of T cells and the effect of hydrocortisone on interleukin-4-induced IgE synthesis by non-T cells, *Clin. Exp. Immunol.*, 90, 286, 1992.

36. Wu, C. Y., Fargeas, C., Nakajima, T., and Delespesse, G., Glucocorticoids suppress the production of interleukin 4 by human lymphocytes, *Eur. J. Immunol.*, 21, 2645, 1991.

37. Byron, K. A., Varigos, G., and Wootton, A. M., Hydrocortisone inhibition of human interleukin 4, *Immunology*, 77, 624, 1992.

38. Settipane, G. A., Pudupakkam, R. K., and McGowan, J. H., Corticosteroid effect on immunoglobulins, *J. Allergy Clin. Immunol.*, 62, 162, 1978.

39. Defrance, T., Aubry, J. P., Rousset, F., Vanbervliet, B., Bonnefoy, J. Y., Aral, N., Takebe, Y., Yokota, T., Lee, F., Arai, K., de Vries, J., and Banchereau, J., Human recombinant interleukin 4 induces Fcε receptors (CD23) on normal human B lymphocytes, *J. Exp. Med.*, 165, 1459, 1987.

40. Sanders, V. M., Fernandez-Botran, R., Uhr, J. W., and Vitetta, E. S., Interleukin 4 enhances the ability of antigen-specific B cells to form conjugates with T cells, *J. Immunol.*, 139, 2349, 1987.

41. Vercelli, D., Jabara, H. H., Lee, B.-W., Woodland, N., Geha, R. S., and Leung, D. Y., Human recombinant interleukin 4 induces FcεR2/CD23 on normal human monocytes, *J. Exp. Med.*, 167, 1406, 1988.

42. Vercelli, D., Jabari, H. H., Arai, K.-I., Yokota., T., and Geha, R. S., Endogenous interleukin 6 plays an obligatory role in interleukin 4-dependent human IgE synthesis, *Eur. J. Immunol.*, 19, 1419, 1989.

43. Bonnefoy, J.-Y., Shields, J., and Mermod, J.-J., Inhibition of human interleukin 4-induced IgE synthesis by a subset of anti-CD23/FcεRII monoclonal antibodies, *Eur. J. Immunol.*, 20, 139, 1990.

44. Rousset, F., de Waal Malefijt, R., Slierendregt, B., Aubry, J.-P., Bonnefoy, J.-Y., Defrance, T., Banchereau, J., and de Vries, J. E., Regulation of Fc receptor for IgE (CD23) and class II MHC antigen expression on Burkitt's lymphoma cell lines by human IL-4 and IFN-γ, *J. Immunol.*, 140, 2625, 1988.

45. Finkelman, F. D., Katona, I. M., Urban, J., Jr., Snapper, C. M., Ohara, J., and Paul, W. E., Suppression of *in vivo* polyclonal IgE responses by monoclonal antibody to the lymphokine B-cell stimulatory factor 1, *Proc. Natl. Acad. Sci. U.S.A.*, 83, 9675, 1986.

46. Kühn, R., Rajewsky, K., and Müller, W., Generation and analysis of interleukin-4 deficient mice, *Science*, 254, 707, 1991.

47. Tepper, R. I., Levinson, D. A., Stanger, B. Z., Campos-Torres, J., Abbas, A. K., and Leder, P., IL-4 induces allergic-like inflammatory disease and alters T cell development in transgenic mice, *Cell*, 62, 457, 1990.

48. Punnonen, J., Aversa, G., Cocks, B. G., McKenzie, A. N. J., Menon, S., Zurawski, G., de Waal Malefyt, R., and de Vries, J. E., Interleukin 13 induces interleukin 4-independent IgG4 and IgE synthesis and CD23 expression by human B cells, *Proc. Natl. Acad. Sci. U.S.A.*, 90, 3730, 1993.

49. Minty, A., Chalon, P., Derocq, J.-M., Dumont, X., Guillemot, J.-C., Kaghad, M., Labit, C., Leplatois, P., Liauzun, P., and Miloux, B., Interleukin 13 is a new human lymphokine regulating inflammatory and immune responses, *Nature*, 362, 248, 1992.

50. Defrance, T., Carayon, P., Billian, G., Guillemot, J.-C., Minty, A., Caput, D., and Ferrara, P., Interleukin 13 is a B cell stimulating factor, *J. Exp. Med.*, 179, 135, 1994.

51. Zurawski, S. M., Vega, F., Jr., Huyghe, B., and Zurawski, G., Receptors for interleukin-13 and interleukin-4 are complex and share a novel component that functions in signal transduction, *EMBO J.*, 12, 2663, 1993.

52. Lopez, A. F., Williamson, D. W., Gamble, J. R., Begley, C. G., Harlan, J. M., Klebanoff, S. J., Waltersdorph, A., Wong, G., Clark, S. C., and Vadas, M. A., Recombinant human granulocyte-macrophage colony-stimulating factor stimulates *in vitro* mature human neutrophil and eosinophil function, surface receptor expression, and survival, *J. Clin. Invest.*, 78, 1220, 1986.

53. Campbell, H. D., Tucker, W. Q. J., Hort, Y., Martinson, M. E., Mayo, G., Clutterbuck, E. J., Sanderson, C. J., and Young, I. G., Molecular cloning, nucleotide sequence, and expression of the gene encoding human eosinophil differentiation factor (interleukin 5), *Proc. Natl. Acad. Sci. U.S.A.*, 84, 6629, 1987.

54. Clutterbuck, E. J., Shields, J. G., and Gordon, J., Recombinant human interleukin 5 is an eosinophil differentiation factor but has no activity in standard human B cell growth factor assays, *Eur. J. Immunol.*, 17, 1743, 1987.

55. Clutterbuck, E., Hirst, E. M. A., and Sanderson, C. J., Human interleukin-5 (IL-5) regulates the production of eosinophils in human bone marrow cultures: comparison and interaction with IL-1, IL-3, IL-6, and GM-CSF, *Blood*, 73, 1504, 1989.

56. Saito, H., Hatake, K., Dvorak, A. M., Lieferman, K. M., Donnenberg, A. D., Arai, N., Ishizaka, K., and Ishizaka, T., Selective differentiation and proliferation of haemopoietic cells induced by recombinant interleukins, *Proc. Natl. Acad. Sci. U.S.A.*, 85, 2288, 1988.

57. Clutterbuck, E. J. and Sanderson, C. J., Regulation of human eosinophil precursor production by cytokines: a comparison of recombinant human interleukin-1 (rhIL-1), rhIL-3, rhIL-5, rhIL-6 and rh granulocyte-macrophage colony-stimulating factor, *Blood*, 75, 1774, 1990.

58. Coffman, R. L., Seymour, B. W. P., Hudak, S., Jackson, J., and Rennick, D., Antibody to interleukin-5 inhibits helminth-induced eosinophilia in mice, *Science*, 245, 308, 1989.

59. Sher, A., Coffman, R. L., Hieny, S., Scott, P., and Cheever, A. W., Interleukin 5 is required for the blood and tissue eosinophilia but not for granuloma formation induced by infection with *Schistosoma mansoni, Proc. Natl. Acad. Sci. U.S.A.*, 87, 61, 1990.

60. Vaux, D. L., Lalor, P. A., Cory, S., and Johnson, G. R., *In vivo* expression of interleukin 5 induces an eosinophilia and expanded Ly-1B lineage populations, *Int. Immunol.*, 2, 965, 1990.

61. Dent, L. A., Strath, M., Mellor, A. L., and Sanderson, C. J., Eosinophilia in transgenic mice expressing interleukin 5, *J. Exp. Med.*, 172, 1425, 1990.

62. Tominaga, A., Takaki, S., Koyama, N., Katoh, S., Matsumoto, R., Migita, M., Hitoshi, Y., Hosoya, Y., Yamauchi, S., Kanai, Y., Miyazaki, J.-I., Usuku, G., Yamamura, K.-I., and Takatsu, K., Transgenic mice expressing a B cell growth and differentiation factor gene (interleukin 5) develop eosinophilia and autoantibody production, *J. Exp. Med.*, 173, 429, 1991.

63. Chang, J. M., Metcalf, D., Lang, R. A., Gonda, T. J., and Johnson, G. R., Nonneoplastic haematopoietic myeloproliferative syndrome induced by dysregulated multi-CSF (IL-3) expression, *Blood*, 73, 1487, 1989.

64. Lang, R. A., Metcalf, D., and Cuthbertson, R. A., Transgenic mice expressing a haemopoietic growth factor gene (GM-CSF) develop accumulations of macrophages, blindness, and a fatal syndrome of tissue damage, *Cell*, 51, 675, 1987.

65. Metcalf, D. and Moore, J. G., Divergent disease patterns in granulocyte-macrophage colony-stimulating factor transgenic mice associated with different transgene insertion sites, *Proc. Natl. Acad. Sci. U.S.A.*, 85, 7767, 1988.

66. Wang, J. M., Rimaldi, A., Biondi, A., Chen, Z. G., Sanderson, C. J., and Mantovani, A., Recombinant human interleukin 5 is a selective eosinophil chemoattractant, *Eur. J. Immunol.*, 19, 701, 1989.

67. Warringa, R. A. J., Koenderman, L., Kok, P. T. M., Kreukniet, J., and Bruijnzeel, P. L. B., Modulation and induction of eosinophil chemotaxis by granulocyte-macrophage colony-stimulating factor and interleukin-3, *Blood*, 77, 2694, 1991.

68. Sehmi, R., Wardlaw, A. J., Cromwell, O., Kurihara, K., Waltmann, P., and Kay, A. B., Interleukin-5 selectively enhances the chemotactic response of eosinophils obtained from normal but not eosinophilic subjects, *Blood*, 79, 2952, 1992.

69. Warringa, R. A. J., Mengelers, H. J. J., Kuijper, P. H. M., Raaijmakers, J. A. M., Bruijnzeel, P. L. B., and Koenderman, L., *In vivo* priming of platelet-activating factor-induced eosinophil chemotaxis in allergic asthmatic individuals, *Blood*, 79, 1836, 1992.

70. Oppenheim, J. J., Zachariae, C. O. C., Mukaida, N., and Matsushima, K., Properties of the novel proinflammatory supergene "intercrine" cytokine family, *Annu. Rev. Immunol.*, 9, 617, 1991.

71. Leonard, E. J. and Yoshimura, T., Neutrophil attractant/activation protein-1 (NAP-1 [interleukin-8]), *Am. J. Respir. Cell Mol. Biol.*, 2, 470, 1990.

72. Warringa, R. A. J., Schweizer, R. C., Maikoe, T., Kuijper, P. H. M., Bruijnzeel, P. L. B., and Koenderman, L., Modulation of eosinophil chemotaxis by interleukin-5, *Am. J. Respir. Cell Mol. Biol.*, 7, 631, 1992.

73. Sehmi, R., Cromwell, O., Wardlaw, A. J., Moqbel, R., and Kay, A. B., Interleukin-8 is a chemoattractant for eosinophils purified from subjects with a blood eosinophilia but not from normal healthy subjects, *Clin. Exp. Allergy*, 23, 1027, 1994.

74. Kameyoshi, Y., Dörschner, A., Mallet, A. I., Christophers, E., and Schröder, J.-M., Cytokine RANTES released by thrombin-stimulated platelets is a potent attractant for human eosinophils, *J. Exp. Med.*, 176, 587, 1992.

75. Rot, A., Krieger, M., Brunner, T., Bischoff, S. C., Schall, T. J., and Dahinden, C. A., RANTES and macrophage inflammatory protein 1α induce the migration and activation of normal human eosinophil granulocytes, *J. Exp. Med.*, 176, 1489, 1992.

76. Alam, R., Stafford, S., Forsythe, P., Harrison, R., Faubion, D., Lett-Brown, M. A., and Grant, J. A., RANTES is a chemotactic and activating factor for human eosinophils, *J. Immunol.*, 150, 3442, 1993.

77. Bischoff, S. C., Krieger, M., Brunner, T., Rot, A., v. Tscharner, V., Baggiolini, M., and Dahinden, C., RANTES and related chemokines activate human basophil granulocytes through different G protein-coupled receptors, *Eur. J. Immunol.*, 23, 761, 1993.

78. Schweizer, R.-C., Welmers, B. A. C., Raaijmakers, J. A. M., Zanen, P., Lammers, J.-W. J., and Koenderman, L., RANTES- and interleukin-8-induced responses in normal human eosinophils: effects of priming with interleukin-5, *Blood*, 83, 3697, 1994.

79. Owen, W. F., Jr., Rothenberg, M. E., Silberstein, D. S., Gasson, J. C., Stevens, R. L., Austen, K. F., and Soberman, R. J., Regulation of human eosinophil viability, density and function by granulocyte/macrophage colony-stimulating factor in the presence of 3T3 fibroblasts, *J. Exp. Med.*, 166, 129, 1987.

80. Rothenberg, M. E., Owen, W. F., Jr., Silberstein, D. S., Woods, J., Soberman, R. J., Austen, K. F., and Stevens, R. L., Human eosinophils have prolonged survival, enhanced functional properties, and become hypodense when exposed to human interleukin 3, *J. Clin. Invest.*, 81, 1986, 1988.

81. Tai, P.-C., Sun, L., and Spry, C. J. F., Effects of IL-5, granulocyte/macrophage colony-stimulating factor (GM-CSF) and IL-3 on the survival of human blood eosinophils *in vitro*, *Clin. Exp. Immunol.*, 85, 312, 1991.

82. Valerius, T., Repp, R., Kalden, J. R., and Platzer, E., Effects of IFN on human eosinophils in comparison with other cytokines: a novel class of eosinophil activators with delayed onset of action, *J. Immunol.*, 145, 2950, 1990.

83. Yamaguchi, Y., Suda, T., Ohna, T., Tominaga, K., Miura, Y., and Kasahara, T., Analysis of the survival of mature human eosinophils: interleukin 5 prevent apoptosis in mature human eosinophils, *Blood*, 78, 2542, 1991.

84. Stern, M., Meagher, L., Savill, J., and Haslett, C., Apoptosis in human eosinophils: programmed cell death in the eosinophil leads to phagocytosis by macrophages and is modulated by IL-5, *J. Immunol.*, 148, 3543, 1992.

85. Wallen, N., Kita, H., Weiler, D., and Gleich, G. J., Glucocorticoids inhibit cytokine-mediated eosinophil survival, *J. Immunol.*, 147, 3490, 1991.

86. Fujisawa, T., Abu-Ghazaleh, R., Kita, H., Sanderson, C. J., and Gleich, G., Regulatory effect of cytokines on eosinophil degranulation, *J. Immunol.*, 144, 642, 1990.

87. Silberstein, D. S. and David, J. R., Tumor necrosis factor enhances eosinophil toxicity to *Schistosoma mansoni* larvae, *Proc. Natl. Acad. Sci. U.S.A.*, 83, 1055, 1986.

88. Slungaard, A., Vercellotti, G. M., Walker, G., and Nelson, R. D., Tumor necrosis factor α/cachectin stimulates eosinophil oxidant production and toxicity towards human endothelium, *J. Exp. Med.*, 717, 2025, 1990.

89. Takafuji, S., Bischoff, S. C., DeWeck, A. L., and Dahinden, C. A., Opposing effects of tumor necrosis factor-α and nerve growth factor upon leukotriene C4 production by human eosinophils triggered with N-formyl-methionyl-leucyl-phenylalanine, *Eur. J. Immunol.*, 22, 969, 1992.

90. Bevilacqua, M. P. and Nelson, R. M., Selectins, *J. Clin. Invest.*, 91, 379, 1993.

91. Bonfanti, R., Furie, B. C., Furie, B., and Wagner, D. D., PADGEM (GMP140) is a component of Weibel–Palade bodies of human endothelial cells, *Blood*, 73, 1109, 1989.

92. McEver, R. P., Beckstead, J. H., Moore, K. L., Marshall-Carlson, L., and Bainton, D. F., GMP-140, a platelet α-granule membrane protein, is also synthesized by vascular endothelial cells and is localized in Weibel–Palade bodies, *J. Clin. Invest.*, 84, 92, 1989.

93. Hattori, R., Hamilton, K. K., Fugates, R. D., McEver, R. P., and Sims, P. J., Stimulated secretion of endothelial von Willebrand factor is accompanied by rapid redistribution to the cell surface of the intracellular granule membrane protein GMP-140, *J. Biol. Chem.*, 264, 7768, 1989.

94. Bevilacqua, M. P., Pober, J. S., Mendrick, D. L., Cotran, R. S., and Gimbrone, M. A., Jr., Identification of an inducible endothelial-leukocyte adhesion molecule, *Proc. Natl. Acad. Sci. U.S.A.*, 84, 9238, 1987.

95. Bevilacqua, M. P., Stengelin, S., Gimbrone, M. A., and Seed, B., Endothelial leukocyte adhesion molecule 1: an inducible receptor for neutrophils related to complement regulatory proteins and lectins, *Science*, 243, 1160, 1989.

96. Foxall, C., Watson, S. R., Dowbenko, D., Fennie, C., Lasky, L. A., Kiso, M., Hasegawa, A., Asa, D., and Brandley, B. K., The three members of the selectin receptor family recognize a common carbohydrate epitope, the sialyl Lewis x oligosaccharide, *J. Cell Biol.*, 117, 895, 1992.

97. Sako, D., Chang, X.-J., Barone, K. M., Vachino, G., White, H. M., Shaw, G., Veldman, G. M., Bean, K. M., Ahern, T. J., Furie, B., Cumming, D. A., and Larsen, G. R., Expression cloning of a functional glycoprotein ligand for P-selectin, *Cell*, 75, 1179, 1993.

98. Lasky, L. A., Singer, M. S., Dowbenko, D., Imal, Y., Henzel, W. J., Grimley, C., Fennie, C., Gillett, N., Watson, S. R., and Rosen, S. D., An endothelial ligand for L-selectin is a novel mucin-like molecule, *Cell*, 69, 927, 1992.

99. Baumhueter, S., Singer, M. S., Henzel, W., Hemmerich, S., Renz, M., Rosen, S. D., and Lasky, L. A., Binding of L-selectin to the vascular sialomucin CD34, *Science*, 262, 436, 1993.

100. Shimizu, Y. and Shaw, S., Mucins in the mainstream, *Nature*, 366, 630, 1993.

101. Lawrence, M. B. and Springer, T. A., Leukocytes roll on a selectin at physiologic flow rates: distinction from and prerequisite for adhesion through integrins, *Cell*, 65, 859, 1991.

102. Abbassi, O., Kishimoto, T. K., McIntire, L. V., Anderson, D. C., and Smith, C. W., E-selectin supports neutrophil adhesion *in vitro* under conditions of flow, *J. Clin. Invest.*, 92, 2719, 1993.

103. Lawrence, M. B. and Springer, T. A., Neutrophils roll on E-selectin, *J. Immunol.*, 151, 6338, 1993.

104. Marlin, S. D. and Springer, T. A., Purified intercellular adhesion molecule-1 (ICAM-1) is a ligand for lymphocyte function-associated antigen 1 (LFA-1), *Cell*, 51, 813, 1987.

105. Elices, M. J., Osborn, L., Takada, Y., Crouse, C., Luhowskyj, S., Helmer, M. E., and Lobb, R. R., VCAM-1 on activated endothelium interacts with the leucocyte integrin VLA-4 at a site distinct from the VLA-4/fibronectin binding site, *Cell*, 60, 577, 1990.

106. Diamond, M. S., Staunton, D. E., Marlin, S. D., and Springer, T. A., Binding of the integrin Mac-1 (CD11b/CD18) to the third immunoglobulin-like domain of ICAM-1 (CD54) and its regulation by glycosylation, *Cell*, 65, 961, 1991.

107. Hogg, N., Harvey, J., Cabanas, C., and Landis, R. C., Control of leukocyte integrin activation, *Am. Rev. Respir. Dis.*, 148, S55, 1993.

108. Lo, S. K., Lee, S., Ramos, R. A., Lobb, R., Rosa, M., Chi-Rosa, G., and Wright, S. D., Endothelial-leukocyte adhesion molecule-1 stimulates the activity of leukocyte integrin CR3 (CD11b/CD18, Mac-1, $\alpha m\beta 2$) on human neutrophils, *J. Exp. Med.*, 173, 1493, 1991.

109. Huber, A. R., Kunkel, S. L., Todd, R. F., III, and Weiss, S. J., Regulation of transendothelial neutrophil migration by endogenous interleukin-8, *Science*, 254, 99, 1991.

110. Tanaka, Y., Adams, D. H., Hubscher, S., Hirano, H., Siebenlist, U., and Shaw, S., T-cell adhesion induced by proteoglycan-immobilized cytokine MIP-1$\beta$, *Nature*, 361, 79, 1993.

111. Zimmerman, G. A., Prescott, S. M., and McIntyre, T. M., Endothelial cell interactions with granulocytes: tethering and signaling molecules, *Immunol. Today*, 13, 93, 1992.

112. Pober, J. S., Gimbrone, M. A., Jr., Lapierre, L. A., Mendrick, D. L., Fiers, W., Rothlein, R., and Springer, T. A., Overlapping patterns of activation of human endothelial cells by interleukin 1, tumor necrosis factor, and immune interferon, *J. Immunol.*, 137, 1893, 1986.

113. Osborn, L., Hession, C., Tizard, R., Vassallo, C., Luhowskyj, S., Chi-Rosso, G., and Lobb, R., Direct expression and cloning of vascular cell adhesion molecule 1, a cytokine-induced endothelial protein that binds to lymphocytes, *Cell*, 59, 1203, 1989.

114. Masinovsky, B., Urdal, D., and Gallatin, W. M., IL-4 acts synergistically with IL-1 to promote lymphocyte adhesion to microvascular endothelium by induction of vascular cell adhesion molecule-1, *J. Immunol.*, 145, 2886, 1990.

115. Thornhill, M. H. and Haskard, D. O., IL-4 regulates endothelial cell activation by IL-1, tumor necrosis factor, or IFN-$\gamma$, *J. Immunol.*, 145, 865, 1990.

116. Wellcome, S. M., Thornhill, M. H., Pitzalis, C., Thomas, D. S., Lanchbury, J. S. S., Panayi, G. S., and Haskard, D. O., A monoclonal antibody that detects a novel antigen on endothelial cells that is induced by tumor necrosis factor, IL-1 or lipopolysaccharide, *J. Immunol.*, 144, 2558, 1990.

117. Bochner, B. S., Luscinskas, F. W., Gimbrone, M. A., Jr., Newman, W., Sterbinsky, S. A., Derse-Anthony, C. P., Klunk, D., and Schleimer, R. P., Adhesion of human basophils, eosinophils, and neutrophils to interleukin 1-activated human vascular endothelial cells: contribution of endothelial cell adhesion molecules, *J. Exp. Med.*, 173, 1553, 1991.

118. Dobrina, A., Menegazzi, R., Carlos, T. M., Nardon, E., Cramer, R., Zacchi, T., Harlan, J. M., and Patriarca, P., Mechanisms of eosinophil adhesion to cultured vascular endothelial cells: eosinophils bind to the cytokine-induced endothelial ligand vascular cell adhesion molecule-1 via the very late activation antigen-4 integrin receptor, *J. Clin. Invest.*, 88, 20, 1991.

119. Schleimer, R. P., Sterbinsky, S. A., Kaiser, J., Bickel, C. A., Klunk, D. A., Tomioka, K., Newman, W., Luscinskas, F. W., Gimbrone, M. A., Jr., McIntyre, B. W., and Bochner, B. S., IL-4 induces adherence of human eosinophils and basophils but not neutrophils to endothelium, *J. Immunol.*, 148, 1086, 1992.

120. Vennegoor, C. J. G. M., van de Wiel-van Kemenade, E., Huijbens, R. J. F., Sanchez-Madrid, F., Melief, C. J. M., and Figdor, C. G., Role of LFA-1 and VLA-4 in the adhesion of cloned normal and LFA-1 (CD11/CD18)-deficient T cells to cultured endothelial cells: indication for a new adhesion pathway, *J. Immunol.*, 148, 1093, 1992.

121. van Kooyk, Y., van de Weil-van Kemenade, E., Weder, P., Hiujbens, R. J. F., and Figdor, C. G., Lymphocyte function-associated antigen 1 dominates very late antigen 4 in binding of activated T cells to endothelium, *J. Exp. Med.*, 177, 185, 1993.

122. Carlos, T., Kovach, N., Schwartz, B., Rosa, M., Newman, B., Wayner, E., Benjamin, C., Osborn, L., Lobb, R., and Harlan, J., Human monocytes bind to two cytokine-induced adhesive ligands on cultured human endothelial cells: endothelial-leukocyte adhesion molecule-1 and vascular cell adhesion molecule-1, *Blood*, 77, 2266, 1991.

123. Jonjic, N., Jílek, P., Bernasconi, S., Peri, G., Martin-Padura, I., Cenzuales, S., Dejana, E., and Mantovani, A., Molecules involved in the adhesion and cytotoxicity of activated monocytes on endothelial cells, *J. Immunol.*, 148, 2080, 1992.

124. Smith, C. W., Marlin, S. D., Rothlein, R., Toman, C., and Anderson, D. C., Cooperative interactions of LFA-1 and Mac-1 with intercellular adhesion molecule-1 in facilitating adherence and transendothelial migration of human neutrophils *in vitro*, *J. Clin. Invest.*, 83, 2008, 1989.

125. Furie, M. B., Tancinco, M. C. A., and Smith, C. W., Monoclonal antibodies to leukocyte integrins CD11a/CD18 and CD11b/CD18 or intercellular adhesion molecule-1 inhibit chemoattractant-stimulated neutrophil transendothelial migration *in vitro*, *Blood*, 78, 2089, 1991.

126. Hakkert, B. C., Kuijpers, T. W., Leeuwenberg, J. F. M., van Mourik, J. A., and Roos, D., Neutrophil and monocyte adherence to and migration across monolayers of cytokine-activated endothelial cells: the contribution of CD18, ELAM-1, and VLA-4, *Blood*, 78, 2721, 1991.

127. Anderson, D. C., Schmalsteig, F. C., Finegold, M. J., Hughes, B. J., Rothlein, R., Miller, L. J., Kohl, S., Tosi, M. F., Jacobs, R. L., Waldrop, T. C., Goldman, A. S., Shearer, W. T., and Springer, T. A., The severe and moderate phenotypes of heritable Mac-1, LFA-1 deficiency: their quantitative definition and relation to leukocyte dysfunction and clinical features, *J. Infect. Dis.*, 152, 668, 1985.

128. Moser, R., Fehr, J., and Bruijnzeel, P. L. B., IL-4 controls the selective endothelium-driven transmigration of eosinophils from allergic individuals, *J. Immunol.*, 149, 1432, 1992.

129. Newman, P. J., Berndt, M. C., Gorski, J., White, G. C., II, Lyman, S., Paddock, C., and Muller, W. A., PECAM-1 (CD31) cloning and relation to adhesion molecules of the immunoglobulin gene superfamily, *Science*, 247, 1219, 1990.

130. Simmons, D. L., Walker, C., Power, C., and Pigott, R., Molecular cloning of CD31, a putative intercellular adhesion molecule closely related to carcinoembryonic antigen, *J. Exp. Med.*, 171, 2147, 1990.

131. Muller, W. A., Weigl, S. A., Deng, X., and Philips, D. M., PECAM-1 is required for transendothelial migration of leukocytes, *J. Exp. Med.*, 178, 449, 1993.

132. Vaporciyan, A. A., DeLisser, H. M., Yan, H.-C., Mendiguren, I. I., Thom, S. R., Jones, M. L., Ward, P. A., and Abelda, S. M., Involvement of platelet-endothelial cell adhesion molecule-1 in neutrophil recruitment *in vivo*, *Science*, 262, 1580, 1993.

133. Huber, H. L. and Koessler, K. K., The pathology of bronchial asthma, *Arch. Intern. Med.*, 30, 689, 1922.

134. James, A. L., Paré, P. D., and Hogg, J. C., The mechanics of airway narrowing in asthma, *Am. Rev. Respir. Dis.*, 139, 242, 1989.

135. Kuwano, K., Bosken, C. H., Pare, P. D., Bai, T. R., Wiggs, B. R., and Hogg, J. C., Small airways dimensions in asthma and in chronic obstructive pulmonary disease, *Am. Rev. Respir. Dis.*, 148, 1220, 1993.

136. Heard, B. E. and Hossain, S., Hyperplasia of bronchial smooth muscle in asthma, *J. Pathol.*, 110, 319, 1972.

137. Wiggs, B. R., Bosken, C., Paré, P. D., James, A., and Hogg, J. C., A model of airway narrowing in asthma and in chronic obstructive pulmonary disease, *Am. Rev. Respir. Dis.*, 145, 1251, 1992.

138. Houston, J. C., de Navasquez, S., and Trounce, J. R., A clinical and pathological study of fatal cases of status asthmaticus, *Thorax*, 8, 207, 1953.

139. Cardell, B. S. and Pearson, R. S. B., Death in asthmatics, *Thorax*, 14, 341, 1959.

140. Messer, J. W., Peters, G. A., and Bennett, W. A., Causes of death and pathologic findings in 304 cases of bronchial asthma, *Dis. Chest*, 38, 616, 1960.

141. McCarter, J. H. and Vazquez, J. J., The bronchial basement membrane in asthma, *Arch. Pathol.*, 82, 328, 1966.

142. Molina, C., Brun, J., Coulet, M., Betail, G., and Delage, J., Immunopathology of the bronchial mucosa in "late-onset" asthma, *Clin. Allergy*, 7, 137, 1977.

143. Roche, W. R., Beasley, R., Williams, J. H., and Holgate, S. T., Subepithelial fibrosis in the bronchi of asthmatics, *Lancet*, 1, 520, 1989.

144. Brewster, C. E. P., Howarth, P. H., Djukanovic, R., Wilson, J., Holgate, S. T., and Roche, W. R., Myofibroblasts and subepithelial fibrosis in bronchial asthma, *Am. J. Respir. Cell Mol. Biol.*, 3, 507, 1990.

145. Monroe, J. G., Haldar, S., Prystowsky, M. B., and Lammie, P., Lymphokine regulation of inflammatory processes: interleukin-4 stimulates fibroblast proliferation, *Clin. Immunol. Immunopathol.*, 49, 292, 1988.

146. Postlethwaite, A. E. and Seyer, J. M., Fibroblast chemotaxis induction by human recombinant interleukin-4: identification by synthetic peptide analysis of two chemotactic domains residing in amino acid sequences 70-88 and 89-122, *J. Clin. Invest.*, 87, 2147, 1991.

147. Postlethwaite, A. E., Holness, M. A., Katai, H., and Raghow, R., Human fibroblasts synthesize elevated levels of extracellular matrix proteins in response to interleukin 4, *J. Clin. Invest.*, 90, 1479, 1992.

148. Vilcek, J., Palombella, V. J., Henrikson-DeStefano, D., Swenson, C., Feinman, R., Hirai, M., and Tsujimoto, M., Fibroblast growth enhancing activity of tumor necrosis factor and its relationship to other polypeptide growth factors, *J. Exp. Med.*, 163, 632, 1986.

149. Postlethwaite, A. E. and Seyer, J. M., Stimulation of fibroblast chemotaxis by human recombinant tumor necrosis factor-α (TNFα) and a synthetic TNFα 31-68 peptide, *J. Exp. Med.*, 172, 1749, 1990.

150. Mauviel, A., Daireaux, M., Rédini, F., Galera, P., Loyau, G., and Pujol, J.-P., Tumor necrosis factor inhibits collagen synthesis in human dermal fibroblasts, *FEBS Lett.*, 236, 47, 1988.

151. Solis-Heruzzo, J. A., Brenner, D. A., and Chojkier, M., Tumor necrosis factor α inhibits collagen gene transcription and collagen synthesis in cultured human fibroblasts, *J. Biol. Chem.*, 263, 5841, 1988.

152. Dayer, J.-M., Beutler, B., and Cerami, A., Cachectin/tumor necrosis factor stimulates collagenase and PGE₂ production by human synovial cells and dermal fibroblasts, *J. Exp. Med.*, 162, 2163, 1985.

153. Brenner, D. A., O'Hara, M., Angel, P., Chojkier, M., and Karin, M., Prolonged activation of jun and collagenase genes by tumor necrosis factor-α, *Nature*, 337, 661, 1989.

154. Piguet, P. F., Grau, G. E., and Vassalli, P., Subcutaneous perfusion of tumor necrosis factor induces proliferation of fibroblasts, capillaries, and epidermal cells, or massive tissue necrosis, *Am. J. Pathol.*, 136, 103, 1990.

155. Ignotz, R. A. and Massagué, J., Transforming growth factor-β stimulates the expression of fibronectin and collagen and their incorporation into the extracellular matrix, *J. Biol. Chem.*, 261, 4337, 1986.

156. Roberts, A. B., Sporn, M. B., Assoian, R. K., Smith, J. M., Roche, N. S., Wakefield, L. M., Heine, U. I., Liotta, L. A., Falanga, V., Kehrl, J. H., and Fauci, A. S., Transforming growth factor type β: rapid induction of fibrosis and angiogenesis *in vivo* and stimulation of collagen formation *in vitro*, *Proc. Natl. Acad. Sci. U.S.A.*, 83, 4167, 1986.

157. Ignotz, R. A., Endo, T., and Massagué, J., Regulation of fibronectin and type I collagen mRNA levels by transforming growth factor-β, *J. Biol. Chem.*, 262, 6443, 1987.

158. Varga, J., Rosenbloom, R., and Jimenez, S. A., Transforming growth factor β (TGFβ) causes a persistent increase in steady-state amounts of type I and type III collagen and fibronectin mRNAs in normal human dermal fibroblasts, *Biochem. J.*, 247, 507, 1987.

159. Balza, E., Borsi, L., Allemanni, G., and Zardi, L., Transforming growth factor β regulates the levels of different fibronectin isoforms in normal human cultured fibroblasts, *FEBS Lett.*, 228, 42, 1988.

160. Roberts, C. J., Birkenmeier, T. M., McQuillan, J. J., Akiyama, S. K., Yamada, S. S., Chen, W.-T., Yamada, K. M., and McDonald, J. A., Transforming growth factor β stimulates the expression of fibronectin and of both subunits of the human fibronectin receptor by cultured human lung fibroblasts, *J. Biol. Chem.*, 263, 4586, 1988.

161. Pearson, C. A., Pearson, D., Shibahara, S., Hofsteenge, J., and Chiquet-Ehrismann, R., Tenascin: cDNA cloning and induction by TGFβ, *EMBO J.*, 7, 2977, 1988.

162. Bassols, A. and Massagué, J., Transforming growth factor β regulates the expression and structure of extracellular matrix chondroitin/dermatan sulfate proteoglycans, *J. Biol. Chem.*, 263, 3039, 1988.

163. Ignotz, R. A., Heinos, J., and Massagué, J., Regulation of cell adhesion receptors by transforming growth factor-β: regulation of vitronectin receptor and LFA-1, *J. Biol. Chem.*, 264, 389, 1989.

164. Laiho, M., Saskela, O., and Keski-Oja, J., Enhanced production and extracellular deposition of the endothelial-type plasminogen activator inhibitor in cultured human lung fibroblasts by transforming growth factor-β, *J. Cell Biol.*, 103, 2403, 1986.

165. Edwards, D. R., Murphy, G., Reynolds, J. J., Whitham, S. E., Docherty, A. J. P., Angel, P., and Heath, J. K., Transforming growth factor beta modulates the expression of collagenase and metalloproteinase inhibitor, *EMBO J.*, 6, 1899, 1987.

166. Laiho, M., Saksela, O., and Keski-Oja, J., Transforming growth factor-β induction of type-I plasminogen activator inhibitor: pericellular distribution and sensitivity to exogenous urokinase, *J. Biol. Chem.*, 262, 17467, 1987.

167. Paulsson, Y., Beckmann, M. P., Westermark, B., and Heidin, C. H., Density-dependent inhibition of cell growth by transforming growth factor β1 in normal human fibroblasts, *Growth Factors*, 1, 19, 1988.

168. Raghow, R., Irish, P., and Kang, A. H., Coordinate regulation of transforming growth factor β gene expression and cell proliferation in hamster lungs undergoing bleomycin-induced pulmonary fibrosis, *J. Clin. Invest.*, 84, 1836, 1989.

169. Phan, S. H., Gharaee-Kermani, M., Wolber, F., and Ryan, U.S., Stimulation of rat endothelial cell transforming growth factor-β production by bleomycin, *J. Clin. Invest.*, 87, 148, 1991.

170. Broekelmann, T. J., Limper, A. H., Colby, T. V., and McDonald, J. A., Transforming growth factor β1 is present at sites of extracellular matrix gene expression in human pulmonary fibrosis, *Proc. Natl. Acad. Sci. U.S.A.*, 88, 6642, 1991.
171. Khalil, N., O'Connor, R. N., Unruh, H. W., Warren, P. W., Flanders, K. C., Kemp, A., Bereznay, O. H., and Greenberg, A. H., Increased production and immunohistochemical localization of transforming growth factor-β in idiopathic pulmonary fibrosis, *Am. J. Respir. Cell Mol. Biol.*, 5, 155, 1991.
172. Gospodarowicz, D., Cheng, J., Lui, G. M., Baird, A., and Bohlen, P., Isolation of brain fibroblast growth factor by heparin-sepharose affinity chromatography: identity with pituitary fibroblast growth factor, *Proc. Natl. Acad. Sci. U.S.A.*, 81, 6963, 1984.
173. Shing, Y., Folkman, J., Sullivan, R., Butterfield, C., Murray, J., and Klagsbrun, M., Heparin affinity: purification of a tumor-derived capillary endothelial cell growth factor, *Science*, 223, 1296, 1984.
174. Moscatelli, D., Presta, M., and Rifkin, D. B., Purification of a factor from human placenta that stimulates capillary endothelial cell protease production, DNA synthesis, and migration, *Proc. Natl. Acad. Sci. U.S.A.*, 83, 2091, 1986.
175. Saksela, O., Moscatelli, D., and Rifkin, D. B., The opposing effects of basic fibroblast growth factor and transforming growth factor-β on the regulation of plasminogen activator activity in capillary endothelial cells, *J. Cell Biol.*, 105, 957, 1987.
176. Davidson, J. M., Klagsbrun, M., Hill, K. E., Buckley, A., Sullivan, R., Brewer, P. S., and Woodward, S. C., Accelerated wound repair, cell proliferation, and collagen accumulation are produced by a cartilage-derived growth factor, *J. Cell Biol.*, 100, 1219, 1985.
177. Pierce, G. F., Tarpley, J. E., Yanigihara, D., Mustoe, T. A., Fox, G. M., and Thomason, A., Platelet-derived growth factor (BB homodimer), transforming growth factor-β1, and basic fibroblast growth factor in dermal wound healing: neovessel and matrix formation and cessation of repair, *Am. J. Pathol.*, 140, 1375, 1992.
178. Brown, P. H., Crompton, G. K., and Greening, A. P., Proinflammatory cytokines in acute asthma, *Lancet*, 338, 590, 1991.
179. Corrigan, C. J., Haczku, A., Gemou-Engesaeth, V., Doi, S., Kikuchi, Y., Takatsu, K., Durham, S. R., and Kay, A. B., CD4 T-lymphocyte activation in asthma is accompanied by increased serum concentrations of interleukin-5: effect of glucocorticoid therapy, *Am. Rev. Respir. Dis.*, 147, 540, 1993.
180. Corrigan, C. J. and Kay, A. B., CD4 T-lymphocyte activation in acute severe asthma: relationship to disease severity and atopic status, *Am. Rev. Respir. Dis.*, 141, 970, 1990.
181. Alexander, A. G., Barkans, J., Moqbel, R., Barnes, N., Kay, A. B., and Corrigan, C. J., Serum interleukin 5 concentrations in atopic and non-atopic patients with glucocorticoid-dependent chronic asthma, *Thorax*, 49, 1231, 1994.
182. Matsumoto, K., Taki, F., Miura, M., Matsuzaki, M., and Tagki, K., Serum levels of soluble IL-2R, IL-4, and soluble FceRII in adult bronchial asthma, *Chest*, 105, 681, 1994.
183. Walker, C., Bode, E., Boer, L., Hansel, T. T., Blaser, K., and Virchow, J.-C., Jr., Allergic and nonallergic asthmatics have distinct patterns of T-cell activation and cytokine production in peripheral blood and bronchoalveolar lavage, *Am. Rev. Respir. Dis.*, 146, 109, 1992.
184. Broide, D. H., Lotz, M., Cuomo, A. J., Coburn, D. A., Federman, E. C., and Wasserman, S. I., Cytokines in symptomatic asthma airways, *J. Allergy Clin. Immunol.*, 89, 958, 1992.
185. Redington, A. E., Lau, L. C. K., Madden, J., Djukanovic, R., Holgate, S. T., and Howarth, P. H., Tumor necrosis factor in asthma: measurement in bronchoalveolar lavage fluid, *Am. J. Respir. Crit. Care Med.*, 151, A703, 1995.
186. Robinson, D. S., Hamid, Q., Ying, S., Tsicopoulos, A., Barkans, J., Bentley, A. M., Corrigan, C., Durham, S. R., and Kay, A. B., Predominant TH2-like bronchoalveolar T-lymphocyte population in atopic asthma, *N. Engl. J. Med.*, 326, 298, 1992.
187. Ying, S., Durham, S. R., Corrigan, C. J., Hamid, Q., and Kay, A. B., Phenotype of cells expressing mRNA for TH2-type (interleukin 4 and interleukin 5) and TH1-type (interleukin 2 and interferon γ) cytokines in bronchoalveolar lavage and bronchial biopsies from atopic asthmatics and normal control subjects, *Am. J. Respir. Crit. Care Med.*, 12, 477, 1995.

188. Ying, S., Robinson, D. S., Varney, V., Meng, Q., Tsicopoulos, A., Moqbel, R., Durham, S. R., Kay, A. B., and Hamid, Q., TNFα mRNA expression in allergic inflammation, *Clin. Exp. Allergy*, 21, 745, 1991.

189. Robinson, D., Hamid, Q., Bentley, A., Ying, S., Kay, A. B., and Durham, S. R., Activation of CD4+ T cells, increased T$_{H2}$-type cytokine mRNA expression, and eosinophil recruitment in bronchoalveolar lavage after allergen challenge in patients with atopic asthma, *J. Allergy Clin. Immunol.*, 92, 313, 1993.

190. Bentley, A. M., Meng, Q., Robinson, D. S., Hamid, Q., Kay, A. B., and Durham, S. R., Increases in activated T lymphocytes, eosinophils, and cytokine mRNA expression for interleukin-5 and granulocyte/macrophage colony-stimulating factor in bronchial biopsies after allergen inhalation challenge in atopic asthmatics, *Am. J. Respir. Cell Mol. Biol.*, 8, 35, 1993.

191. Bradding, P., Feather, I. H., Howarth, P. H., Mueller, R., Roberts, J. A., Britten, K., Bews, J. P. A., Hunt, T. C., Okayama, Y., Heusser, C. H., Bullock, G. R., Church, M. K., and Holgate, S. T., Interleukin 4 is localized to and released by human mast cells, *J. Exp. Med.*, 176, 1381, 1992.

192. Bradding, P., Roberts, J. A., Britten, K. M., Montefort, S., Djukanovic, R., Mueller, R., Heusser, C. H., Howarth, P. H., and Holgate, S. T., Interleukins-4, -5, and -6 and tumor necrosis factor-α in normal and asthmatic airways: evidence for the human mast cell as a source of these cytokines, *Am. J. Respir. Cell Mol. Biol.*, 10, 471, 1994.

193. Broide, D. H., Gleich, G. J., Cuomo, A. J., Coburn, D. A., Federman, E. C., Schwartz, L. B., and Wasserman, S. I., Evidence of ongoing mast cell and eosinophil degranulation in symptomatic airways, *J. Allergy Clin. Immunol.*, 88, 637, 1991.

194. Ohkawara, Y., Yamauchi, K., Tanno, Y., Tamura, G., Ohtani, H., Nagura, H., Ohkuda, K., and Takishima, T., Human lung mast cells and pulmonary macrophages produce tumor necrosis factor-α in sensitized lung tissue after IgE receptor triggering, *Am. J. Respir. Cell Mol. Biol.*, 7, 385, 1992.

195. Horsmanheimo, L., Harvima, I. T., Järvikallio, A., Harvima, R. J., Naukkarinen, A., and Horsmanheimo, M., Mast cells are one major source of interleukin-4 in atopic dermatitis, *Br. J. Dermatol.*, 131, 348, 1994.

196. Okayama, Y., Quint, D., and Hunt, T. C., Expression of IL-4 mRNA in human dermal mast cells in response to Fce receptor cross-linkage in the presence of SCF, *J. Allergy Clin. Immunol.*, 91 (Abstr.), 256, 1993.

197. Jaffe, J. S., Schulman, E. S., and Wang, Y., IgE-dependent secretion of IL-5 by lung fragments and human lung mast cells, *J. Allergy Clin. Immunol.*, 93 (Abstr.), 225, 1994.

198. Beil, W. J., Login, G. R., Galli, S. J., and Dvorak, A. M., Ultrastructural immunogold localization of tumor necrosis factor-α to the cytoplasmic granules of rat peritoneal mast cells with rapid microwave fixation, *J. Allergy Clin. Immunol.*, 94, 531, 1994.

199. Aalbers, R., de Monchy, J. G. R., Kauffman, H. F., Smith, M., Hoekstra, Y., Vrugt, B., and Timens, W., Dynamics of eosinophil infiltration in the bronchial mucosa before and after the late asthmatic reaction, *Eur. Respir. J.*, 6, 840, 1993.

200. Bradding, P., Mediwake, R., Feather, I. H., Madden, J., Church, M. K., Holgate, S. T., and Howarth, P. H., TNFα is localised to nasal mucosal mast cells and is released in acute allergic rhinitis, *Clin. Exp. Allergy*, 25, 406, 1995.

201. Lopez, A. F., Sanderson, C. J., Gamble, J. R., Campbell, H. D., Young, I. G., and Vadas, M. A., Recombinant human interleukin 5 is a selective activator of human eosinophil function, *J. Exp. Med.*, 167, 219, 1988.

202. Dubois, G. R. and Bruijnzeel, P. L. B., IL-4-induced migration of eosinophils in allergic inflammation, *Ann. N.Y. Acad. Sci.*, 725, 268, 1993.

203. Tepper, R. I., Pattengale, P. K., and Leder, P., Murine interleukin-4 displays potent anti-tumor activity *in vivo*, *Cell*, 57, 503, 1989.

204. Lukacs, N. W., Strieter, R. M., Chensue, S. W., and Kunkel, S. L., Interleukin-4-dependent pulmonary eosinophil infiltration in a murine model of asthma, *Am. J. Respir. Cell Mol. Biol.*, 10, 526, 1994.

205. Le Gros, G., Ben-Sasson, S. Z., Seder, R., Finkelman, F. D., and Paul, W. E., Generation of interleukin 4 (IL-4)-producing cels *in vivo* and *in vitro*: IL-2 and IL-4 are required for *in vitro* generation of IL-4 producing cells, *J. Exp. Med.*, 172, 921, 1990.

206. Swain, S. L., Weinberg, A. D., English, M., and Huston, G., IL-4 directs the development of Th2-like helper effectors, *J. Immunol.*, 145, 3796, 1990.

207. Gauchat, J.-F., Henchoz, S., Mazzel, G., Aubry, J.-P., Brunner, T., Blasey, H., Life, P., Talabot, D., Flores-Romo, L., Thompson, J., Kishi, K., Butterfield, J., Dahinden, C., and Bonnefoy, J.-Y., Induction of human IgE synthesis in B cells by mast cells and basophils, *Nature*, 365, 340, 1993.

208. Del Prete, G. F., De Carli, M., D'Elios, M. M., Maestrelli, P., Ricci, M., Fabbri, L., and Romagnani, S., Allergen exposure induces the activation of allergen-specific Th2 cells in the airway mucosa of patients with allergic respiratory disorders, *Eur. J. Immunol.*, 23, 1445, 1993.

209. Corrigan, C. J., Baiqing, L., Durham, S. R., and Kay, A. B., Allergen-specific T lymphocytes selectively accumulate in the airways of atopic nonasthmatics, *Am. J. Respir. Crit. Care Med.*, 149 (Abstr.), A951, 1994.

210. Kupfer, A., Mosmann, T. R., and Kupfer, H., Polarized expression of cytokines in cell conjugates of helper T cells and splenic B cells, *Proc. Natl. Acad. Sci. U.S.A.*, 88, 775, 1991.

211. Krug, N., Madden, J., Redington, A. E., Lackie, P., Schauer, U., Holgate, S. T., Frew, A. J., and Howarth, P. H., T cell cytokine profile evaluated at the single cell level in subjects with asthma and control subjects: comparison between peripheral blood and bronchoalveolar lavage fluid, *Am. J. Respir. Cell Mol. Biol.*, 14, 319, 1996.

212. Broide, D. H., Paine, M. M., and Firestein, G. S., Eosinophils express interleukin 5 and granulocyte-macrophage colony-stimulating factor mRNA at sites of allergic inflammation in asthmatics, *J. Clin. Invest.*, 90, 1414, 1992.

213. Dubucquoi, S., Desreumaux, P., Janin, A., Klein, O., Goldman, M., Tavernier, J., Capron, A., and Capron, M., Interleukin 5 synthesis by eosinophils: association with granules and immunoglobulin-dependent secretion, *J. Exp. Med.*, 179, 703, 1994.

214. Redington, A. E., Bradding, P., Douglass, J. A., Teran, L. M., Roberts, J. A., Holgate, S. T., and Howarth, P. H., Bronchial epithelial cytokine production in asthmatics and non-asthmatics, *Thorax*, 48 (Abstr.), 1081, 1993.

215. Sousa, A. R., Poston, R. N., Lane, S. J., Nakhosteen, J. A., and Lee, T. H., Detection of GM-CSF in asthmatic bronchial epithelium and decrease by inhaled corticosteroids, *Am. Rev. Respir. Dis.*, 147, 1557, 1993.

216. Woolley, K. L., Adelroth, E., Woolley, M. J., Ellis, R., Jordana, M., and O'Byrne, P. M., Granulocyte-macrophage colony-stimulating factor, eosinophils, and eosinophil cationic protein in mild asthmatics and nonasthmatics, *Eur. Respir. J.*, in press, 1996.

217. Devalia, J. L., Wang, J. H., Sapsford, R. J., and Davies, R. J., Expression of RANTES in human bronchial epithelial cells is downregulated by beclomethasone dipropionate (BDP), *Clin. Exp. Allergy*, 10 (Abstr.), 992, 1994.

218. Sousa, A. R., Lane, S. J., Nakhosteen, J. A., Yoshimura, T., Lee, T. H., and Poston, R. N., Increased expression of the monocyte chemoattractant protein-1 in bronchial tissue from asthmatic subjects, *Am. J. Respir. Cell Mol. Biol.*, 10, 142, 1994.

219. Marini, M., Soloperto, M., Mazzetti, M., Fasoli, A., and Mattoli, S., Interleukin-1 binds to specific receptors on human bronchial epithelial cells and upregulates granulocyte/macrophage colony-stimulating factor synthesis and release, *Am. J. Respir. Cell Mol. Biol.*, 4, 519, 1991.

220. Cromwell, O., Hamid, Q., Corrigan, C. J., Barkans, J., Meng, Q., Collins, P. D., and Kay, A. B., Expression and generation of interleukin-8, IL-6 and granulocyte-macrophage colony-stimulating factor by bronchial epithelial cells and enhancement by IL-1β and tumour necrosis factor-α, *Immunology*, 77, 330, 1992.

221. Churchill, L., Friedman, B., Schleimer, R. P., and Proud, D., Production of granulocyte-macrophage colony-stimulating factor by cultured human tracheal epithelial cells, *Immunology*, 75, 189, 1992.

222. Marini, M., Vittori, E., Hollemborg, J., and Mattoli, S., Expression of the potent inflammatory cytokines, granulocyte-macrophage colony-stimulating factor and interleukin-6 and interleukin-8, in bronchial epithelial cells of patients with asthma, *J. Allergy Clin. Immunol.*, 89, 1001, 1992.

223. Kwon, O. J., Jose, P. J., Robbins, R. A., Schall, T. J., Williams, T. J., and Barnes, P., J., Glucocorticoid inhibition of RANTES expression in human lung epithelial cells, *Am. J. Respir. Cell Mol. Biol.*, 12, 488, 1995.

224. Devalia, J. L., Campbell, A. M., Sapsford, R. J., Rusznak, C., Quint, D., Godard, P., Bousquet, J., and Davies, R. J., Effect of nitrogen dioxide on synthesis of inflammatory cytokines expressed by human bronchial epithelial cells *in vitro*, *Am. J. Respir. Cell Mol. Biol.*, 9, 271, 1993.

225. Becker, S., Koren, H. S., and Henke, D. C., Interleukin-8 expression in normal nasal epithelium and its modulation by infection with respiratory syncytial virus and cytokines tumor necrosis factor, interleukin-1, and interleukin-6, *Am. J. Respir. Cell Mol. Biol.*, 8, 20, 1993.

226. Rot, A., Neutrophil attractant/activation protein-1 (interleukin-8) induces *in vitro* neutrophil migration by haptotactic mechanism, *Eur. J. Immunol.*, 23, 303, 1993.

227. Paralkar, V. M., Vukicevic, S., and Reddi, A. H., Transforming growth factor β type 1 binds to collagen IV of basement membrane matrix: implications for development, *Dev. Biol.*, 143, 303, 1991.

228. Fava, R. A. and McClure, D. B., Fibronectin-associated transforming growth factor, *J. Cell Physiol.*, 131, 184, 1987.

229. Yamaguchi, Y., Mann, D. M., and Ruoslahti, E., Negative regulation of transforming growth factor-β by the proteoglycan decorin, *Nature*, 346, 281, 1990.

230. Border, W. A., Noble, N. A., Yamamoto, T., Harper, J. R., Yamaguchi, Y., Pierschbacher, M. D., and Ruoslahti, E., Natural inhibitor of transforming growth factor-β protects against scarring in experimental kidney disease, *Nature*, 360, 361, 1992.

231. Redington, A. E., Madden, J., Djukanovic, R., Holgate, S. T., and Howarth, P. H., Transforming growth factor-beta levels in bronchoalveolar lavage fluid are increased in asthma, *J. Allergy Clin. Immunol.*, 95 (Abstr.), 377, 1995.

232. Redington, A. E., Madden, J., Frew, A. J., Djukanovic, R., Roche, W. R., Holgate, S. T., and Howarth, P. H., Basic fibroblast growth factor in asthma: immunolocalization in bronchial biopsies and measurement in bronchoalveolar lavage fluid at baseline and following allergen challenge, *Am. J. Respir. Crit. Care Med.*, 151 (Abstr.), A702, 1995.

233. Sommer, A. and Rifkin, D. B., Interaction of heparin with human basic fibroblast growth factor: protection of the angiogenic protein from proteolytic degradation by a glycosaminoglycan, *J. Cell Physiol.*, 138, 215, 1989.

234. Gospodarowicz, D. and Cheng, J., Heparin protects basic and acidic FGF from inactivation, *J. Cell Physiol.*, 128, 475, 1986.

235. Thompson, R. W., Whalen, G. F., Saunders, K. B., Hores, T., and D'Amore, P. A., Heparin-mediated release of fibroblast growth factor-like activity into the circulation of rabbits, *Growth Factors*, 3, 221, 1990.

236. Bashkin, P., Razin, E., Eldor, A., and Vlodavsky, I., Degranulating mast cells secrete an endoglycosidase that degrades heparan sulfate in subendothelial extracellular matrix, *Blood*, 75, 2204, 1990.

237. Barnes, P. J., Chung, K. F., and Page, C. P., Platelet-activating factor as a mediator of allergic disease, *J. Allergy Clin. Immunol.*, 81, 919, 1988.

238. Spence, D. P. S., Johnston, S. L., Calverley, P. M. A., Dhillon, P., Higgins, C., Ramhamadany, E., Turner, S., Winning, A., Winter, J., and Holgate, S. T., The effect of the orally active platelet-activating factor antagonist WEB 2086 in the treatment of asthma, *Am. J. Respir. Crit. Care Med.*, 149, 1142, 1994.

Chapter 3

# INFLAMMATION AND CYTOKINES IN AIRWAY WALL REMODELLING

John W. Wilson and Xun Li

## CONTENTS

0-8493-7813-3/97/$0.00+$.50
© 1997 by CRC Press, Inc.

## I. OVERVIEW

Considerable advances have been made in understanding the process of inflammation in response to injury since the discovery of cytoactive chemicals in healing tissues. Our understanding of the tissue response had for centuries been limited by the resolving power of the light microscope and the ability of generations of pathologists to accurately interpret their findings. Understanding of the processes that initiate and perpetuate inflammation was hindered until the relatively recent advent of the instruments we depend on today, the animal model, the clinical trial, and the immunology laboratory.

The concept of the cytokine as a chemical released by an activated cell, which may act on the same or another cell, occupies a central place in current thinking of inflammatory mechanisms in asthma, so much so, in fact, that many studies have been directed at reevaluation of the specific changes seen in the bronchial wall in asthma, so that they may be explained by the actions of one or more specific cytokines.

Molecular biologic techniques have radically changed the traditional view of a dominant cell or cytokine in airway inflammation. Clearly, all airway cells possess the genetic information to code for all known cytokines. The expression of these genes is highly regulated, such that familiar patterns are now being described in the setting of active asthma. Rather than there being a limited number of cytokines controlling a few cells in asthmatic airway inflammation, it is highly likely that many cytokines are produced, by virtually all cells of the airway, at variable rates and times, governed by a myriad of promoting and inhibitory factors.

Despite the widely diverse response and redundancy of cytokine actions, specific patterns have appeared that may be associated with the tissue changes that are characteristic of asthma. The definition of these patterns and their regulating events is vitally important for the understanding of asthma, bronchial wall remodelling, and the design of future interventional strategies.

## II. AIRWAY INFLAMMATION IN ASTHMA

Airway inflammation is now recognised as being a fundamental component of asthma.[1-3] Although the cellular response and tissue changes seen in the airway are well described, no clear relationship exists between measurable parameters of inflammation and asthma symptoms, airflow obstruction, or airway hyperreactivity. Indices of airway inflammation in human asthma have been derived either directly or indirectly from studies on peripheral blood, bronchial lavage, bronchial biopsy, post-mortem and resection specimens, and animal models.

## A. PERIPHERAL BLOOD

Asthma severity has been linked to various measurable parameters in peripheral blood, including eosinophil count,[4,5] activated lymphocytes,[6-8] IgE levels,[9] and cytokines.[8,10,11] Although having the advantage of accessibility, peripheral blood provides an indirect view of events in the airway and may well be confounded by atopy.

## B. BRONCHIAL LAVAGE

The interpretation of bronchial lavage data has been limited by difficulty assessing dilutional factors[12] and lack of uniform standardisation of technique.[13,14] Mast cells have been shown to be increased in some studies,[5,15-17] but not universally.[18,19] Eosinophils were found to be elevated in most studies,[5,15-21] but not in one.[22] Occasionally, studies have found increased numbers of lymphocytes in asthmatic bronchial lavage.[21,23] However, suppressible lymphocyte activation has been more consistently demonstrated.[7,24] Total cells, macrophages, and neutrophils have not been found to be elevated in asthmatic lavage. The selective elevation of some cell types seems to represent one of the following: site of lavage (i.e., bronchial vs. alveolar), selective traffic from the submucosa into the lumen, or dislodgement of nonadherent cells from the epithelial surface. Although statistical correlations have been made between cell numbers in lavage and indices of asthma, no clear relationship exists between lavage cell numbers and specific features of the submucosa taken at simultaneously performed biopsy.[22]

## C. BRONCHIAL BIOPSY

Endobronchial biopsy in asthma has the distinct advantages of accurate characterisation of asthmatic subjects and the possibility of repeated intervention. Early studies involved the more invasive procedure of rigid bronchoscopy.[25,26] However, fibreoptic bronchoscopy has made endobronchial biopsy a relatively safe and tolerable procedure.[22,23] Limitations of this technique include epithelial sampling without submucosal tissue, epithelial damage, and crush artefact. Identification of specific cell types is usually unreliable in standard haematoxylin and eosin-stained sections (Figure 1). Specific monoclonal antibodies enable the accurate enumeration of cells (Figures 2 and 3).

Biopsy studies in asthma have identified epithelial denudation,[26] subepithelial collagen deposition,[27] eosinophil infiltration and mast cell activation,[19,28] T-lymphocyte activation,[29] capillary dilatation,[30] the presence of interleukin 4 (IL-4) and tumour necrosis factor α (TNFα),[31] and the expression of mRNA for IL-5 using *in situ* hybridisation.[32]

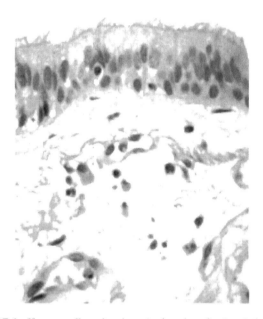

**FIGURE 1**   Haematoxylin and eosin–stained section of asthmatic bronchus.

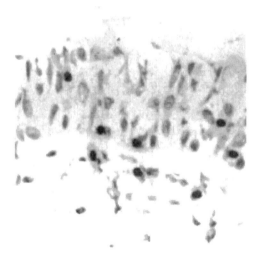

**FIGURE 2**   Asthmatic airway stained with immunoperoxidase to detect CD3+ lymphocytes.

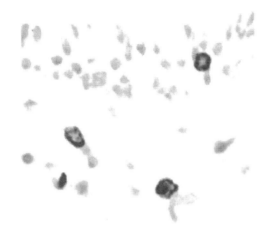

**FIGURE 3**   Asthmatic airway stained with immunoperoxidase to detect tryptase-containing mast cells.

## D.  POST-MORTEM STUDIES

Until recently, general descriptions of the pathology of asthma were biased towards the more severe cases and included descriptions of mucus plugging, eosinophil infiltration of the airway and lumen, mucous gland hypertrophy, and smooth muscle hyperplasia.[25,30,33-35] In a landmark study by Dunnill,[30] there was apparent thickening of the epithelial basement membrane. This study also identified expansion of the capillary bed of the airway wall in fatal asthma. More-recent studies have also identified inflammatory cells adhering to peripheral vessels in fatal asthma.[36] Although smooth muscle hyperplasia/hypertrophy has been described in a number of studies,[33,36,37] specific quantitation of airway muscle volume and the simple relationship between hypertrophy and hyperplasia have not been completely resolved. Convincingly, all studies have reported a marked inflammatory response and epithelial shedding associated with airway mucus plugging in fatal asthma.

## E.  ANIMAL MODELS

Many different animal models have been studied, with a view to gaining a better perspective of the human asthmatic response. A number of advantages make these systems attractive and include access to subjects with restricted genetic diversity, favourable environmental control, easily repeatable intervention, a well-characterised genotype and phenotype, as well as ready availability.

Unfortunately, no single animal system accurately pertains to the human, because of either fundamentally different physiological or immunological responses. Many of these limitations have been reviewed by Hirschman and Downes.[38] In the mouse, the immunological system is well described and specific subsets of T-lymphocytes are characterised by their cytokine secretion profile.[39-41] Guinea pigs may be used effectively as small animal models of asthma, either by tracheostomy or plethysmography.[42,43] The immunology of the guinea pig is, however, less well defined, and there is a tendency towards exaggerated eosinophilic responses.[43] A rat model of asthma has been developed.[44] However, rodent models may preferentially respond to serotonin rather than to histamine.[45] Models of antigen-induced bronchoconstriction are also available in large animals using the parasite *Ascaris suum* responses in the dog (sheep and monkey are also well described[38]). These larger animals, although easier to study physiologically, are limited by genetic diversity and less-predictable immunological responses.

## III. CYTOKINES AND INFLAMMATION

Antigen-induced asthma is caused by a type I hypersensitivity reaction in which antigen cross-links IgE molecules on the surface of mast cells, leading to cell activation, inflammatory mediator release, and the production of inflammatory cytokines. As a result, bronchoconstriction occurs with an early asthmatic response (EAR, 30 min to 4 h) and/or a late asthmatic response (LAR, 3 to 12 h). The EAR has been attributed to the cumulative response to bronchoconstricting, mast cell-derived mediators, such as histamine, sulphidopeptide leukotrienes, prostaglandins $D_2$ ($PGD_2$), $PGF_{2\alpha}$, kinins, and platelet-activating factor (PAF).[46] The late response to allergen has been best described in skin, where T-lymphocyte activation occurs in association with eosinophil and neutrophil influx and oedema.[47,48] The direct application of these responses to clinical asthma is uncertain, given the "nonatopic" nature of asthma in some patients, the probable overlap of EAR and LAR in others, and the difficulty in identifying specific causative allergens in most patients. It is not surprising, then, that direct application of the findings of such well-described models to biopsies taken from patients with stable, mild asthma does not result in accurate correlations with disease activity. Furthermore, factors that regulate and limit the acute response are not well described. It is likely, therefore, that biopsy samples from patients with mild stable asthma show a combination of a contemporary acute response with underlying chronic features. Studies in mild asthma, acute severe asthma and allergen-provoked asthma have provided the evaluable evidence to date, describing the role of cytokines in asthma. It is tempting to speculate that linkage between cytokine genes on chromosome 5 — IL-3, -4, -5, -9, -13, and granulocyte/macrophage colony-stimulating factor (GM-CSF) — and bronchial hyperreactivity form the genetic basis for asthma.[49]

## A. DETECTION OF CYTOKINES

Circulating cytokines may be measured in the peripheral blood of patients with asthma. The interpretation of levels is somewhat limited by the sensitivity of available assays and the relevance of circulating cytokines to local cellular microenvironmental events in the airway. Brown et al.[10] found that GM-CSF was elevated in the sera of patients with acute severe asthma. Corrigan and Kay[9] found that interferon-γ (IFNγ) was increased in acute severe asthma, and fell with treatment. IL-5 levels have been found to be elevated in the sera of stable asthmatics, although levels determined by ELISA were not related to severity.[50]

Elevated levels have also been found in patients requiring oral prednisolone therapy for exacerbations of disease.[11] There is evidence that a "spill over" of cytokines occurs in the peripheral blood of patients with more severe asthma.

Cytokines have been measured with some success in bronchoalveolar lavage (BAL) fluid from subjects with atopic asthma.[51] IL-4 and IL-5 were detected in lavage from atopic asthmatic subjects, while intrinsic asthmatic subjects showed IL-2 and IL-5, but not IL-4. In BAL fluid examined 24 h after allergen challenge, GM-CSF levels were found to be elevated in atopic asthmatic subjects.[52] In this study, *in situ* hybridisation of BAL cells suggested that GM-CSF mRNA was expressed by lymphocytes. The same group examined cytokine concentrations in BAL fluid from symptomatic and asymptomatic asthma subjects. IL-2 and IL-1β were detected in both groups, while symptomatic subjects returned increased concentrations of IL-6, TNFα, and GM-CSF. Interestingly, IL-1α and IL-4 were not detected in either group. The absence of IL-4 and the finding of TNFα may seem contradictory to the Th2 hypothesis of lymphocyte activity in asthma. Once again, the role of specific cytokines may only be inferred indirectly and is somewhat hampered by dilutional factors and collection techniques.

The use of *in situ* hybridisation to determine the cytokine-producing potential of specific airway cells has been fundamental in formulating the Th2 hypothesis. Original work by Robinson and co-workers[53] identified the presence of signals for IL-2, IL-3, IL-4, IL-5, and GM-CSF mRNA in atopic asthmatic subjects at higher levels than could be found in nonsmoking, nonatopic control subjects. The finding of increased expression of IL-2 could not be easily explained in this model, nor could cytokine expression be specifically localised to lymphocytes. Subsequently, TNFα mRNA was also found to be elevated in BAL fluid from atopic asthmatic subjects.[54] In response to this conflicting information, the same group analysed data based on airway responsiveness and asthmatic symptoms.[55] Their findings further supported the Th2 hypothesis by showing that increased expression of mRNA for IL-3, IL-4, IL-5, and GM-CSF occurred in those patients with symptoms, but that IL-2 or IFNγ mRNA did not. They also inferred that higher proportions of IL-4 and IL-5 mRNA-positive cells in BAL fluid were indicative of more severe airway obstruction and bronchial hyperreactivity. The interpretation of these findings rests heavily on identification of specific cell types producing positive mRNA signals. Although possible, no studies have conclusively used double-labelling techniques to identify cytokine mRNA expression by *in situ* hybridisation in immunohistochemically labelled cells. Presumptive evidence may soon be available from cell-sorting studies using flow cytometric methods. Possibly, larger numbers of T-lymphocytes have the capacity to generate Th2 cytokines, while only mast cells are capable of storing product for release on activation.

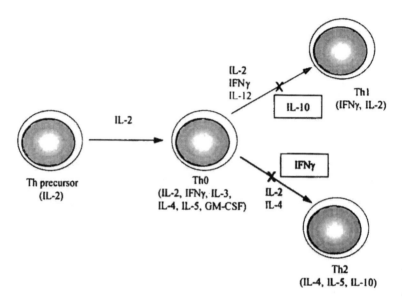

Induction of Th subsets.

## B. Th1 VS. Th2 CYTOKINE PROFILES

Mosmann et al.[39-41] have provided evidence for two distinct subsets of murine T cell clones, Th1 and Th2, based on the spectrum of cytokines they produce. Evidence for the existence of Th2 cytokines in human asthma has been presented by Kay and colleagues,[32,53,54,56] who have examined bronchial lavage cells and bronchial biopsies from mild asthmatics, using *in situ* hybridisation techniques. T cell clones derived from human lymphocyte cultures do not generally conform to the Th1/Th2 categorisation.[57] However, the accumulated evidence from sampling studies in asthma indicates that local factors may well regulate the emergence of specific Th2 clones. It is likely that infection or antigenic triggers such as tuberculin may induce a Th1 response, while allergen exposure favours a Th2 response. A Th1 response producing IFNγ and IL-2 may induce B cell proliferation and differentiation with production of IgG2a. IFNγ otherwise blocks IgE production. Bactericidal activity of macrophages is enhanced by Th1 release of IFNγ and TNFβ.[58,59] The release of IFNγ inhibits proliferation of mast cells and eosinophils, normally influenced by the Th2 cytokines IL-3, IL-4, IL-5, and IL-10 and by IL-3, IL-5, and GM-CSF, respectively.[60]

Th2 lymphocytes produce IL-5, which supports eosinophil proliferation and activation. Also, IL-4, IL-5, and IL-10 induce B-lymphocyte differentiation with a bias towards the production of IgE. IL-4 and IL-10 are also inhibitory to cytokine production by Th1 cells.[61] There would, therefore, seem to be a tendency to perpetuation of one type of response, with reciprocal inhibition of the other.

### TABLE 1
### T-lymphocyte "Subsets" in Asthma

| Th0 | Th1 | Th2 |
|-----|-----|-----|
| IL-2 | IL-2 | |
| | IL-3 | IL-3 |
| | GM-CSF | GM-CSF |
| IL-4 | | IL-4 |
| | | IL-5 |
| | | IL-6 |
| | | IL-10 |
| | | IL-13 |
| IFNγ | IFNγ | |
| | TNFα | |
| | TNFβ | |

## C. MAST CELL-DERIVED CYTOKINES

Mast cells have traditionally been known as effectors of type I hypersensitivity reactions, capable of releasing newly generated or preformed mediators of acute inflammation from electron-dense granules. IL-3, IL-4, IL-10, and stem cell factor (SCF) are likely to be responsible for the proliferation and survival of mast cells in tissues.[46,62] Also, IgE-dependent degranulation of mast cells may be enhanced by IL-3, IL-5, IL-8, GM-CSF, and SCF.[63,63] Mast cells are also capable of producing cytokines, including IL-1, IL-3, IL-4, IL-5, IL-8, IL-9, IL-13, GM-CSF, transforming growth factor β (TGFβ), and TNFα.[64] Recent work from Bradding and co-workers[31] on biopsies from asthmatic subjects has shown mast cells to be capable of producing IL-4, IL-5, IL-6, and TNFα. Interestingly, TNFα was significantly upregulated in asthma, while virtually all cells staining for IL-4, IL-6, and TNFα were found to be mast cells. Ackerman et al.[65] also used monoclonal antibodies to localise cytokines to cells within the asthmatic bronchial mucosa. Cytokines were not localised solely to cells identified as lymphocytes[66] or solely to mast cells.[31] In this study, cytokines were localised to both T-lymphocytes and mast cells. Although the evidence would appear to be conflicting, it is likely that all airway cells retain the potential to produce cytokines and that specific, permissive conditions will allow the expression of cytokine genes and the elaboration of protein products. Resolution of this issue awaits the development of dual-staining techniques capable of detecting mRNA expression by *in situ* hybridisation and cytokine products by immunolocalisation in specific cell types. It is to be hoped that the application of double-staining techniques to airway tissues will not only resolve the identity of cytokine-producing cells, but also address the issue of the significance of mRNA expression in relation to cytokine product elaboration.

## IV. SPECIFIC INFLAMMATORY CYTOKINES

Inflammatory cell activity within the wall of the airway is under the influence of specific cytokines that regulate their proliferation, differentiation, migration, activation, mediator release, and eventual apoptosis (or programmed cell death). One possible function of any cell within the airway is to produce its own array of cytokines. They may generally be considered as interleukins, colony-stimulating factors, and growth factors. Those with proinflammatory activity implicated in asthma are shown in Table 2.

### A. INTERLEUKIN 1

The polypeptide interleukin family comprises a range of nonimmunoglobulin molecules with hormonelike actions in health and disease.[67-70] IL-1 is a single chain polypeptide released by activated tissue macrophages and monocytes (as well as many body cells, including keratinocytes, endothelial cells, and neutrophils) that exists in two partially homologous forms (IL-1α and IL-1β) that have similar proinflammatory actions and bind to the same receptor.[67,68] Previously known as endogenous pyrogen, IL-1 probably has little role in the healthy state but may have wide-ranging actions in disease. mRNA for IL-1 appears 2 h after stimulation of resting monocytes, while detectable protein appears within 3 h.[71] It acts to stimulate the release of TNFα and acute-phase reactants from the liver during acute inflammation and activates tissue lymphocytes to replicate on exposure to antigen. This action assists in the clearance of organisms from the reticuloendothelial system.[72] Other actions include the induction of REM sleep, fever, adrenocorticotrophic hormone (ACTH) release, neutrophilia, and a fall in zinc and bound-iron levels.[67,68] There are two separate but structurally related proteins, IL-1α and IL-1β. Both genes have been coded and proteins sequenced, identifying a gene locus on chromosome 2, producing mature peptides of 155 amino acids.[73,74] The two peptides have 26% amino acid homology,[75] share the same cell surface receptors,[76] and exhibit many similar actions.[77] Although many cell types are capable of producing IL-1, including monocyte/macrophages, fibroblasts, β-lymphocytes, stromal cells, smooth muscle cells, and neutrophils,[78] it is likely that macrophages represent the major source of IL-1 in the airway. The release of IL-1 by these cells may occur on exposure to a range of stimuli, including

## TABLE 2
## Proinflammatory Cytokines in Asthma

| Cytokine | Source | Actions | Ref. |
|---|---|---|---|
| IL-2 | T cells | T cell growth factor, eosinophil chemoattractant | 199, 200 |
| IL-3 | T cells<br>Mast cells<br>Eosinophils | Eosinophil and neutrophil differentiation and activation, *in vitro* survival, priming chemotaxis (eosinophils), and mast cell survival and degranulation | 89–91 |
| GM-CSF | T cells<br>Mast cells<br>Macrophage<br>Epithelial<br>Eosinophils | Eosinophil and neutrophil differentiation and activation, *in vitro* survival, chemotaxis (eosinophils), mast cell degranulation | 90, 96, 201, 202 |
| IL-4 | T cells<br>Mast cells | Essential for IgE synthesis, T cell growth factor, mast cell survival | 111, 134, 203 |
| IL-5 | T cell<br>Mast cells<br>Eosinophils | Eosinophil differentiation, maturation, and activation, endothelial adhesion, priming for chemoattraction, cofactor for IgE synthesis, mast cell degranulation | 40, 119, 131, 135, 193, 203 |
| IL-6 | Macrophages<br>Fibroblasts<br>T cells | T cell activation costimulus, macrophage and eosinophil activation | 204, 205 |
| IL-8 | Monocytes<br>Fibroblasts | Neutrophil and T cell chemoattractant, neutrophil activation, inhibition of IgE synthesis, primes for eosinophil chemotaxis, mast cell degranulation | 108, 206, 207 |
| IL-10 | T cells<br>Monocytes<br>B cells | Inhibition of Th1 cytokine production (action on APC), mast cell growth | 157 |
| IL-12 | T cells | NK cells, T cell growth, inhibits IgE synthesis | 209 |
| TNFα | Th1<br>Macrophages<br>Epithelium | Endothelial cell activation, induction of adhesion glycoproteins, fibroblast stimulation (indirect) | 210, 306 |

*Note:* APC, antigen-presenting cell.

IL-1, TNFα, GM-CSF, phorbol ester, and viral gene products, which have been reviewed extensively by Aksamit and Hunninghake.[79] IL-1 secretion may be significantly enhanced by the presence of other cytokines, including IL-2 and IFNα.[80] Other than its role in inducing the acute-phase response to bacterial endotoxin, IL-1 has the capacity to induce the release of PAF and enhance the expression of adhesion glycoproteins on endothelial cells (ELAM-1 and ICAM-1). Of relevance to airway wall remodelling is the fact that IL-1 may induce fibroblast proliferation[81] and increase collagen production.[78] Acting as a fundamental stimulant to T cell activation, it may induce the production of IL-2 and the IL-2 receptor.[30]

Although a clinically evident acute-phase response is not associated with acute asthma in atopic subjects, the local actions of IL-1 are compatible with the findings of increased polymorph adherence to airway vessels and remodelling of the airway wall seen in asthma.

## B. INTERLEUKIN 2

IL-2 is a polypeptide of 153 amino acids, produced by activated T-lymphocytes, which acts to promote division of T-, B-, and NK-lymphocytes.[67,68] The production of IL-2 by lymphocytes is an index event in the activation process.[302] IL-2 binds to a low-affinity receptor (55 kDa, TAC) which may combine with an intermediate-affinity element in the cell membrane (75 kDa) to form the dimeric high-affinity receptor.[303] Receptor studies have shown IL-2 to be the major stimulus for T cell activation and replication.[82] Identification of the low-affinity portion of the IL-2 receptor using anti-TAC antibodies has been used to identify T cell activation in the airway in asthma and its suppression after inhaled steroid therapy.[7,24] IL-2 has been measured at low concentration in bronchial lavage fluid from asthmatic subjects,[51] while mRNA has been detected in bronchial lavage cells.[53] Broide et al.[83] found IL-2 in bronchial lavage fluid from both symptomatic and asymptomatic asthmatic subjects, with no significant difference in levels. A pivotal role for T-lymphocytes as a key source of cytokines in the bronchial mucosa is therefore highly dependent on the elaboration and maintenance of IL-2 levels. Cyclosporin A acts as an immune suppressant by inhibiting IL-2 gene expression,[84] and this agent has been shown to act effectively in the treatment of chronic severe asthma.[85] Whether or not the specific therapy aimed at deactivation of lymphocytes through modulation of the IL-2 receptor would be an effective treatment for asthma remains a matter for speculation.

## C. INTERLEUKIN 3

IL-3 is a haemopoietic growth factor, produced by activated T-lymphocytes, with the capacity to stimulate bone marrow progenitor cells (myeloid, monocyte/macrophage, megakaracyte, erythroid lineages, and pleuripotent stem cells) to replicate and differentiate before release to the periphery.[86,87] The gene for IL-3 is located on chromosome 5 and codes for a 152 amino acid protein.[88] *In vitro* studies have provided evidence to suggest that IL-3 may be intimately involved in mast cell homeostasis. Mast cell survival and degranulation may be enhanced by the addition of IL-3.[89] Mast cells also have the capacity to produce IL-3 following IgE-dependent stimulation.[90,91] Eosinophils are also apparently activated on exposure to IL-3.[92] IL-3, therefore, has an activating and proinflammatory effect on airway inflammatory cells. mRNA signal for IL-3 has been detected in bronchial lavage cells in asthma[53] particularly in those patients with symptoms.[55] Interestingly, although IL-3 controls the maturation and release of neutrophils, these cells do not generally feature in asthma. It suggests, therefore, that IL-3 most likely acts as a cofactor for mast cell and eosinophil activation in asthma, rather than acting dominantly as a stimulus for replication within the bronchial mucosa.

## D. GRANULOCYTE/MACROPHAGE COLONY-STIMULATING FACTOR

GM-CSF is a glycoprotein of 127 amino acids encoded by a gene on the long arm of chromosome 5. It is produced by a range of cells resident within the airway, including T-lymphocytes, macrophages, epithelial cells, fibroblasts, eosinophils, and mast cells.[90,93-98] It acts to prime, activate, and induce replication of cells of the myeloid lineage, including eosinophils, as well as mast cells and fibroblasts.[62,99-102] Of great relevance to airway inflammation in asthma is the ability of GM-CSF to induce eosinophil chemotaxis, eosinophil proliferation, hypodensity and activation, as well as degranulation.[97,102,104-106] GM-CSF also enhances mast cell activation by C5a or anti-IgE antibodies[62] and induces fibroblast replication and differentiation.[102,107] Although not readily detectable in serum, eosinophil survival-enhancing activity from the peripheral blood from asthmatic subjects has been blocked by treatment with anti-GM-CSF antibodies and anti-IL-5 antibodies, while supernatant fluid from cultured T cells supported eosinophil survival but was blocked by anti-GM-CSF antibody alone.[108] mRNA for GM-CSF has been detected in bronchial lavage cells from stable asthma,[53] while elevated GM-CSF levels were detectable in bronchial lavage fluid from symptomatic asthmatic subjects.[83] The same group identified GM-CSF in bronchial lavage fluid 24 h after allergen challenge in atopic asthmatic subjects and found that mRNA was expressed within lavage lymphocytes.[52]

Again, it is clear that the function of any one cytokine cannot be viewed in isolation. GM-CSF both activates and promotes long-term survival of neutrophils.[109,110,304] Despite the apparent importance of GM-CSF in regulating inflammation in the bronchial mucosa, activated neutrophils are not a characteristic feature of chronic asthma; hence, it must be assumed that GM-CSF acts predominantly as a permissive cofactor, particularly with IL-5 in the regulation of eosinophil infiltration and function.

## E. INTERLEUKIN 4

Principally known as an activator and regulator of B-lymphocyte proliferation, IL-4 is also trophic for T cells, mast cells, and other lineages.[111-113] The human IL-4 gene on chromosome 5 codes for a 153 amino acid protein.[114,115] In the airway, IL-4 may potentially enhance IgE production, enhance T cell activation, and stimulate mast cells.[116-118]

Mast cells are also capable of producing IL-4,[119] while a specific activated form has been identified in bronchial biopsies from patients with mild asthma[31,120] (Plate 1*). The unique origin of IL-4 within the airway is not certain. T-lymphocytes cultured from bronchial lavage cells from atopic asthmatic cases

---

* Plate 1 follows page 80.

that have been subject to *in situ* hybridisation indicate that T-lymphocytes might also produce IL-4 in the bronchial mucosa.[121] Robinson et al.[56] have suggested that mast cells secrete IL-4 to prime T-lymphocytes, producing a Th2 pattern of cytokine response, based on suggestive *in vitro* evidence.[122,123] They also clearly demonstrated that cells expressing mRNA for IL-4 can be suppressed by treatment with oral steroids. IL-4 may induce CD23 expression on B-lymphocytes and upregulate class II major histocompatibility complex (MHC) antigen expression.[124,125] Of importance in the regulation of the airway cytokine network, is the counterregulatory effect of IFNγ. It is likely that IFNγ may act to functionally antagonise IL-4.[124,126]

## F. INTERLEUKIN 5

The relative specificity of the inflammatory response described in the asthmatic airway has outlined the important relationship among mast cells, eosinophils, and their supporting cytokines. The hypothesis supporting an important role for IL-5 in asthma rests on the selective action of IL-5 in several stages in eosinophil development and activation.[127-129] The gene for IL-5 is located on chromosome 5 and codes for a sequence of 134 amino acids, with a mature functional protein of 115 amino acids.[130] IL-5 acts on eosinophils to increase adhesion to endothelial surfaces through the elaboration of adhesion glycoproteins CD11a, CD11b, and CD18 binding to ICAM-1.[129] It induces the morphological changes of activation in eosinophils and stimulates the production of the superoxide anion.[131] The characteristic finding of eosinophilic infiltration in the airway in asthma poses two fundamental questions that are as yet not fully answered. First, as IL-3, GM-CSF, and IL-5 each has the capacity to induce differentiation and activate eosinophils *in vitro*, is IL-5 of greater relevance to asthma, given that (1) IL-5 has no significant influence on neutrophils and (2) neutrophil infiltration and activation, which might occur under the influence of IL-3 and GM-CSF, are not major features in asthma? Second, which cell or cells in the airway wall are the source(s) of IL-5?

Concerning the first question, it would seem apparent that the neutrophil is involved in animal models of asthma[132] and occupational asthma.[133] Neutrophils have been found to be increased in lavage fluid in one study of asthmatic subjects.[21] There is otherwise little evidence to support their role in asthma[1] Other possibilities for selective eosinophil recruitment, therefore, include upregulation of receptors for IL-3, GM-CSF, and IL-5 on eosinophils in preference to neutrophils or, alternatively, upregulation of IL-5 receptors where they exist, that is, on eosinophils and B-lymphocytes. Finally, it must be remembered that evidence to date suggests that cytokine-producing cells elaborate a wide range of factors after activation, therefore, subscribing specific patterns (e.g., Th1 vs. Th2) to lymphocytes in asthma may be premature at present.[58]

When considering which cells produce IL-5 in asthma, it is known that T-lymphocytes, mast cells, fibroblasts, and eosinophils may all act as sources.[51,134,135] Using *in situ* hybridisation techniques, Robinson and colleagues[55,56] have accrued evidence indicating that the T-lymphocyte may well be the predominant source of IL-5 in asthma. Using correlation analysis, this group has shown that of ten subjects with atopic asthma, six produced specific signals for IL-5 mRNA, while none of nine control subjects was positive.[32] This study found a correlation between the expression of IL-5 in asthma and numbers of activated lymphocytes and eosinophils. Indirect evidence has also come from positive correlations between IL-5 activity and CD4 lymphocyte activation in bronchial lavage fluid.[51] In allergen-induced asthma, bronchial lavage at 24 h after challenge returned increased numbers of eosinophils and activated CD4-positive lymphocytes, together with increased numbers of cells expressing IL-4, IL-5, and GM-CSF mRNA detected by *in situ* hybridisation.[66] In patients with symptomatic asthma treated with oral prednisolone or placebo, numbers of bronchial lavage eosinophils were reduced in association with numbers of cells expressing mRNA for IL-4 and IL-5.[136] Cell-separation techniques applied to T-lymphocytes retrieved at bronchial lavage have indicated that IL-5 mRNA is predominantly expressed by T-lymphocytes in those with atopic mild asthma.[53] These studies have been confirmed by others, who have found IL-5 to be produced by bronchial lavage T cells obtained 24 h after allergen challenge.[121]

Current information suggests that active T-lymphocytes are highly likely to produce IL-5 in the asthmatic airway. Until further cell-separation studies or improved double-staining techniques are available, the collaboration of other cell types of IL-5 production awaits confirmation. A recent study by Ackerman et al.[65] has indicated that both T-lymphocytes and mast cells have the capability of producing IL-5 in biopsies from patients with atopic asthma.

## G. INTERLEUKIN 6

Previously known as interferon β2 or B cell differentiation factor, IL-6 is produced by T-lymphocytes, fibroblasts, and macrophages.[137,138] The gene for IL-6, located on chromosome 7, codes for a protein of 212 amino acids and releases a mature protein of 184 amino acids.[139] The production of IL-6 is regulated by other cytokines, including IL-1, TNFα, platelet-derived growth factor B (PDGFB), and TGFβ.[140-142] Although IL-6 has been shown to induce immunoglobulin synthesis by B-lymphocytes, it does not stimulate B cell proliferation or IgE production.[143,144] Both CD4+ and CD8+ T cells proliferate in response to IL-6.[145] This function of IL-6 may well be dependent on IL-1 and IL-2 receptor activation,[146,147] although only early in the activation process. The extensive biologic activities of IL-6 have been reviewed by Zitnic and Elias.[148] Lung fibroblast and alveolar macrophage production of IL-6 has been most studied in the respiratory context. Lung fibroblasts, when stimulated by inflammatory cytokines, such as IL-1, TNFα, or TGFβ, produce IL-6.[149,150] Alveolar macrophages, on the other hand, tend to produce IL-6 in response to lipopolysaccharide endotoxin, rather than cytokine stimulation.[151] Of importance to asthma is the finding of raised levels of IL-6 in bronchial lavage from symptomatic asthmatic patients,[83] and the markedly elevated levels of IL-6

found in bronchial lavage from ozone-treated subjects.[152] Interestingly, eosinophils also synthesise and secrete IL-6.[153] These findings indicate that IL-6
most likely acts as an indicator of injury and repair, rather than as a major
orchestrator of immune responses in the airway.

## H. INTERLEUKIN 10

IL-10 is a broadly expressed cytokine (predominantly T-lymphocytes,
B-lymphocytes, and monocytes), having a powerfully suppressive effect on
Th1 cytokines.[154,155] It acts to suppress TNFα production by macrophages, as
well as dramatically enhancing the growth of mast cells when cocultured with
IL-3 or IL-4.[60] Evidence to date suggests that IL-10 is capable of completely
suppressing the T cell proliferative response to antigen.[156] The wide range of
actions of IL-10 suggests that it acts overall as a Th2 cytokine, enhancing the
allergic response.[157] Although IL-10 has been detected in biologic samples, its
specific role in asthma is currently unknown.

## I. INTERFERON γ

IFNγ has a broad range of biologic activity to inhibit viral and cell proliferation.[158] This cytokine is produced primarily by activated Th1-lymphocytes
inducing macrophage expression of MHC antigens (allowing more-efficient
presentation of antigen), LFA-1 (CD11a/CD18) expression, production of
oxidation species, as well as release of IL-1 and TNFα.[159-162] IFNγ also stimulates endothelial cells to increase ICAM-1 expression, potentially enhancing
the adhesion of inflammatory cells.[163,164] The gene for IFNγ is located on
chromosome 12 and codes for a 166 amino acid protein, released as a 143 amino
acid product.[165,166] The secreted protein is structurally unrelated to IFNα or
IFNβ, suggesting a distinctly different origin. The receptor for IFNγ is distinct
from receptors for IFNα and IFNβ[167] and is widely distributed on different
cell types. Of relevance to atopic asthma is the finding that IFNγ may suppress
the induction of IgE production by IL-4.[126] This antiallergic action of IFNγ is
consistent with its classification as a Th1 cytokine.

In addition to its established role in inflammatory responses, IFNγ also
exhibits duality of function in the pathogenesis of fibrosis. It may well act
early in fibrogenesis to promote macrophage activation and secretion of fibrogenic cytokines.[168] Together with TNFα, it may act as a cofactor to stimulate
collagen production by human skin fibroblasts.[169] Alternatively, it has the
capacity to inhibit fibroblast chemotaxis and proliferation and is able to suppress collagen production.[170,171]

In stable asthma, IFNγ has been detected in bronchial lavage fluid at low
levels, by comparison with IL-4 and IL-5.[51] mRNA for IFNγ was not elevated
in BAL fluid from patients with mild asthma.[53] In patients with acute severe
asthma admitted to hospital, serum levels of IFNγ were elevated and correlated
with lung function and fell after corticosteroid treatment.[8] Oral prednisolone
was also shown to reduce serum IFNγ in acute severe asthma[11] Interestingly,
oral prednisolone caused a reduction in the proportion of cells in bronchial

CHAPTER 3, PLATE 1  Immunoperoxidase staining of asthmatic airway for IL-4.

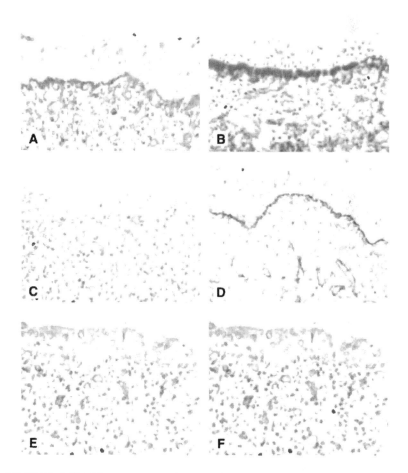

CHAPTER 4, PLATE 1  Immunoreactivity of collagen subtypes in the airway submucosa: A. collagen type I, B. collagen type III, C. collagen type IV, D. collagen type V, E. laminin, F. fibronectin.

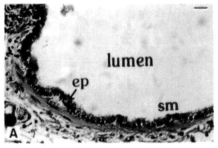

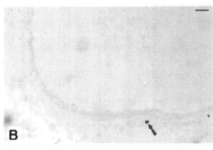

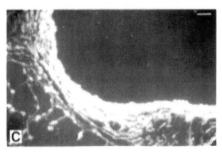

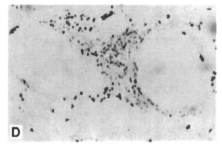

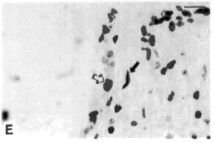

**CHAPTER 7, PLATE 1** Repeated ovalbumin challenges induce BrdU incorporation into airway epithelial and smooth muscle cells.

**Control (A,B,C):**
A. Representative light photomicrograph of a medium-sized airway demonstrating airway epithelium (ep), smooth muscle (sm), and lumen (400x).

B. Immunocytochemical staining of the identical airway with an anti-BrdU antibody (arrow indicate positive staining).

C. DAPI staining reveals that airway epithelial and smooth muscle cell nuclei are intact.

**OA-challenged (D,E):**
D. Immunocytochemical staining of a medium-sized airway with an anti-BrdU antibody (250x).

E. Identical section viewed at 600x. Filled arrow indicates positive anti-BrdU nuclear staining of an airway myocyte; open arrow indicates positive staining of an airway epithelial cell. (From Panettieri et al., *Am. J. Physiol.*, 259, L365, 1990. With permission.)

lavage fluid expressing mRNA for IL-4 and IL-5, but increased the number of cells expressing mRNA for IFNγ.[136] Why prednisolone treatment should reduce serum IFNγ but increase bronchoalveolar IFNγ mRNA expression is unclear. Although IFNγ may seem a potential antagonist of Th2 cytokines,[122] including the functional antagonism of IL-4 in the promotion of IgE synthesis, IFNγ was unable to induce a clinical response or suppress IgE concentrations in allergic rhinitis.[172] IFNγ is therefore a powerful macrophage activator; however, its precise role in regulating airway inflammatory responses is unknown. Possibly, its significance may rest with modulation of fibroblast function and collagen production.

## J. TUMOUR NECROSIS FACTOR

The descriptions TNFα and TNFβ describe two structurally unrelated protein products of separate genes located close together on chromosome 6.[173-175] TNFα is produced predominantly by macrophages and was originally described in the serum of mycobacterium-primed, endotoxin-treated mice, which had the ability to induce haemorrhagic necrosis in experimental skin tumours after intravenous or intralesion injection.[176] Also called *cachectin*, human TNFα was identified and cloned in 1986.[177] TNFβ, which has cytotoxic activity, is produced predominantly by lymphocytes.[178]

TNFα is produced at low levels under physiological conditions; however, it may act together with IL-1 in infection-induced hypotension and shock.[179] Experimental models of septic shock have shown a rapid rise in TNF levels after the injection of either lipopolysaccharide endotoxin or Gram-negative bacteria.[180]

Conceptually, TNFα may be involved in airway inflammation through its ability to activate endothelial cells and induce cytokine production by other cell types. TNFα may enhance vascular permeability after either systemic administration[181] or, interestingly, intratracheal administration.[182] It is highly likely that the peripheral neutropenia and lymphopenia seen after the injection of TNFα are due to the upgraded expression of endothelial–leukocyte adhesion molecules.[183] TNF has a broad range of functions that are consistent with inflammation seen in the airway wall in asthma. These include the induction of microvascular permeability, cytotoxic effect of mast cells after anti-IgE-induced degranulation, and eosinophil cytotoxicity.[184-186] Through the enhanced expression of leukocyte–endothelial cell adhesion molecules, including E-selectin, VCAM-1, and ICAM-1, the infiltration of cells into the bronchial wall may be facilitated.[187-189] In models of bronchial reactivity, TNFα has been shown to increase bronchial responsiveness in rats and sheep.[190,191]

TNFα has been shown to be produced by monocytes/macrophages, T cells, and mast cells.[143,178,192] Recent work has shown TNFα mRNA and product to be produced by human eosinophils.[194] Holgate and co-workers[31] have used immunostaining techniques to identify TNFα in bronchial biopsies from asthmatic and control subjects. This study found TNFα to be localised almost entirely to mast cells, where a sevenfold increase in the expression of TNFα was seen in the asthmatic biopsies. Bronchial lavage studies have also indicated increased levels of TNFα in asthma.[83]

TNFα is capable of inducing tissue remodelling, including angiogenesis and fibrogenesis. In models of angiogenesis it is at least as potent as fibroblast growth factor, epidermal growth factor, TGFα, or angiogenin, both *in vitro* and *in vivo*.[195] TNFα may directly stimulate fibroblasts[196] and indirectly stimulate fibrogenesis through the elaboration of PDGF and TGFβ.[179]

Although TNFα has a wide range of functions, including its supported roles as a proinflammatory cytokine in asthma and as an agent capable of mediating bronchial wall remodelling, there is some evidence that its action may be biphasically dose dependent.[197,198] It would seem that TNFα acts to influence the local microenvironment at low levels, given that little systemic evidence of activity is identified in clinical asthma.

## V. CELLULAR ELEMENTS

### A. T-LYMPHOCYTES

The determination of T cell phenotype is dependent upon the migration of T-lymphocyte precursors to the thymus, where microenvironmental influences induce expression of cells positive for both CD4 and CD8 antigens. Through the influence of supporting epithelial cells expressing MHC antigens, mature T cells emerge from the thymus capable of recognising self-MHC molecules and expressing the T cell receptor.[211,212] Mature, differentiated T-lymphocytes expressing CD4 or CD8 antigens then migrate to specific organs (such as the spleen, lymph nodes, and tonsils). Although evidence for specific "bronchus associated lymphoid tissue" aggregates is lacking, post-mortem studies have shown increased numbers of lymphocytes in the airway in fatal asthma,[30,33] while "atypical intra-epithelial lymphocytes" have been described in mild asthma.[213] Populations of lymphocytes within asthmatic airways seem to show normal CD4 and CD8 numbers in both BAL[7] and in bronchial mucosa.[29] A study by Fukuda et al.,[214] aimed at identifying the significance of lymphocyte subpopulations in the bronchial mucosa of patients with symptomatic asthma found that CD3+/CD4+/CD25+ cells and natural killer cells were represented in higher numbers in symptomatic asthmatic subjects, compared with asymptomatic asthmatic and control subjects. This situation is different in asthmatic subjects challenged with allergen, where CD4 lymphocytes fall in the peripheral blood initially[6] and are found to be increased in BAL.[215] Subjects that were found to exhibit an early asthmatic response to antigen, without a persisting late response, seem to be protected by the migration of CD8+ lymphocytes into the bronchial lumen.[215]

Lymphocytes may be further characterised according to their activation status. Early in activation, CD4+ lymphocytes express mRNA for specific cytokines and upregulate surface markers including HLA-DR, CD25 (IL-2R), and very late activation-1 (VLA-1).[7,80,216] Although HLA-DR and CD25 may be expressed on B-lymphocytes, macrophages, and eosinophils, as well as T-lymphocytes, double-labelling techniques have enabled the enumeration of activated cells of a specific type in both bronchial biopsies[29] and bronchial lavage.[7] Peripheral blood T-lymphocyte activation has been seen in asthmatic subjects challenged with allergen[6] in acute severe asthma[216] and in mild atopic asthma.[7,51] Walker and colleagues[217] have identified an association between T-lymphocyte activation and eosinophilia in bronchial lavage with asthma severity, suggesting that lymphocyte deactivation might be associated with clinical improvement.

Much information is now available regarding the ability of T-lymphocytes within the airway to produce immunoregulatory cytokines.[1,56,218] Probably, CD4+ lymphocytes producing cytokines do so with defined patterns of elaboration (see Section III.B). The antigen-recognising T cell receptor may be specifically involved in acquisition of airway reactivity. Transfer of Vβ T-lymphocytes in a mouse model of airway hyperreactivity led to the development of IgE production, cutaneous sensitivity, and isolated tracheal hyperreactivity.[307-309]

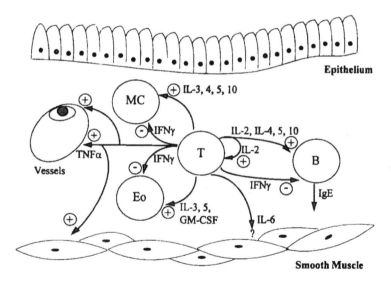

T-lymphocytes. Th1 produces IL-2, IL-3, GM-CSF, IFNγ, TNFα, and TNFβ; Th2 produces IL-3, IL-4, IL-5, IL-6, IL-10, IL-13, and GM-CSF.

Treatment with inhaled corticosteroids leads to reduced numbers and deactivation of bronchial lavage lymphocytes[24] in association with a reduction in airway eosinophil infiltration and mast cell activation.[219,220] Depletion rather than inactivation of CD4+ lymphocytes may be achieved in animal models by treatment with anti-CD4 antibodies. Gavett et al.[221] found that administration of anti-CD4 to mice sensitised with sheep red blood cells before challenge resulted in a reduction in airway hyperreactivity and pulmonary eosinophilia in a dependent manner. As well as producing inflammatory cytokines,

B-lymphocytes are capable of producing growth factors that support airway fibrosis. Either directly or indirectly, these factors may support fibroblast proliferation and collagen production.[222]

Activated lymphocytes have clearly been identified in the peripheral blood, bronchial lavage, and bronchial mucosa of asthmatics. Lymphocyte deactivation can be satisfactorily achieved with either inhaled or oral corticosteroids, which have been shown to result in loss of typical inflammatory changes in the airway and associated improvement in asthma symptoms, lung function, and airway reactivity. These cells are capable of producing inflammatory cytokines and play a central role in the inflammatory response characteristic of asthma.

## B. MAST CELLS

Mast cells are of myeloid origin and contain characteristic electron-dense granules which may release inflammatory mediators at sites of allergic inflammation.[2,223,224] Mast cells have been described in bronchial lavage in asthma.[22,225-231] Early biopsy and post-mortem studies reported a decrease in active disease.[232,233] They have been described in bronchial biopsies in asthma and, although not necessarily increased in number, are in an activated state.[2,19] Following activation, mast cells may degranulate upon exposure to immunologic (IgE, cross-linking anti-IgE) or nonimmunologic stimuli (C5a, cyclic AMP, hyperosmolar conditions). Under these conditions, which may be enhanced by cytokines[58] such as IL-3, IL-5, IL-8, GM-CSF, or SCE, mast cells release both preformed mediators (histamine, tryptase, chymase, bradykinin) and newly formed mediators (prostaglandins, sulphidopeptide leukotrienes, and PAF). Mast cells also express the c-*kit* proto-oncogene (a member of the tyrosine kinase receptor class) which binds SCF. This immunologically discernible receptor both induces mediator release from mast cells upon activation and enhances IgE-dependent mediator release.[62,234] After IgE receptor crosslinking, IL-1, TNF$\alpha$, and IL-8 are produced relatively early, while the production of IL-3, IL-4, IL-5, and GM-CSF is somewhat delayed.[64]

Subtypes of mast cells exist, based on their enzyme content. All human mast cells contain tryptase although only some contain chymase ($M_{TC}$). Those without chymase have tryptase alone ($M_T$).[235-238] Chymase-containing mast cells are normally less than 7% of the total; however, that may be as high as 87% in patients with cystic fibrosis.[239] Mast cells containing tryptase may be found in the lamina propria, particularly in association with mucosal glands.

Normally representing less than 1% of cells in bronchial lavage fluid, mast cells may occupy up to 2% of cells in lavage fluid from patients with asthma.[19,22] In the bronchial mucosa, mast cells are usually less prevalent than eosinophils, lymphocytes, or macrophages, generally comprising less than 5% of nucleated cells in sections from asthmatic airways.

Holgate and co-workers[31] have identified IL-4, IL-5, IL-6, and TNF$\alpha$ in mucosal biopsies from asthmatic subjects, predominantly within mast cells,

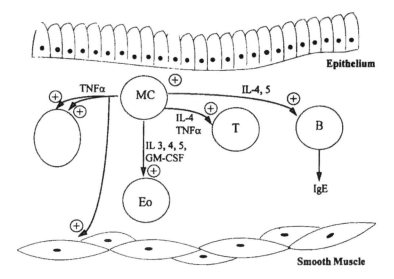

Mast cells produce IL-1, IL-3, IL-4, IL-5, IL-6, IL-7, IL-8, IL-9, IL-10, IL-13, GM-CSF, TNFα, and TGFβ.

rather than T-lymphocytes. They hypothesise that mast cells have the capacity to store cytokines, which can remain detectable by immunolocalisation techniques, thus differing from those produced by T-lymphocytes, which do not. Extensive use of *in situ* hybridisation techniques by Kay and co-workers[53,56,66] has indicated that the T-lymphocyte is the predominant cell expressing mRNA for Th2 cytokines. To accommodate these two positions, it may be possible that activated lymphocytes produced Th2 cytokines during a limited response which may take hours to generate[80] until modulated by the rising concentrations of IFNγ. Mast cells, with the ability to store preformed mediators, and apparently cytokines, might therefore account for more instantaneous cytokine release in response to antigen. Further studies of the human response to antigen incorporating both immunolocalisation and *in situ* hybridisation techniques will be required to resolve this issue.

## C. EOSINOPHILS

Derived from myeloid progenitors in the bone marrow, mature eosinophils circulate briefly in the peripheral blood and home to sites of inflammation, particularly parasitic or allergic in nature. Eosinophils have been described in large numbers, infiltrating the walls of airways in fatal asthma,[33,240] as well as in mild asthma.[2,22,241] Eosinophilia described in peripheral blood and bronchial lavage has been related to airway hyperreactivity.[4,5,242,243] Eosinophil production and maturation have been shown to be regulated by GM-CSF, IL-3, and IL-5.[86,244-247] Eosinophils may be activated, resulting in a reduction in cell density, by the binding of surface FcεRII,[248,249] PAF,[250-252] GM-CSF,[253] and

IL-5.[128,246] Activated eosinophils release toxic proteins capable of causing airway tissue damage, including major basic protein (MBP), eosinophil-derived neurotoxin (EDN), eosinophil cationic protein (ECP), and eosinophil peroxidase.[241,247] In the activated state, eosinophils increase expression of surface VLA-4, Mac-1, as well as CD69, HLA-DR, and ICAM-1, but lose L-selectin. As well, eosinophils are capable of generating phospholipid mediators including leukotriene $C_4$ (LTC$_4$), PAF,[311] and superoxide. Until relatively recently, eosinophils were considered to be effector cells in asthma, without the capacity to generate cytokines.[241] Evidence now exists to show that eosinophils produce a range of cytokines, including IL-3,[91] IL-5,[135] IL-6,[153] IL-8,[312] TGFβ, and GM-CSF.[96] Eosinophil infiltration of tissues, therefore, seems to provide both the means for acute tissue injury through the release of granule contents and the regulation of inflammation through the elaboration of cytokines. Specifically, autoregulation may occur through the production of IL-3, IL-5, and GM-CSF.

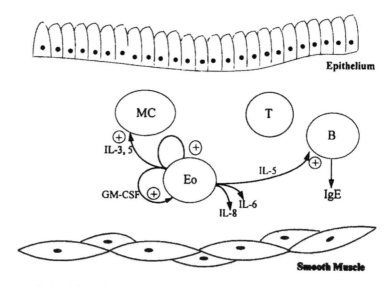

Eosinophils produce IL-1, IL-2, IL-3, IL-5, IL-6, IL-8, GM-CSF, and TGFβ.

Fundamental to understanding the role of the eosinophil in asthma is its relationship to bronchial hyperresponsiveness. Airway hyperreactivity has been found to correlate with peripheral eosinophil counts,[4] BAL eosinophilia,[5] and bronchial mucosal eosinophil count.[313] The role of the eosinophil in the induction of hyperresponsiveness has been clearly described in recent studies, where the induction of airway hyperresponsiveness in sensitised rhesus monkeys was blocked by the administration of an antibody to ICAM-1, which markedly inhibited eosinophil accumulation in the airways.[164] Using a mouse model of airway reactivity arising from sensitisation to sheep red blood cells, Gavett and co-workers[221] used a monoclonal antibody to deplete CD4+ T-lymphocytes, thus abrogating both airway eosinophilia and hyperreactivity seen after antigen exposure. More-direct studies of the role of IL-5 have shown that the administration of IL-5 *in vivo* may induce hyperresponsiveness in mice[314] and that treatment of mice with antibodies to IL-5 will inhibit antigen-induced eosinophil infiltration of the trachea.[315] In human studies of allergen response in the airways, eosinophils were increased in BAL fluid after 24 h, while T cell activation and numbers of cells expressing mRNA for IL-5 were also increased.[66] In peripheral blood there is a transient eosinopenia at 6 h,[316] followed by an eosinophilia up to 24 h after challenge.[254] Interestingly, this eosinophilia only occurs in those patients with asthma who develop a late asthmatic response and correlates with basal airway hyperresponsiveness.[254] Airway eosinophils are profoundly sensitive to treatment with corticosteroids, and their disappearance is associated with an improvement in airway hyper-responsiveness.[24,220] Although compelling, the link between eosinophilia and bronchial hyperreactivity is not absolute, as cyclosporin A may inhibit antigen-induced eosinophil and lymphocyte influx into the airway without significantly altering bronchial hyperreactivity.[255] Much evidence implicating the eosinophil in airway hyperreactivity has led to speculation regarding the importance of the cytokine IL-5. Although IL-5 has provided a logistic explanation for the presence of eosinophilia and eosinophil activation in airway inflammation, the mechanism by which eosinophils might affect bronchial hyperresponsiveness remains elusive.

## D. MACROPHAGES

Macrophages are phagocytic cells, derived from bone marrow precursors, that circulate as monocytes in peripheral blood, then migrate into tissues, where they undergo relatively specific differentiation in response to local environmental factors.[256] Recent interest in the role of the macrophage in asthma has arisen because of the recognition of the "activated macrophage," the ability of macrophages to be stimulated by the low-affinity IgE receptor (FcεRII), and the ability of macrophages to release a wide range of inflammatory cytokines.

Macrophages taken from animals that have developed resistance to intracellular parasites showed increased ability to kill coincubating organisms.[257,258] Activated macrophages were found to possess different functional and metabolic qualities.[259,260] Activation may occur through exposure to IFNγ,[260,261] GM-CSF,[261,262] or through the binding of allergen to surface FcεRII.[263-265] Once activated, macrophages are capable of producing an extraordinary range of over 100 secretory products.[260] Eicosanoids released by macrophages include prostaglandins $PGD_2$, $PGE_2$, and $PGF_{2\alpha}$ and thromboxans.[266,267] These prostaglandins have the ability to induce bronchoconstriction,[268] while $PGD_2$ and $PGF_{2\alpha}$ have been shown to increase mucous secretion from bronchial wall explants.[267,269] Also, macrophages produce the potent, long-acting broncho-constrictors $LTC_4$, $LTD_4$, and $LTE_4$.[270-272] Leukotrienes are detectable in bronchial lavage fluid from patients with asthma and from fragments of asthmatic lung challenged *in vitro*.[268] PAF is released in greater amounts from alveolar macrophages derived from asthmatic subjects and may be detected in bronchial lavage fluid in asthma.[273] PAF has a range of actions in human subjects consistent with a role in airway inflammation, including eosinophil chemoat-traction,[248,274] bronchoconstriction,[275] the induction of airway inflammation,[317] and prolonged airway hyperresponsiveness.[276] Of special interest is the ability of macrophages to release a specific, restricted range of mediators on exposure to allergen. This rather more selective response may help explain the specific tissue changes seen in atopic states, rather than an "all or none" release of mediators.

Macrophages produce and release IL-1, IL-10, GM-CSF, and TNFα. In addition, macrophages produce a range of molecules with the capacity to stimulate histamine release from basophils and mast cells via an interaction with surface IgE.[277] Histamine-releasing factors (HRF) are also released by lymphocytes and platelets.[278,279] Following antigen challenge in the upper airway, basophils and HRFs are increased.[280]

A number of differences have been described between normal and asthmatic peripheral blood monocytes. Monocytes from asthmatic subjects bear more FcεRII receptors, which may be suppressed by corticosteroids.[265,281] They also show enhanced complement receptor expression.[282]

## E. FIBROBLASTS

The process of healing following tissue injury is associated with sequential platelet-induced haemostasis associated with polymorph and fibroblast infiltration, the laying down of extracellular matrix, angiogenesis, and cellular regeneration within the tissue. There are a number of facets of fibroblast biology that have direct relevance to airway inflammation in asthma. Rather than considering fibroblasts to be associated with chronic inflammation and scar formation alone, it is clear that fibroblasts are associated with the acute response to injury and exhibit a widely heterogeneous phenotype.

The acute response has been relatively well characterised. Gauldie et al. proposed a "cascade," whereby quiescent fibroblasts may be stimulated by IL-1 or TNFα (released by monocytes) to produce copious amounts of inflammatory cytokines, including IFNβ-1, IL-6, IL-8, GM-CSF, M-CSF, and monocyte chemotactic factors.[150,283-286] Possibly, such stimulation results in a permanent phenotypic change in the inflamed airway, resulting in persistent cytokine production.[287]

Myofibroblasts within the airway wall have been described as cells staining with an antibody capable of identifying colonic pericrypt sheath cells,[288] but not containing α-smooth muscle actin.[289] Cells identified as α-actin negative, to distinguish them from PR2D3-positive cells within the media of bronchial vessels, were found to be increased in number in association with thickening of sub-basement membrane collagen.[289] A range of factors have been identified as potential stimulants for myofibroblast growth, including mast cell histamine, heparin, and cytokines,[90,119,290,291] eosinophil-derived fibroblast stimulants,[292] lymphocyte-derived factors, macrophage-derived factors,[293] and, possibly, endothelin.[294]

Although fibroblasts are capable of tissue migration, their location within the airway during chronic stable asthma may well dictate their functional capacity. Although easily identified beneath the true basement membrane by electronmicroscopy,[289] similar cells are found deeper within the submucosa (Figure 4). Staining of bronchial biopsies from patients with asthma with PR2D3 shows positive cells within bronchial and vascular smooth muscle, as well as a concentration below the bronchial epithelium. As much as 50% of cells express α-smooth muscle actin, indicating a proportion of myofibroblasts to be heterogeneous in phenotype with the ability to express this protein.[289,295] The distribution of myofibroblasts deeper in the submucosa is reduced when compared with the subepithelial region (Figure 5).

Of interest is the difference in the distribution of collagen within the airway in asthma compared with controls. The determinants of fibroblast function dictate the production of scar-type collagen in response to tissue injury (types III, V) are at present unknown; however, as the number of myofibroblasts present in the submucosa correlates directly with subepithelial collagen deposition,[289] it is likely that fibroblast activity under the influence of profibrogenic cytokines will also prove to be of great importance.[168]

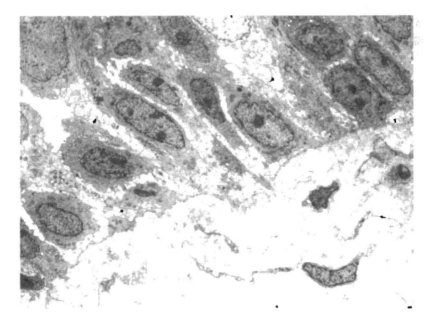

**FIGURE 4** Electronmicrograph of subepithelial collagen and myofibroblast (lower right corner).

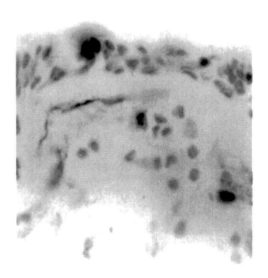

**FIGURE 5**   Immunoperoxidase staining of subepithelial myofibroblast.

## F.  BRONCHIAL EPITHELIUM

The concept of airway inflammation supported by cytokine production following injury rests upon an ongoing stimulus for the inflammatory response. The bronchial epithelium represents the most obvious site for injury in the asthmatic airway. Reported epithelial changes include (1) typical desquamated cells in asthmatic sputum (Creola bodies), (2) epithelial sloughing in autopsy specimens[30] and bronchial lavage specimens,[22] (3) damage and sloughing in bronchial biopsies,[26] (4) goblet cell metaplasia,[25] as well as (5) mast cell and eosinophil infiltration.[19] The finding of increased scar-type collagen tissue deposited beneath the epithelial basement membrane suggests a local stimulus for injury, possibly arising from epithelium.[27] Furthermore, numbers of epithelial cells retrieved by bronchial lavage have been used as an index of epithelial injury and correlated with airway responsiveness.[2,22] Barnes[1] has described a number of the mechanisms by which injury to the epithelial barrier may lead to tissue structural changes characteristic of asthma. These include the loss of a protective barrier preventing exposure to irritants and allergens; reduced production of nitric oxide which may act directly on smooth muscle limiting relaxation; loss of epithelial enzymes capable of degrading inflammatory mediators such as tachykinins, bradykinin, and endothelin; increased exposure of sensory nerve endings to airway stimuli, thereby provoking inflammation by an axon reflex;[296] and increased release of epithelial-derived inflammatory mediators, such as chemotactic 15-lipoxygenase products, bronchodilating $PGE_2$, and bronchoconstricting endothelin. The epithelium is also capable of producing a range of cytokines and growth factors including IL-6, IL-8, GM-CSF, TNFα, PDGF, and insulin-like growth factor (IGF-1).[218] Stimulation of human cultured bronchial epithelial cells has shown the capacity to produce: GM-CSF when stimulated by IL-1,[98,297] IL-6, and IL-8; GM-CSF when stimulated by IL-1β and TNFα;[202] TNFα and IL-8 which may be suppressed by glucocorticoid exposure;[298] and, interestingly, GM-CSF, TNFα, and IL-8 after exposure to the air pollutant nitrogen dioxide.[299] IL-6, IL-8, and GM-CSF have been detected in bronchial epithelial cells from patients with asthma. Both IL-1 and TNFα may influence cellular traffic by increasing expression of adhesion molecules (ICAM-1) on epithelial cells.[300] Furthermore, ample evidence exists for the accumulation of mast cells and eosinophils in the epithelium in asthma.[19]

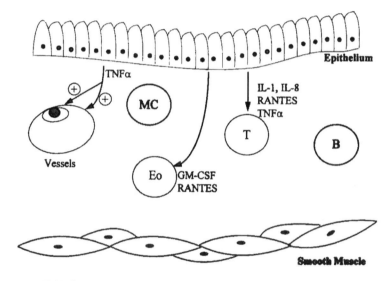

Epithelial cells produce IL-1, IL-6, IL-8, GM-CSF, TNFα, and RANTES.

It would seem that the airway epithelium is clearly capable of exhibiting its own response to injury, initiated by asthmogenic factors such as viruses, allergens, and pollutants. This response may promote chemotaxis and cell adherence, as well as releasing cytokines capable of stimulating inflammatory mediator release from infiltrating cells. Such a response would seem to be proinflammatory and destructive to the airway epithelium. The action of corticosteroids in asthma may well include a capacity to suppress this autostimulatory feedback loop.

## VI. FUTURE TRENDS

The recent expansion in knowledge of the immune response has had a significant impact on our interpretation of the characteristic injury seen in the airway in asthma. We now understand that cytokines orchestrate the cellular events associated with tissue injury and airway remodelling, fundamental to the physiological finding of reversible airflow obstruction. Given the new tools of molecular biology, immunolocalisation and bronchial biopsy, what are the important, answerable questions ahead of us?

Which cell makes which cytokine? This is a fundamental issue in the same way that "which cell causes asthma?" was a decade ago. The specific origins of certain cytokines and their regulating factors will identify the targets for future asthma treatments. Currently, we are using broad-based anti-inflammatory therapy, with low specificity and limited efficacy in severe disease. It is likely that most cell types will be capable of producing most cytokines; however, which cells act most influentially will become clearer when double-labelling techniques are better developed and subset analysis of cells becomes more easily performed in tissues.

Which cytokines are important in asthma? Current evidence is providing a simple picture of the relative importance of specific cytokines. Any early interpretation of importance must be tempered by the factors that make specific cytokines detectable. Easily localised factors are more commonly studied, better described, and seem to readily become central to current dogma. Theoretical interpretations are based on cytokine actions *in vitro* and in animal models. Caution should therefore be applied when formulating roles for factors within the human airway. Cytokine and cytokine receptor antagonists are currently available, and their place in asthma therapy awaits elucidation. What lessons have we learnt from molecular biology in asthma? From suggesting a genetic linkage to atopy, to describing the regulation of cytokines by drugs, molecular biologic techniques have proved to be very powerful when directed to specific issues. The current limitation is in the ability to ask the right questions, hopefully avoiding the pitfalls of overinterpretation.

How do cytokines cause specific changes in the airway wall recognised as remodelling? This probably occurs via two mutually dependent events. Cells releasing inflammatory mediators are responsible for tissue injury, which then stimulates the process of repair, probably dependent on the action of specific growth factors. Some inflammatory cytokines themselves may act directly to take part in this process. The result, a combination of smooth muscle hyperplasia/hypertrophy, cellular influx, vascular expansion, and scar-tissue formation, may be better reversed with the use of appropriate anti-inflammatory therapy.

How do the resultant cellular events in asthma translate to physiological airflow obstruction? Currently, few studies are capable of examining more than simple correlations between lung function and airway reactivity and the complex indices of airway inflammation. We have been limited to unifactorial analysis of cellular and cytokine function in asthma, while we are nonetheless aware that multiple cell types and cytokines are involved in airway inflammation. Multifactorial analysis with modelling capable of predicting treatment responses is logically a most desirable option.

# ACKNOWLEDGMENTS

The authors wish to acknowledge the assistance of Ms. Barbara Welton with the preparation of the manuscript.

# REFERENCES

1. Barnes, P. J., Inflammation, in *Bronchial Asthma: Mechanisms and Therapeutics*, Weiss, E. B. and Stein, M., Eds., 3rd ed., Little, Brown, Boston, 1993, 80.
2. Djukanovic, R., Roche, W. R., Wilson, J. W., Beasley, C. R., Twentyman, O., and Holgate, S. T., The role of mucosal inflammation in asthma. State of the art review, *Am. Rev. Respir. Dis.*, 142, 434, 1990.
3. U.S. Department of Health, National Institutes of Health, National Asthma Education Program, Expert Panel Report: *Guidelines for the Diagnosis and Management of Asthma*, Bethesda, Publication No. 91-3042, 1991.
4. Taylor, K. J. and Luksza, A. R., Peripheral blood eosinophil counts and bronchial responsiveness, *Thorax*, 42, 452, 1987.
5. Wardlaw, A. J., Dunnette, S., Gleich, G. J., Collins, J. V., and Day, A. B., Eosinophils and mast cells in bronchoalveolar lavage in subjects with mild asthma. Relationship to bronchial hyperreactivity, *Am. Rev. Respir. Dis.*, 137, 62, 1988.
6. Gerblich, A. A., Campbell, A. E., and Schugler, M. R., Changes in T-lymphocyte subpopulations after antigenic bronchial provocation in asthmatics, *N. Engl. J. Med.*, 310, 1349, 1984.
7. Wilson, J. W., Djukanovic, R., Howarth, P. H., and Holgate, S. T., Lymphocyte activation in bronchoalveolar lavage and peripheral blood in atopic asthma, *Am. Rev. Respir. Dis.*, 145, 958, 1992.
8. Corrigan, C. J. and Kay, A. B., CD4 T-lymphocyte activation in acute severe asthma. Relationship to disease severity and atopic status, *Am. Rev. Respir. Dis.*, 141, 970, 1990.
9. Burrows, B., Martinez, F. D., Halonen, M., Barbere, R. A., and Clin, M. G., Association of asthma with serum IgE levels and skin-test reactivity to allergens, *N. Engl. J. Med.*, 320, 271, 1989.
10. Brown, P. H., Crompton, G. K., and Greening, A. P., Proinflammatory cytokines in acute asthma, *Lancet*, 338, 590, 1991.
11. Corrigan, c. J., Haczku, A., Gemou-Engesaeth, V., Doi, S., Kikuchi, Y., Takatsu, K., Durham, S. R., and Kay, A. B., CD4 T-lymphocyte activation in asthma is accompanied by increased serum concentrations of interleukin-5: effect of glucocorticoid therapy, *Am. Rev. Respir. Dis.*, 147, 540, 1993.
12. Walters, E. H. and Gardiner, P. V., Bronchoalveolar lavage as a research tool, *Thorax*, 46, 613, 1991.
13. American Thoracic Society, Summary and recommendations of a workshop on the investigative use of fibreoptic bronchoscopy and bronchoalveolar lavage in asthmatics, *Am. Rev. Respir. Dis.*, 132, 180, 1985.
14. NIH Workshop Summary and Guidelines, Investigative use of bronchoscopy, lavage, and bronchial biopsies in asthma and other airways diseases, *Eur. Respir. J.*, 5, 115, 1992.
15. Kirby, J. G., Hargreave, F. E., Gleich, G. J., and O'Byrne, P. M., Bronchoalveolar cell profiles of asthmatic and nonasthmatic subjects, *Am. Rev. Respir. Dis.*, 136, 379, 1987.
16. Flint, K. C., Leung, K. B. P., Hudspith, B. N., Brostoff, J., Pearce, F. L., and Johnson, N. M., Bronchoalveolar mast cells in extrinsic asthma: a mechanism for the initiation of antigen specific bronchoconstriction, *Br. Med. J.*, 291, 923, 1985.

17. Casale, T. B., Wood, D., Richerson, H. B., Trapp, S., Metzger, W. J., Zavala, D., and Hunninghake, G. W., Elevated bronchoalveolar lavage fluid histamine levels in allergic asthmatics are associated with methacholine bronchial responsiveness, *J. Clin. Invest.*, 79, 1197, 1987.
18. Agius, R. M., Godfrey, R. C., and Holgate, S. T., Mast cell histamine content of human bronchoalveolar lavage, *Thorax*, 40, 760, 1985.
19. Djukanovic, R., Wilson, J. W., Britten, K. M., Wilson, S. J., Walls, A. F., Roche, W. R., Howarth, P. H., and Holgate, S. T., Quantitation of mast cells and eosinophils in the bronchial mucosa of symptomatic atopic asthmatics and healthy controls using immuno-histochemistry, *Am. Rev. Respir. Dis.*, 142, 863, 1990.
20. Lam, S., Chan, H., LeRiche, J. C., Chan-Yeung, M., and Salari, H., Release of leukotrienes in patients with bronchial asthma, *J. Allergy Clin. Immunol.*, 81, 711, 1988.
21. Godard, P., Bousquet, J., Lebel, B., and Michel, F. B., Bronchoalveolar lavage in the asthmatic, *Bull. Eur. Physiopathol. Respir.*, 23, 73, 1987.
22. Beasley, R., Roche, W. R., Roberts, J. A., and Holgate, S. T., Cellular events in the bronchi in mild asthma and after bronchial provocation, *Am. Rev. Respir. Dis.*, 139, 806, 1989.
23. Djukanovic, R., Wilson, J. W., Lai, C. K. W., Holgate, S. T., and Howarth, P. H., The safety aspects of fiberoptic bronchoscopy, bronchoalveolar lavage and endobronchial biopsy in asthma, *Am. Rev. Respir. Dis.*, 143, 772, 1991.
24. Wilson, J. W., Djukanovic, R., Howarth, P. H., and Holgate, S. T., Inhaled beclomethasone dipropionate downregulates airway lymphocyte activation in atopic asthma, *J. Respir. Crit. Care Med.*, 149, 86, 1994.
25. Glynn, A. A. and Michaels, L., Bronchial biopsy in chronic bronchitis and asthma, *Thorax*, 15, 142, 1960.
26. Laitinen, L. A., Heino, M., Laitinen, A., Kava, T., and Haahtela, T., Damage of the airway epithelium and bronchial reactivity in patients with asthma, *Am. Rev. Respir. Dis.*, 131, 599, 1985.
27. Roche, W. R., Beasley, R., Williams, J. H., and Holgate, S. T., Subepithelial fibrosis in the bronchi of asthmatics, *Lancet*, 1, 520, 1989.
28. Djukanovic, R., Lai, C. K., Wilson, J. W., Britten, K. M., Wilson, S. J., Roche, W. R., Howarth, P. H., and Holgate, S. T., Bronchial mucosal manifestations of atopy: a comparison of markers of inflammation between atopic asthmatics, atopic nonasthmatics and healthy controls, *Eur. Respir. J.*, 5, 538, 1992.
29. Azzawi, M., Bradley, B., Jeffery, P. K., Frew, A. J., Wardlaw, A. J., Knowles, G., Assonti, B., Collins, J. V., Durkam, S., and Kay, A. B., Identification of activated T lymphocytes and eosinophils in bronchial biopsies in stable atopic asthma, *Am. Rev. Respir. Dis.*, 142, 1407, 1990.
30. Dunnill, M. S., The pathology of asthma with special reference to changes in the bronchial mucosa, *J. Clin. Pathol.*, 13, 27, 1960.
31. Bradding, P., Roberts, J. A., Britten, K. A., Montefort, S., Djukanovic, R., Mueller, R., Huesser, C. H., Howarth, P. H., and Holgate, S. T., Interleukin-4, -5, and -6 and tumor necrosis factor-$\alpha$ in normal and asthmatic airways: evidence of the human mast cell as a source of these cytokines, *Am. J. Resp. Cell Mol. Biol.*, 10, 471, 1994.
32. Hamid, Q., Azzawi, M., Ying, S., Moqbel, R., Wardlaw, A. J., Corrigan, C. J., Braddley, B., Durham, S. R., Collins, J. V., Jeffery, P. K., Quint, D. J., and Kay, A. B., Expression of mRNA for interleukin-5 in mucosal bronchial biopsies from asthma, *J. Clin. Invest.*, 87, 1541, 1991.
33. Dunnill, M. S., Massarella, G. R., and Anderson, J. A., A comparison of the quantitative anatomy of the bronchi in normal subjects, in status asthmaticus, in chronic bronchitis and in emphysema, *Thorax*, 24, 176, 1969.
34. Kountz, W. B. and Alexander, H. L., Death from bronchial asthma, *Arch. Pathol.*, 5, 1003, 1928.
35. Cutz, E., Levison, H., and Cooper, D. M., Ultrastructure of airways in children with asthma, *Histopathology*, 2, 407, 1978.

36. Saetta, M., Di Stefano, A., Rosina, C., Thiene, G., and Fabbri, L. M., Quantitative structural analysis of peripheral airways and arteries in sudden fatal asthma, *Am. Rev. Respir. Dis.*, 143, 138, 1991.

37. Bai, T. R., Abnormalities in airway smooth muscle in fatal asthma, *Am. Rev. Respir. Dis.*, 141, 552, 1990.

38. Hirschman, C. A. and Downes, H., Experimental asthma in animals, in *Bronchial Asthma: Mechanisms and Therapeutics*, Weiss, E. B. and Stein, M., Eds., 3rd ed., Little, Brown, Boston, 1993, 80.

39. Mosmann, T. R., Cherwinski, H., Bond, M. W., Giedlin, M. A., and Coffman, R. L., Two types of murine helper T cell clone. I. Definition according to profiles of lymphokine activities and secreted proteins, *J. Immunol.*, 136, 2348, 1986.

40. Mosmann, T. R. and Coffman, R. L., Th1 and Th2 cells: different patterns of lymphokine secretion lead to different functional properties, *Annu. Rev. Immunol.*, 7, 145, 1989.

41. Street, N. E. and Mosmann, T. R., Functional diversity of T lymphocytes due to secretion of different cytokine patterns, *FASEB J.*, 5, 171, 1991.

42. Douglas, J. S., Dennis, M. W., Ridgway, P., et al., Airway dilatation and constriction in spontaneous breathing guinea pigs, *J. Pharmacol. Exp. Ther.*, 180, 98, 1972.

43. Hutson, P. A., Holgate, S. T., and Church, M. K., The effect of cromolyn sodium and albuterol on early and late phase bronchoconstriction and airway leucocyte infiltration after allergen challenge of nonanesthetised guinea pigs, *Am. Rev. Respir. Dis.*, 138, 1157, 1988.

44. Holroyde, M. C., Smith, S. Y., and Holme, G., Analysis of antigen-induced changes in pulmonary mechanics in sensitized inbred rats, *Can. J. Physiol. Pharmacol.*, 60, 644, 1982.

45. Piechuta, H., Smith, M. E., Share, N. N., and Holme, G., The respiratory response of sensitized rats to challenge with antigen aerosols, *Immunology*, 38, 385, 1979.

46. Holgate, S. T. and Finnerty, J. P., Recent advances in understanding the pathogenesis of asthma and its clinical applications, *Q. J. Med.*, 66, 5, 1988.

47. Frew, A. J. and Kay, A. B., The relationship between infiltrating CD4+ lymphocytes, activated eosinophils and the magnitude of the allergen-induced late-phase cutaneous reaction in man, *J. Immunol.*, 141, 4158, 1988.

48. Frew, A. J. and Kay, A. B., Eosinophils and T-lymphocytes in late-phase allergic reactions, *J. Allergy Clin. Immunol.*, 85, 533, 1990.

49. Postma, D. S., Bleecker, E. R., Amelung, P. J., Holroyd, K. J., Xu, J., Panhuysen, C. I. M., Meyers, D. A., and Levitt, R. C., Genetic susceptibility to asthma — bronchial hyperresponsiveness coinherited with a major gene for atopy, *N. Engl. J. Med.*, 333, 894, 1995.

50. Motojima, S., Akutsu, I., Fukuda, T., Makino, S., and Takutsa, K., Clinical significance of measuring levels of sputum and serum ECP and serum IL-5 in bronchial asthma, *Allergy*, 48, 98, 1993.

51. Walker, C., Bode, E., Boer, L., Hansel, T. T., Blaser, K., and Virchow, J.-C., Jr., Allergic and nonallergic asthmatics have distinct patterns of T-cell activation and cytokine production in peripheral blood and bronchoalveolar lavage, *Am. Rev. Respir. Dis.*, 146, 109, 1992.

52. Broide, D. H. and Firestein, G. S., Endobronchial allergen challenge in asthma: demonstration of cellular source of granulocyte macrophage colony-stimulating factor by *in situ* hybridisation, *J. Clin. Invest.*, 88, 1048, 1991.

53. Robinson, D. S., Hamid, Q., Ying, S., Tsicopoulos, A., Barkans, J., Bentley, A. M., Corrigan, C., Durham, S. R., and Kay, A. B., Predominant Th2-like bronchoalveolar T lymphocyte population in atopic asthma, *N. Engl. J. Med.*, 326, 298, 1992.

54. Ying, S., Robinson, D. S., Varney, V., Meng, Q., Tsicopoulos, A., Moqbel, R., Durham, S. R., Kay, A. B., and Hamid, Q., TNFα mRNA expression in allergic inflammation, *Clin. Exp. Allergy*, 21, 745, 1991.

55. Robinson, D. S., Ying, S., Bentley, A. M., Meng, Q., North, J., Durham, S. R., Kay, A. B., and Hamid, Q., Relationships among numbers of bronchoalveolar lavage cells expressing mRNA for cytokines, asthma symptoms, and airway methacholine responsiveness in atopic asthma, *J. Allergy Clin. Immunol.*, 92, 397, 1993.

56. Robinson, D. S., Durham, S. R., and Kay, A. B., Cytokines in asthma, *Thorax*, 48, 845, 1993.
57. Paliard, X., de Waal Malefijt, R., Yssel, H., Blanchard, D., Chretien, I., Abrams, J., de Vries, J., and Spits, H., Simultaneous production of IL-2, IL-4 and IFN-c by activated human CD4+ and CD8+ T cell clones, *J. Immunol.*, 141, 849, 1988.
58. Nicod, L. P., Cytokines 1 — overview, *Thorax*, 48, 660, 1993.
59. Zanders, E. D., IgE, in *Encyclopedia of Immunology*, Vol. 1, Roitt, J. M., Ed., Academic Press, London, 1992, 737.
60. Thompson-Snipes, L. A., Dhar, V., Bond, M. W., Mosmann, T. R., Moore, K. W., and Rennick, D. M., Interleukin 10: a novel stimulatory factor for mast cells and their progenitors, *J. Exp. Med.*, 173, 507, 1991.
61. Quesniaux, V. F. J., Interleukins 9, 10 and 12 and kit ligand: a brief overview, *Res. Immunol.*, 143, 385, 1992.
62. Siraganian, R. P., Mast cells, in *Encyclopedia of Immunology*, Vol. 2, Roitt, J. M., Ed., Academic Press, London, 1992, 1035.
63. Columbo, M., Horowitz, E. M., Botana, L. M., MacGlashan, D. W., Bochner, B. S., Gillis, S., Zsebo, K. M., Giollis, S. J., and Lichtenstien, L. M., The rat c-kit receptor ligand, rhSCF, induces mediator release from human cutaneous mast cells and enhances IgE-dependent mediator release from both skin mast cells and peripheral blood basophils, *J. Immunol.*, 149, 599, 1992.
64. Gordon, J. R., Burd, P. R., and Galli, S. J., Mast cells as a source of multifunctional cytokines, *Immunol. Today*, 11, 458, 1991.
65. Ackerman, V., Marini, M., Vittori, E., Bellini, A., Vassali, G., and Mattoli, S., Detection of cytokines and their cell sources in bronchial biopsy specimens from asthmatic patients, *Chest*, 105, 687, 1994.
66. Robinson, D. S., Hamid, Q., Bentley, A. M., Ying, S., Kay, A. B., and Durham, S. R., Activation of CD4+ T cells and increased Th2-type cytokine mRNA expression, and eosinophil recruitment in bronchoalveolar lavage fluid after allergen inhalation challenge in patients with atopic asthma, *J. Allergy Clin. Immunol.*, 92, 313, 1993.
67. Hamblin, A. S., Lymphokines, in *In Focus Series*, Male, D. and Rickwood, D., Eds., IRL Press, Oxford, 1988.
68. Dinarello, C. A. and Meir, J. W., Lymphokines, *N. Engl. J. Med.*, 317, 940, 1987.
69. Balkwill, F. R. and Burke, F., The cytokine network, *Immunol. Today*, 10, 299, 1989.
70. Powrie, F. and Coffman, R. L., Cytokine regulation of T-cell function: potential for therapeutic intervention, *Immunol. Today*, 14, 270, 1993.
71. Windle, J. J., Shin, H. S., and Morrow, J. F., Induction of interleukin-1 messenger RNA and induction in oocytes, *J. Immunol.*, 132, 1317, 1984.
72. Pepys, M. B. and Baltz, M., Acute phase proteins with special reference to c-reactive protein and related proteins (pentaxins) and serum amyloid A protein, *Adv. Immunol.*, 34, 141, 1983.
73. Gubler, U., Chua, A. O., Stern, A. S., Hellman, C. P., Vitek, M. P., DeChiara, T. M., Benjamin, W. R., Collier, K. G., Dukovich, M., Familletti, P. C., Fiedler-Nagy, C., Jensen, J., Kaffka, K., Kilian, P., Stremlo, D., Weittreich, B. H., Woehle, D., Mizel, S. B., and Lomedico, P. T., Recombinant human interleukin 1: Purification and biological characterization, *J. Immunol.*, 136, 2492, 1986.
74. Auron, P. E., Webb, A. C., Rosenwasser, L. J., Mucci, S. F., Rich, A., Wolff, S. M., and Dinarello, C. A., Nucleotide sequence of human monocyte interleukin 1 precursor cDNA, *Proc. Natl. Acad. Sci. U.S.A.*, 81, 7907, 1984.
75. Clark, B. D., Collins, K. L., Gandy, M. S., Webb, A. C., and Auron, P. E., Genomic sequence for human prointerleukin 1 beta: possible evolution from a reverse transcribed prointerleukin 1 alpha gene, *Nucleic Acids Res.*, 14, 7897, 1986.
76. Dower, S. K., Kronheim, S. R., Hopp, T. P., Cantrell, M., Deeley, M., Gillis, S., Henney, C. S., and Urdal, D. L., The cell surface receptors for interleukin-1 alpha and interleukin-1 beta are identical, *Nature*, 324, 266, 1986.

77. Wood, D. D., Bayne, E. K., Goldring, M. B., Gowen, M., Hamerman, D., Humes, J. L., Ihrie, E. J., Lipsky, P. E., and Staruch, M.-J., The four biochemically distinct species of interleukin-1 all exhibit similar biological activities, *J. Immunol.*, 134, 895, 1985.
78. Dinarello, C. and Savage, N., Interleukin-1 and its receptor, *Crit. Rev. Immunol.*, 9, 1, 1989.
79. Aksamit, T. R. and Hunninghake, G. W., Interleukin-1, in *Cytokines of the Lung*, Kelley, J., Ed., Marcel Dekker, New York, 1993, 185.
80. Danis, V. A., Kulesz, A. J., Nelson, D. S., and Brooks, P. M., Cytokine regulation of human monocyte interleukin-1 (IL-1) production in vitro. Enhancement of IL-1 production by interferon (IFN) gamma, tumour necrosis factor-alpha, IL-2 and IL-1, and inhibition by IFN-alpha, *Clin. Exp. Immunol.*, 80, 435, 1990.
81. Schmidt, J. A., Mizel, S. B., Cohen, D., and Green, I., Interleukin-1, a potential regulator of fibroblast proliferation, *J. Immunol.*, 128, 2177, 1982.
82. Cantrell, D. A. and Smith, K. A., Transient expression of IL-2 receptors. Consequences for T-cell growth, *J. Exp. Med.*, 158, 1895, 1983.
83. Broide, D. H., Lotz, D., Cuomo, A. J., Coburn, D. A., Federman, E. C., and Wasserman, S. I., Cytokines in symptomatic asthma airways, *J. Allergy Clin. Immunol.*, 89, 958, 1992.
84. Flanagan, W. M., Corthesy, B., Bram, R. J., and Crabtree, G. R., Nuclear association of T-cell transcription factor blocked by FK 506 and cyclosporin A, *Nature*, 352, 803, 1991.
85. Alexander, A. G., Barnes, N. C., and Kay, A. B., Trial of cyclosporin A in corticosteroid-dependent chronic severe asthma, *Lancet*, 329, 324, 1992.
86. Metcalf, D., Begley, C. G., Johnson, G. R., Nicola, N. A., Vadas, M. A., Lopez, A. F., Williamson, D. J., Wong, G. G., Clark, S. C., and Wang, E. A., Biologic properties in vitro of a recombinant human granulocyte-macrophage colony-stimulating factor, *Blood*, 67, 37, 1986.
87. Nicola, N. A. and Vadas, M., Hemopoietic colony-stimulating factors, *Immunol. Today*, 5, 76, 1984.
88. Yang, Y.-C., Ciarletta, A. B., Temple, P. A., Chung, M. P., Kovacic, S., Witek-Giann, J. S., Leary, A. C., Kriz, R., Donahue, R. E., Wong, G. G., and Clark, S. C., Human IL-3 (multi-CSF): identification by expression cloning of a novel hematopoietic growth factor related to murine IL-3, *Cell*, 47, 3, 1986.
89. Schrader, J. W., The panspecific hemopoietin of activated T lymphocytes (interleukin-3), *Annu. Rev. Immunol.*, 7, 377, 1986.
90. Wodnar-Filipowicz, A., Heusser, C. H., and Moroni, C., Production of the haemopoietic growth factors GM-CSF and interleukin-3 by mast cells in response to IgE receptor-mediated activation, *Nature*, 339, 150, 1989.
91. Kita, H., Ohnishi, T., Okubo, Y., Weiler, D., Abrams, J. S., and Gleich, G. J., Granulocyte/macrophage colony-stimulating factor and interleukin 3 release from human peripheral blood eosinophils and neutrophils, *J. Exp. Med.*, 174, 745, 1991.
92. Rothenberg, M. E., Owen, W. F., Jr., Silberstein, D. S., Woods, J., Soberman, R. J., Austen, K. F., and Stevens, R. L., Human eosinophils have prolonged survival, enhanced functional properties, and become hypodense when exposed to interleukin 3, *J. Clin. Invest.*, 81, 1986, 1988.
93. Clark, S. C. and Kamen, R., The human hemotopoietic colony-stimulating factors, *Science*, 236, 1229, 1987.
94. Yamato, K., El-Hajjaoui, Z., Kuo, J. F., and Koeffler, K. P., Granulocyte-macrophage colony stimulating factor: signals for its mRNA accumulation, *Blood*, 74, 1314, 1989.
95. Howell, c. J., Pujol, J.-L., Crea, A. E. G., Davidson, R., Gearing, A. J. H., Godard, P. H., and Lee, T. H., Identification of an alveolar macrophage-derived activity in bronchial asthma that enhances leukotriene C4 generation by human eosinophils stimulated by ionophore A23187 as a granulocyte-macrophage colony-stimulating factor, *Am. Rev. Respir. Dis.*, 140, 1340, 1989.
96. Moqbel, R., Hamid, Q., Ying, S., Barkans, J., Hartnell, A., Tsicopoulos, A., Wardlaw, A. J., and Kay, A. B., Expression of mRNA and immunoreactivity for the granulocyte/macrophage colony-stimulating factor in activated human eosinophils, *J. Exp. Med.*, 174, 749, 1991.

97. Cromwell, O., Hamid, Q., Corrigan, C. J., Barkans, J., Meng, Q., Collins, P. D., et al., Expression and generation of IL-6, IL-8, and GM-CSF by human bronchial epithelial cells and enhancement by IL-1β and TNFα, *Immunology,* 77, 330, 1992.

98. Marini, M., Soloperto, M., Mezzetti, M., Fasoli, A., and Mattoli, S., Interleukin 1 binds to specific receptors on human bronchial epithelial cells and upregulates granulocyte-macrophage colony-stimulating factor synthesis and release, *Am. J. Respir. Cell Mol. Biol.,* 4, 519, 1991.

99. Owen, W. F., Jr., Rothenberg, M. E., Silberstain, D. S., Gasson, J. C., Stevens, R. L., Austen, K. F., and Soberman, R. J., Regulation of human eosinophil viability, density, and function by granulocyte/macrophage colony-stimulating factor in the presence of 3T3 fibroblasts, *J. Exp. Med.,* 166, 129, 1987.

100. Kaushansky, K., Lin, N., and Adamson, J. W., Interleukin-1 stimulates fibroblasts to synthesize granulocyte-macrophage and granulocyte colony-stimulating factors, *J. Clin. Invest.,* 81, 92, 1988.

101. Silberstein, D. S., Eosinophils, in *Encyclopedia of Immunology,* Vol. 2, Roitt, J. M., Ed., Academic Press, London, 1992, 512.

102. Rubbia-Brandt, L., Sappino, A., and Gabbiani, G., Locally applied GM-CSF induces the accumulation of alpha smooth muscle actin containing fibroblasts, *Virchows Arch. (B),* 60, 73, 1991.

103. Sonoda, Y., Arai, N., and Ogawa, M., Humoral regulation of eosinophilopoiesis in vitro: analysis of the targets of interleukin 3, granulocyte/macrophage colony-stimulating factor (GM-CSF), and interleukin-5, *Leukemia,* 3, 14, 1989.

104. Fujisawa, T., Abu-Ghazaleh, R., Kita, H., Sanderson, C. J., and Gleich, G. J., Regulatory effect of cytokines on eosinophil degranulation, *J. Immunol.,* 144, 642, 1990.

105. Warringa, R. J., Moqbel, R., Cromwell, O., and Kay, A. B., Platelet activating factor. A potent chemotactic and chemokinetic factor for human eosinophils, *J. Clin. Invest.,* 78, 1701, 1986.

106. Vancheri, C., Gauldie, J., Bienenstock, J., Cox, G., Scicchitano, R., Stanisz, A., and Jordana, M., Human lung fibroblast-derived granulocyte-macrophage colony stimulating factor (GM-CSF) mediates eosinophil survival in vitro, *Am. J. Respir. Cell Mol. Biol.,* 1, 289, 1989.

107. Dedhar, S., Gaboury, L., Galloway, P., and Eaves, C., Human granulocyte-macrophage colony-stimulating factor is growth factor active on a variety of cell types of non-hemopoietic origin, *Proc. Natl. Acad. Sci. U.S.A.,* 85, 9253, 1988.

108. Walker, C., Virchow, J.-C., Bruijnzeel, P. L. B., and Blaser, K., T cell subsets and their soluble products regulate eosinophilia in allergic and nonallergic asthma, *J. Immunol.,* 146, 1829, 1991.

109. Arnaout, M. A., Wang, E. A., Clark, S. C., and Sief, C. A., Human recombinant granulocyte-macrophage colony stimulating factor increases cell to cell adhesion and surface expression of adhesion promoting surface glycoproteins on mature granulocytes, *J. Clin. Invest.,* 78, 597, 1986.

110. Fleischman, J., Golde, D. W., Weisbart, R. H., and Gasson, J. C., Granuloycte-macrophage colony stimulating factor enhances phagocytosis of bacteria by human neutrophils, *Blood,* 68, 708, 1986.

111. Paul, W. E. and Ohara, J., B-cell stimulatory factor-1/interleukin 4, *Annu. Rev. Immunol.,* 5, 429, 1987.

112. Noma, Y., Sideras, T., Naito, T., Bergstedt-Lindquist, S., Azuma, C., Severinson, E., Tanabe, T., Kinashi, T., Matsuda, F., Yaoita, Y., and Honjo, T., Cloning of cDNA encoding the murine IgG induction factor by a novel strategy using SP6 promoter, *Nature,* 319, 640, 1986.

113. Lee, F., Yokota, T., Ostsuka, T., Meyerson, P., Villaret, D., Coffman, R., Mosmann, T., Rennick, D., Roehm, N., Smith, C., Zlotnik, A., and Arai, K., Isolation and characterisation of mouse interleukin cDNA clone that expresses B-cell stimulatory factor 1 activities and T-cell- and mast-cell-stimulating activities, *Proc. Natl. Acad. Sci. U.S.A.,* 83, 2061, 1986.

114. Yokota, T., Otsuka, T., Mosmann, T., Banchereau, J., De France, T., Blanchard, D., de Vries, J. E., Lee, F., and Arai, K., Isolation and characterization of a human interleukin cDNA clone, homologous to mouse B-cell stimulatory factor 1, that expresses B-cell- and T-cell-stimulating activities, *Proc. Natl. Acad. Sci. U.S.A.*, 83, 5894, 1986.
115. van Leeuwen, B. H., Martinson, M. E., Webb, G. C., and Young, I. G., Molecular organisation of the cytokine gene cluster, involving the human IL-3, IL-4, IL-5, and GM-CSF genes, on chromosome 5, *Blood*, 73, 1142, 1989.
116. Widmer, M. B., Acres, R. B., Sassenfeld, H. M., and Grabstein, K. H., Regulation of cytolytic cell populations from peripheral blood by B cell stimulatory factor 1 (interleukin 4), *J. Exp. Med.*, 166, 1447, 1987.
117. Hamaguchi, Y., Kanakura, Y., Fujita, J.-I., Takeda, S., Nakamo, T., Tarui, S., Honjo, T., and Kitamura, Y., Interleukin 4 as an essential factor for in vitro clonal growth of murine connective tissue-type mast cells, *J. Exp. Med.*, 165, 268, 1987.
118. Crawford, R. M., Finbloom, D. S., Ohara, J., Paul, W. E., and Meltzer, M. S., B cell stimulatory factor-1 (interleukin 4) activates macrophages for increased tumoricidal activity and expression of Ia antigens, *J. Immunol.*, 139, 135, 1987.
119. Plaut, M., Pierce, J. H., Watson, C. J., Hanley-Hyde, J., Nordan, R. P., and Paul, W. E., Mast cell lines produce lymphokines in response to cross linkage of FcER1 by calcium ionophores, *Nature*, 339, 64, 1989.
120. Bradding, P., Feather, I., Howarth, P. H., Mueller, R., Roberts, J. A., Britten, K., Bews, J. P. A., Hunt, T. C., Okayama, Y., Heusser, C. H., Bullock, G. R., Church, M. K., and Holgate, S. T., Interleukin 4 immunoreactivity is localised to and released by human mast cells, *J. Exp. Med.*, 176, 1382, 1992.
121. Sedgwick, J. B., Calhoun, W. J., Gleich, G. J., Kita, H., Abrams, J. S., Schwartz, L. B., Volovitz, B., Ben-Yaakov, M., and Busse, W. W., Immediate and late airway response of allergic rhinitis patients to segmental antigen challenge, *Am. Rev. Respir. Dis.*, 144, 1274, 1991.
122. Gajewski, T. F. and Fitch, F. W., Anti-proliferative effect of IFN-γ in immune regulation. III. Differential selection of Th1 and Th2 murine T helper T lymphocyte clones using recombinant IL-2 and IFNγ, *J. Immunol.*, 143, 15, 1988.
123. Maggi, E., Parronchi, P., Manetti, R., Simonell, C., Piccinni, M. P., Rugiu, F. S., De Carli, M., Ricci, M., and Romagnani, S., Reciprocal regulatory effects of INF-gamma and IL-4 on the in vitro development of human Th1 and Th2 clones, *J. Immunol.*, 148, 2142, 1992.
124. Defrance, T., Aubry, J. P., Rousset, F., Vanbervliet, B., Bonnefoy, J. Y., Arai, N., Takebe, Y., Yokota, T., Lee, F., Arai, K., de Vries, J., and Banchereall, J., Human recombinant interleukin 4 induces Fcε receptors (CD23) on normal B lymphocytes, *J. Exp. Med.*, 165, 1459, 1987.
125. Rousset, F., Malefijt, R. W., Slierendregt, B., Aubry, J. P., Bonnefoy, J. Y., Defrance, T., Banchereau, J., and de Vries, J. E., Regulation of Fc receptor for IgE (CD23) and class II MHC antigen expression on Burkitt's lymphoma cell lines by human IL-4 and IFN-gamma, *J. Immunol.*, 140, 2625, 1988.
126. Pene, J., Rousset, F., Briere, F., Chretien, I., Widemanm, J., Bonnefoy, J. Y., and De Vries, J. E., Interleukin 5 enhances interleukin 4-induced IgE production by normal human B cells. The role of soluble antigen, *Eur. J. Immunol.*, 18, 929, 1988.
127. Clutterbuck, E. J., Hirst, E. M., and Sanderson, C. J., Human interleukin-5 (IL-5) regulates the production of eosinophils in human bone marrow cultures: comparison and interaction with IL-1, IL-3, IL-6 and GM-CSF, *Blood*, 73, 1504, 1989.
128. Lopez, A. F., Sanderson, C. J., Gamble, J. R., Campbell, H. D., Young, I. G., and Vadas, M. A., Recombinant human interleukin 5 is a selective activator of human eosinophil function, *J. Exp. Med.*, 167, 119, 1988.
129. Walsh, G. M., Wardlaw, A. J., Hartnell, A., Sanderson, C. J., and Kay, A. B., Interleukin-5 enhances the in vitro adhesion of human eosinophils, but not neutrophils, in a leucocyte integrin (CD11/18)-dependent manner, *Int. Arch. Allergy Appl. Immunol.*, 94, 174, 1991.

130. Campbell, H. D., Tucker, W. Q. J., Hort, Y., Martinson, M. E., Mayo, G., Clutterbuck, E. J., Sanderson, C. J., and Young I. G., Molecular cloning, nucleotide sequence, and expression of the gene encoding human eosinophil differentiation factor (interleukin 5), *Proc. Natl. Acad. Sci. U.S.A.*, 84, 6629, 1987.

131. Sanderson, C. J., Campbell, H. D., and Young I. G., Molecular and cellular biology of eosinophil differentiation factor (interleukin 5) and its effects on human and mouse B cells, *Immunol. Rev.*, 102, 29, 1988.

132. O'Byrne, P. M., Walters, E. H., Gold, B. D., Aizawa, H. A., Fabbri, L. M., Alpert, S. E., Nadel, J. A., and Holtzman, M. J., Neutrophil depletion inhibits airway hyperresponsiveness induced by ozone exposure in dogs, *Am. Rev. Respir. Dis.*, 130, 214, 1984.

133. Fabbri, L. M., Boschetto, P., Zocca, E., Milani, G., Pivirotto, F., Plebani, M., Burlina, A., Licata, B., and Mapp, C. E., Bronchoalveolar neutrophilia during late asthmatic reactions induced by toluene diisocyanate, *Am. Rev. Respir. Dis.*, 136, 36, 1987.

134. Palut, M., Pierce, J. H., Watson, C. J., Hanley-Hyde, J., Nordan, R. P., and Paul, W. E., Mast cell lines produce lymphokines in response to cross-linkage of FceR-1 or to calcium ionophores, *Nature*, 339, 64, 1989.

135. Desreumaux, P., Janin, A., Colombel, J. F., Prin, L., Plumas, J., Emilie, D., Torpier, G., Capron, A., and Capron, M., Interleukin-5 messenger RNA expression by eosinophils in the interstinal mucosa of patients with coeliac disease, *J. Exp. Med.*, 175, 293, 1992.

136. Robinson, D. S., Hamid, Q., Ying, S., Bentley, A. M., Assoufi, B., North, J., Durham, S. R., and Kay, A. B., A prednisolone treatment in asthma is associated with modulation of bronchoalveolar lavage all IL-4, IL-5 and IFNγ cytokine gene expression, *Am. Rev. Respir. Dis.*, 148, 401, 1993.

137. Kelley, J., Cytokines of the lung, *Am. Rev. Respir. Dis.*, 141, 765, 1990.

138. Tosato, G., Seamon, K. B., Goldman, N. D., Sehgal, P. V., May, L. T., Washington, G. C., Jones, K. D., and Pike, S. E., Monocyte-derived human B-cell growth factor identified as interferon-$\beta_2$ (BSF-2, IL-6), *Science*, 239, 502, 1988.

139. Hirano, R., Akiro, S., Taga, T., and Kishimoto, T., Biological and clinical aspects of interleukin 6, *Immunol. Today*, 11, 443, 1990.

140. Ray, A., Tatter, S. B., Santhanam, U., Halfgott, D. C., May, L. T., and Sehgal, P. B., Regulation of expression of interleukin-6. Molecular and clinical studies, *Ann. N.Y. Acad. Sci.*, 557, 353, 1989.

141. Walther, Z., May, L. T., and Sehgal, P. B., Transcriptional regulation of the interferon-beta 2/B cell differentiation factor (BSF-2)/hepatocyte stimulating factor gene in human fibroblasts by other cytokines, *J. Immunol.*, 140, 974, 1987.

142. Kohase, M., May, L. T., Tamm, I., Vilcek, J., and Sehgal, P. B., A cytokine network in human diploid fibroblasts: interactions of beta-interferons, tumor necrosis factor, platelet-derived growth factor, and interleukin-1, *Mol. Cell Biol.*, 7, 273, 1988.

143. Muraguchi, A., Hirano, T., Tang, B., Matsuda, T., Horii, Y., Nakajima, K., and Kishimoto, T., The essential role of B cell stimulatory factor 2 (BSF-2/IL-6) for the terminal differentiation of B-cells, *J. Exp. Med.*, 167, 332, 1988.

144. Beagley, K. W., Eldridge, J. H., Lee, F., Kiyono, H., Everson, M. P., Koopman, W. J., Hirano, T., Kishimoto, T., and McGhee, J. R., Interleukins and IgA synthesis — human and murine interleukin 6 induce high rate IgA secretion in IgA committed B cells, *J. Exp. Med.*, 169, 2133, 1989.

145. Uyttenhove, C., Coulie, P. G., and Van Snick, J., T cell growth and differentiation induced by interleukin HP1/IL-6, the murine hybridoma/plasmacytoma growth factor, *J. Exp. Med.*, 167, 1417, 1988.

146. Houssiau, F. A., Coulie, P. G., and van Snick, J., Distinct roles of IL-1 and IL-6 in human T cell activation, *J. Immunol.*, 143, 2520, 1989.

147. Baroja, M. L., Ceuppens, J. L., Van Damme, J., and Billiau, A., Cooperation between an anti-T cell (anti-CD28) monoclonal antibody and monocyte-produced IL-6 in the induction of T cell responsiveness to IL-2, *J. Immunol.*, 141, 1502, 1988.

148. Zitnik, R. J. and Elias, J. A., Interleukin-6 and the lung, in *Cytokines of the Lung. Lung Biology in Health and Disease*, Vol. 61, Kelley, J. and Lenfant, C., Eds., Marcel Dekker, New York, 1993, 229.

149. Elias, J. A. and Lentz, V., Interleukin-1 and tumor necrosis factor synergistically stimulate fibroblast interleukin-6 production and stabilise interleukin-6 messenger RNA, *J. Immunol.*, 145, 161, 1990.

150. Elias, J. A., Lentz, V., and Cummings, P., Transforming growth factor-beta regulation of IL-6 production by unstimulated and IL-1 stimulated human fibroblasts, *J. Immunol.*, 146, 3437, 1991.

151. Kotloff, R. M., Little, J., and Elias, J. A., Human alveolar macrophage and blood monocyte interleukin-6 production, *Am. J. Respir. Cell Mol. Biol.*, 3, 497, 1990.

152. Devlin, R. B., McDonnell, W. F., Mann, R., Becker, S., House, D. E., Schreinemachers, D., and Koren, H., Exposure of humans to ambient levels of ozone for 6.6 hours causes cellular and biochemical changes in the lung, *Am. J. Respir. Cell Mol. Biol.*, 4, 72, 1991.

153. Hamid, Q., Barkans, J., Meng, Q., Ying, S., Abrams, J. S., Kay, A. B., and Moqbel, R., Human eosinophils synthesise and secrete interleukin-6 in vitro, *Blood*, 80, 1496, 1992.

154. Fiorentino, D. F., Bond, M. W., and Mosman, T. R., Two types of mouse T helper cell. IV. Th2 clones secrete a factor that inhibits cytokine production by Th1 clones, *J. Exp. Med.*, 170, 2081, 1989.

155. Fiorentino, D. F., Zlotnick, A., Mosmann, T. R., Howard, M., Moore, K. W., and O'Garra, A., IL-10 acts on the antigen presenting cell to inhibit cytokine production by Th1 cells, *J. Immunol.*, 146, 3444, 1991.

156. De Wall Malefyt, R., Haanen, J., Spits, H., Roncarolo, M. G., te Velde, A., Figdor, C., Johnson, K., Kastelein, R., Yssel, H., and de Vries, J. E., Interleukin-10 and viral-IL-10 strongly reduce antigen-specific human T-cell proliferation by diminishing the antigen-presenting capacity of monocytes via downregulation of class-II major histocompatibility complex expression, *J. Exp. Med.*, 174, 915, 1991.

157. Howard, M. and O'Gara, A., Biological properties of interleukin 10, *Immunol. Today*, 13, 198, 1992.

158. Wheelock, E. F., Interferon-like virus-inhibitor induced in human leukocytes by phytohemagglutinin, *Science*, 149, 310, 1965.

159. Adams, D. O., Macrophage activation, in *Encyclopedia of Immunology*, Roitt, J. M., Ed., Vol. 2, Academic Press, London, 1992, 1020.

160. Wewers, M. D., Cytokines and macrophages, in *Cytokines in Health and Disease*, Kunkel, S. L. and Remick, D. G., Eds., Marcel Dekker, New York, 1992, 327.

161. Vogel, S. N. and Friedman, R. M., Interferon and macrophages: activation and cell surface changes, in *Interferons: Vol. 2. Interferon and the Immune System*, Vilcek, J. and DeMaeyer, E., Eds., Elsevier, Amsterdam, 1984, 35.

162. Kelley, V. E., Fiers, W., and Strom, T. B., Cloned human interferon-γ, but not interferon-β or α, induces expression of HLA-DR determinants by fetal monocytes and myeloid leukemic cell lines, *J. Immunol.*, 132, 240, 1984.

163. Stauton, D. E., Dustin, M. L., and Springer, T. A., Functional cloning of ICAM-2, a cell adhesion ligand for LFA-1 homologous to ICAM-2, *Nature*, 339, 61, 1989.

164. Wegner, C. D., Gundel, R. H., Reilly, P., Haynes, N., Letts, L. G., and Rothlein, R., Intercellular adhesion molecule-1 (ICAM-1) in the pathogenesis of asthma, *Science*, 247, 456, 1990.

165. Naylor, S. L., Sakaguchi, A. Y., Shows, T. B., Law, M. L., Goeddel, D. V., and Gray, P. W., Human immune interferon gene is located on chromosome 12, *J. Exp. Med.*, 157, 1020, 1983.

166. Gray, P. W. and Goeddel, D. V., Structure of the human immune interferon gene, *Nature*, 298, 859, 1982.

167. Celada, A., Gray, P. W., Rinderknecht, E., and Schreiber, R. D., Evidence for a gamma-interferon receptor that regulates macrophage tumoricidal activity, *J. Exp. Med.*, 160, 55, 1984.

168. Kovacs, E. J., Fibrogenic cytokines: the role of immune mediators in the development of scar tissue, *Immunol. Today,* 12, 17, 1991.

169. Scharffetter, K., Heckmann, M., Hatamochi, A., Maunch, C., Stein, B., Reithmuller, G., Ziegler-Heitbrock, H. W., and Krieg, T., Synergistic effect of tumor necrosis factor-alpha and interferon-gamma on collagen synthesis of human skin fibroblasts *in vitro, Exp. Cell Res.,* 181, 409, 1989.

170. Adelmann-Grill, B. C., Hein, R., Wach, F., and Krieg, T., Inhibition of fibroblast chemotaxis by recombinant human interferon gamma and interferon alpha, *J. Cell. Physiol.,* 130, 270, 1987.

171. Elias, J. A., Jimenez, S. A., and Freundlich, B., Recombinant gamma, alpha and beta interferon regulation of human lung fibroblast proliferation, *Am. Rev. Respir. Dis.,* 135, 62, 1987.

172. Li, J. T. C., Yunginger, J. W., Reed, C. E., Jaffe, H. S., Nelson, D. R., and Gleich, G. J., Lack of suppression of IgE production by recombinant interferon gamma: a controlled clinical trial in patients with allergic rhinitis, *J. Allergy Clin. Immunol.,* 85, 934, 1990.

173. Gray, P. W., Aggarwal, B. B., Benton, C. V., Bringman, T. S., Henzel, W. J., Jarrett, J. A., Leung, D. W., Moffat, B., Ng, P., Svedensky, L. P., Palladino, M. A., and Nedwin, G. E., Cloning and expression of cDNA for human lymphotoxin, a lymphokine with tumor necrosis activity, *Nature,* 312, 721, 1984.

174. Nawroth, P., Bank, I., Handley, D., Cassimeris, J., Chess, L., and Stern, D., TNF interacts with endothelial cell receptors to induce release of IL-1, *J. Exp. Med.,* 163, 1363, 1986.

175. Aggarwal, B., Essalu, T., and Hass, P., Characterization of receptors for human TNF and their regulation by gamma IFN, *Nature,* 318, 665, 1985.

176. Carswell, E. A., Old, L. J., Kassel, R. L., Green, S., Fiore, N., and Williamson, B., An endotoxin-induced serum factor that causes necrosis of tumors, *Proc. Natl. Acad. Sci. U.S.A.,* 72, 3666, 1975.

177. Beutler, B., Krochin, N., Milsark, I. W., Leudke, C., and Cerami, A., Control of TNF synthesis: mechanisms of endotoxin resistance, *Science,* 232, 977, 1986.

178. Pennica, D., Nedwin, G. E., Hayflick, J. S., Seeburg, P. H., Derynck, R., Palladino, M. A., Kohr, W. J., Aggarwal, B. B., and Goeddel, D. V., Human tumor necrosis factor. Precursor structure, expression, and homology to lymphotoxin, *Nature,* 312, 724, 1984.

179. Tracey, K. J., Vlassara, H., and Cerami, A., Cachectin/TNF, *Lancet,* 1, 1122, 1989.

180. Ulich, T. R., Guo, K., Irwin, B., Remick, D. G., and Davatelis, G. N., Endotoxin-induced cytokine gene expression in vivo. II. Regulation of TNF and IL-1 expression and suppression, *Am. J. Pathol.,* 137, 1173, 1990.

181. Tracey, K. J., Beutler, B., Lowry, S. F., Merryweather, J., Wope, S., Milsark, J. W., Hariri, R J., Fahey, T. J., Zentella, A., Albert, J. D., Shires, G. T., and Cerami, A., Shock and tissue injury induced by recombinant cachectin, *Science,* 234, 470, 1986.

182. Ulich, T. R., Watson, L. R., Yin, S. M., Guo, K. Z., Wang, P., Thang, H., and del Castillo, J., The intratracheal administration of endotoxin and cytokines. I. Characterization of LPS-induced IL-1 and TNF mRNA expression and the LPS-IL-1-, and TNF-induced inflammatory infiltrate, *Am. J. Pathol.,* 138, 1485, 1991.

183. Ulich, T. R., del Castillo, J., Ni, R. X., Bikhazi, N., and Calvin, L., Mechanisms of TNF-induced lymphopenia, neutropenia, and biphasic neutrophilia: a study of lymphocyte recirculation and hematologic interactions of TNF with endogenous mediators of leukocyte trafficking, *J. Leukocyte Biol.,* 45, 155, 1989.

184. Silberstein, D. S. and Davis, J. R., Tumour necrosis factor enhances eosinophil toxicity to *Schistosoma mansoni* larvae, *Proc. Natl. Acad. Sci. U.S.A.,* 83, 1055, 1986.

185. Slungaard, A., Vercellotte, G. M., Walker, G., Nelson, R. D., and Jacob, H. E., Tumour necrosis factor/cachectin stimulates eosinophil oxidant production and toxicity towards human endothelium, *J. Exp. Med.,* 171, 2025, 1990.

186. Benyon, R. C., Bissonette, E. Y., and Befus, A. D., Tumor necrosis factor alpha-dependent cytotoxicity of human skin mast cells in enhanced by anti-IgE antibodies, *J. Immunol.,* 147, 2253, 1991.

187. Bevilacqua, M. P., Stengelin, S., Gimbrone, M. A., and Seed, B., Endothelial leucocyte adhesion molecule-1: an inducible receptor for neutrophils related to complement regulatory proteins and lectins, *Science,* 243, 1160, 1989.
188. Osborn, L., Hession, C., Tizard, R., Vassallo, C., Luhowskyi, R., Chi-Rosso, C., and Lobb, R., Direct expression and cloning of vascular cell adhesion molecule-1, a cytokine-induced endothelial protein that binds to lymphocytes, *Cell,* 59, 1203, 1989.
189. Pober, J. S., Gimbrone, M. A., Lapierre, L. A., Mendrick, D. L., Fiers, W., Rothlein, R., and Springer, T. A., Overlapping patterns of activation of human endothelial cells by interleukin 1, tumour necrosis factor, and immune interferon, *J. Immunol.,* 137, 1893, 1986.
190. Wheeler, A. P., Jesmok, G., and Brigham, K. L., Tumour necrosis factor's effect on lung mechanics, gas exchange and airway reactivity in sheep, *J. Appl. Physiol.,* 68, 2542, 1990.
191. Kips, J. C., Tavernier, J., and Pauwels, R. A., Tumor necrosis factor (TNF) causes bronchial hyperresponsiveness in rats, *Am. Rev. Respir. Dis.,* 145, 332, 1992.
192. Anderson, U. and Matsuda, T., Human interleukin 6 and tumour necrosis factor-α production studied at a single cell level, *Eur. J. Immunol.,* 19, 1157, 1989.
193. Walsh, L. J., Trinchieri, G., Waldorf, H. A., Whittaker, D., and Murphy, G. F., Human dermal mast cells contain and release tumour necrosis factor α, which induces endothelial leucocyte adhesion molecule-1, *Proc. Natl. Acad. Sci. U.S.A.,* 88, 4220, 1991.
194. Costa, J. J., Matossian, K., Resnick, M. B., Beil, W. J., Wong, D. T. W., Gordon, J. R., Dvorak, A. M., Weller, P. F., and Galli, S. J., Human eosinophils can express the cytokines tumour necrosis factor-α and macrophage inflammatory protein-1α, *J. Clin. Invest.,* 91, 2673, 1993.
195. Leibovich, S. J., Polverini, P. J., Shepard, M. H., Wiseman, D. M., Shively, V., and Nusewir, N., Macrophage-induced angiogenesis is mediated by TNFα, *Nature,* 329, 630, 1987.
196. Kohase, M., Henriksen-DeStefano, D., May, L. T., Vilcek, J., and Sehgal, P. B., Induction of β2-interferon by TNF: a homeostatic mechanism in the control of cell proliferation, *Cell,* 45, 659, 1986.
197. Otsuka, Y., Nagano, K., Nagano, K., Hori, K., Ohishi, J., Hayashi, H., Watanabe, N., and Niitsu, Y., Inhibition of neutrophil migration by TNF, *J. Immunol.,* 145, 2639, 1990.
198. Stewart, A. G., Tomlinson, P. R., Wilson, J. W., and Harris, T., Tumour necrosis factor α modulates mitogenic responses of human cultured airway smooth muscle, *Am. J. Respir. Cell Mol. Biol.,* 12, 110, 1995.
199. Smith, K. A., Interleukin 2, *Annu. Rev. Immunol.,* 2, 319, 1984.
200. Rand, T. H., Silberstein, D. S., Kornfeld, H., and Weller, P. E., Human eosinophils express functional interleukin-2 receptors, *J. Clin. Invest.,* 88, 825, 1991.
201. Groopman, J. E., Molina, J.-M., and Scadden, D. T., Hemotopoietic growth factors biology and clinical applications, *N. Engl. J. Med.,* 321, 1449, 1989.
202. Cromwell, O., Hamid, Q., Corrigan, C. J., Barkans, J., Meng, Q., and Collins, P. D., Expression and generation of IL-6, IL-8 and GM-CSF by human bronchial epithelial cells and enhancement by IL-1β and TNF-α, *Immunology,* 77, 330, 1992.
203. Pene, J., Rousset, F., Briere, F., Chretien, I., Bonnefoy, J. Y., Spits, H., Yokota, T., Arai, N., Arai, K., Banchereau, J., et al., IgE production by normal lymphocytes is induced by interleukin 4 and suppressed by interferons γ and α and prostaglandin E₂, *Proc. Natl. Acad. Sci. U.S.A.,* 85, 6880, 1988.
204. Turner, M., Londer, M., and Feldmann, M., Human T-cells from autoimmune and normal individuals can produce tumor necrosis factor, *Eur. J. Immunol.,* 17, 1807, 1987.
205. Revel, M., Host defence against infections and inflammation: role of the multifunctional IL-6/IFN-beta 2 cytokine, *Experientia,* 45, 549, 1989.
206. Kimata, H., Yoshida, A., Ishioka, C., Lindley, I., and Mikawa, H., Interleukin 8 (IL-8) selectively inhibits immunoglobulin E production induced by IL-4 in human B cells, *J. Exp. Med.,* 176, 1227, 1992.
207. Larsen, C. G., Anderson, A. O., and Appella, E., The neutrophil-activating protein (NAP-1) is also chemotactic for T lymphocytes, *Science,* 243, 1464, 1989.

208. Zachariae, C. O. C. and Matsushima, K., Interleukin 8, in *Encyclopedia of Immunology*, Vol. 2, Roitt, J. M., Ed., Academic Press, London, 1992, 922.

209. Kiniwa, M., Gateley, M., Chizzonite, R., Fargeas, C., and Delespesse, G., Recombinant interleukin-12 suppresses the synthesis of immunoglobulin E by interleukin-4 stimulated human lymphocytes, *J. Clin. Invest.*, 90, 262, 1992.

210. Old, L. J., Tumour necrosis factor (TNF), *Science*, 230, 630, 1985.

211. Swain, S. L., T cell subsets and the recognition of MHC class, *Immunol. Rev.*, 74, 129, 1983.

212. Toyonaga, B. and Mak, T. W., Genes of the T-cell antigen receptor in normal and malignant T cells, *Annu. Rev. Immunol.*, 5, 585, 1987.

213. Jeffery, P. K., Wardlaw, A. J., Nelson, F. C., Collins, J. V., and Kay, A. B., Bronchial biopsies in asthma: an ultrastructural, quantitative study and correlation with hyperreactivity, *Am. Rev. Respir. Dis.*, 140, 1745, 1989.

214. Fukuda, T., Ando, N., Numao, T., Akutsu, I., Nakajima, H., and Makino, S., Lymphocyte subsets in bronchial mucosa of symptomatic and asymptomatic asthmatics, *J. Allergy Clin. Immunol.*, 87, 302, 1991.

215. Gonzalez, M. C., Diaz, P., Galleguillos, F. R., Ancic, P., Cromwell, O., and Kay, A. B., Allergen-induced recruitment of bronchoalveolar (OKT4) and suppressor (OKT8) cells in asthma: relative increases inn responders, *Am. Rev. Respir. Dis.*, 136, 600, 1987.

216. Corrigan, C. J., Hartnell, A., and Kay, A. B., CD4 T-lymphocyte activation in acute severe asthma, *Lancet*, 1, 1129, 1988.

217. Walker, C., Kaegi, M. K., Braun, P., and Blaser, K., Activated T cells and eosinophilia in bronchoalveolar lavages from subjects with asthma correlated with disease severity, *J. Allergy Clin. Immunol.*, 88, 935, 1991.

218. Barnes, P. J., Cytokines as mediators of chronic asthma, *Am. J. Respir. Crit. Care Med.*, 150, S42, 1994.

219. Adelroth, E., Rosenhall, L., Johansson, S.-A., Linden, M., and Venge, P., Inflammatory cells and eosinophilic activity in asthmatics investigated in asthmatic by bronchoalveolar lavage. The effects of antiasthmatic treatment with budesonide or terbutaline, *Am. Rev. Respir. Dis.*, 142, 91, 1990.

220. Djukanovic, R., Wilson, J. W., Britten, K. M., Wilson, S. J., Walls, A. F., Roche, W. R., Howarth, P. H., and Holgate, S. T., The effect of inhaled corticosteroids on airway inflammation and symptoms of asthma, *Am. Rev. Respir. Dis.*, 145, 669, 1992.

221. Gavett, S. H., Chen, X., Finkelman, F., and Wills-Karp, M., Depletion of murine CD4+ T lymphocytes prevents antigen-induced airway hyperreactivity and pulmonary eosinophilia, *Am. J. Respir. Cell Mol. Biol.*, 10, 587, 1994.

222. Holgate, S. T., Djukanovic, R., Howarth, P. H., Montefort, S., and Roche, W. R., The T cell and the airway's fibrotic response in asthma, *Chest*, 103, 125S, 1993.

223. Schleimer, R. P., MacGlashan, D. W., Schulman, E. S., et al., Human mast cells and basophils — structure, function, pharmacology and biochemistry, *Clin. Rev. Allergy*, 1, 327, 1983.

224. Lai, C. K. W. and Holgate, S. T., The mast cell in asthma, in *Clinical Immunology and Allergy: the Allergic Basis of Asthma*, Kay, A. B., Ed., Balliere Tindall, London, 1988, 37.

225. Tomioka, M., Ida, S., Shindoh, Y., Ishihara, T., and Takishima, T., Mast cells in bronchoalveolar lumen of patients with bronchial asthma, *Am. Rev. Respir. Dis.*, 129, 1000, 1984.

226. Agius, R. M., Godfrey, R. C., and Holgate, S. T., Mast cell and histamine content of human bronchoalveolar lavage, *Thorax*, 40, 760, 1985.

227. Flint, K. C., Leung, K. B. P., Hudspith, B. N., Brostoff, J., Pearce, F. L., and Johnson, N. M., Bronchoalveolar mast cells in extrinsic asthma: a mechanism for the initiation of antigen specific bronchoconstriction, *Br. Med. J.*, 291, 923, 1985.

228. Pearce, F. L., Flint, K. C., Leung, K. B. P., Hudspith, B. N., Seager, K., Hammond, M. D., Brostoff, J., Geraint-James, D., and Johnson, N. M., Some studies on human pulmonary mast cells obtained by bronchoalveolar lavage and by enzymatic dissociation of whole lung tissue, *Int. Arch. Allergy Appl. Immunol.*, 82, 507, 1987.

229. Casale, T. B., Wood, D., Richerson, H. B., Zehr, B., Zavala, D., and Hunninghake, G. W., Direct evidence of a role for mast cells in the pathogenesis of antigen-induced broncho-constriction, *J. Clin. Invest.*, 80, 1507, 1987.

230. Kirby, J. G., Hargreave, F. E., Gliech, G. J., and O'Byrne, P. M., Bronchoalveolar cell profiles of asthmatic and nonasthmatic subjects, *Am. Rev. Respir. Dis.*, 136, 379, 1987.

231. Wenzel, S. E., Fowler, A. A., and Schwartz, L. B., Activation of pulmonary mast cells by bronchoalveolar allergen challenge: *in vivo* release of histamine and tryptase in atopic subjects with and without asthma, *Am. Rev. Respir. Dis.*, 137, 1002, 1988.

232. Salvato, G., Some histological changes in chronic bronchitis and asthma, *Thorax*, 23, 168, 1968.

233. Heard, B. E., Nunn, A. J., and Kay, A. B., Mast cells in human lungs, *J. Pathol.*, 157, 59, 1989.

234. Denburg, J. A., Basophil and mast cell lineages *in vitro* and *in vivo*, *Blood*, 79, 846, 1992.

235. Osman, I. A. R., Garrett, J. R., and Smith, R. E., Enzyme histochemical discrimination between tryptase and chymase in mast cells of human gut, *J. Histochem. Cytochem.*, 37, 415, 1989.

236. Irani, A. M., Craig, S. S., DeBlois, G., Elson, C. O., Schechter, N. M., and Schwartz, L. B., Deficiency of the tryptase-positive, chymase-negative mast cell type in gastrointestinal mucosa of patients with defective T lymphocyte function, *J. Immunol.*, 138, 4381, 1987.

237. Irani, A. A., Schechter, N. M., Craig, S. S., DeBlois, G., and Schwartz, L. B., Two types of human mast cells that have distinct neutral protease compositions, *Proc. Natl. Acad. Sci. U.S.A.*, 83, 4464, 1986.

238. Irani, A. M., Brandford, T. R., Kepley, C. L., Schechter, N. M., and Schwartz, L. B., Detection of MCT and MCTC types of human mast cells by immunohistochemistry using new mono-clonal anti-tryptase and anti-chymase antibodies, *J. Histochem. Cytochem.*, 37, 1509, 1989.

239. Schwartz, L. B., Irani, A. M., Roller, K., Castells, C., and Schechter, N. M., Quantitation of histamine, tryptase and chymase in dispersed human T and TC mast cells, *J. Immunol.*, 138, 2611, 1987.

240. MacDonald, I. G., The local and constitutional pathology of bronchial asthma, *Ann. Intern. Med.*, 6, 253, 1932.

241. Gleich, G. J., The eosinophil and bronchial asthma: current understanding, *J. Allergy Clin. Immunol.*, 85, 422, 1990.

242. Fukuda, T., Dunnette, S. L., Reed, C. E., Ackerman, S. J., Peters, M. S., and Gleich, G. J., Increased numbers of hypodense eosinophils in the blood of patients with bronchial asthma, *Am. Rev. Respir. Dis.*, 132, 981, 1985.

243. Bousquet, J., Chanez, P., Lacoste, J. Y., Barneon, G., Ghavanioan, N., Enander, I., Venge, P., Ahlstedt, S., Simony-Lafontaine, J., Godard, P., and Michel, F. B., Eosinophilic inflam-mation in asthma, *N. Engl. J. Med.*, 323, 1033, 1990.

244. Lopez, A. F., To, L. B., Yang, Y. C., Gamble, J. R., Shannon, M. F., Burns, G. F., Dyson, P. G., Juttner, C. A., Clark, S., and Vadas, M. S., Stimulation of proliferation, differentia-tion, and function of human cells by primate interleukin 3, *Proc. Natl. Acad. Sci. U.S.A.*, 84, 2761, 1987.

245. Thorne, K. J. I., Richardson, B. A., Taverne, J., Williamson, D. J., Vadas, M. A., and Butterworth, A. E., A comparison of eosinophil-activating factor (EAF) with other mono-kines and lymphokines, *Eur. J. Immunol.*, 16, 1143, 1986.

246. Yamaguchi, Y., Hayashi, Y., Sugawa, Y., Miura, Y., Kasahara, T., Kitamura, S., Torisu, M., Mita, S., Tominaga, A., and Takatsu, K., High purified murine interleukin 5 (IL-5) stim-ulates eosinophil function and prolongs *in vitro* saliva, *J. Exp. Med.*, 167, 1737, 1988.

247. Gleich, G. J., Flavahan, N. A., Fujisawa, T., and Vanhoutte, P. M., The eosinophil as a mediator of damage to respiratory epithelium: a model for bronchial hyperreactivity, *J. Allergy Clin. Immunol.*, 81, 776, 1988.

248. Capron, M., Spiegelberg, H. L., Prin, L., Bennich, H., Butterworth, A. E., Pearce, R. J., Ouaissi, M. A., and Capron, A., Role of IgE receptors in effector function of eosinophils, *J. Immunol.*, 232, 462, 1984.

249. Capron, M., Tomassini, M., Torpier, G., Kusnierz, J. P., MacDonald, S., and Capron, A., Selectivity of mediators released by eosinophils, *Int. Arch. Allergy Clin. Immunol.*, 88, 54, 1989.

250. Kroegel, C., Yukawa, T., Dent, G., Chanez, P., Chung, K. F., and Barnes, P. J., Platelet activating factor induces eosinophil peroxidase release from human eosinophils, *Immunology*, 64, 559, 1988.

251. Kroegel, C., Yukawa, T., Dent, G., Chanez, P., Chung, K. F., and Barnes, P. J., Stimulation of degranulation from human eosinophils by platelet activating factor, *J. Immunol.*, 142, 3518, 1989.

252. Yukawa, T., Kroegel, C., Evans, P., Fukuda, T., Chung, K. F., and Barnes, P. J., Density heterogeneity of eosinophil leukocytes: induction of hypodense eosinophils by platelet activating factor, *Immunology*, 68, 140, 1989.

253. Lopez, A. F., Williamson, D. F., Gamble, J. R., Begley, C. G., Harlan, J. M., Klebanoff, S. J., Waltersdorph, A., Wong, G., Clark, S. C., and Vadas, M. A., Recombinant human granulocyte-macrophage colony-stimulating factor stimulates *in vitro* mature human neutrophil and eosinophil function, surface receptor expression, and survival, *J. Clin. Invest.*, 78, 1220, 1986.

254. Durham, S. R. and Kay, A. B., Eosinophils, bronchial hyperreactivity and late-phase asthmatic reactions, *Clin. Allergy*, 15, 411, 1985.

255. Elwood, W., Lotvall, J. O., Barnes, P. J., and Chung, K. F., Effect of dexamethasone and cyclosporin A on allergen-induced airway hyperresponsiveness and inflammatory cell responses in sensitized Brown-Norway rats, *Am. Rev. Respir. Dis.*, 145, 1289, 1992.

256. Johnston, R. B., Jr., Current concepts: immunology. Monocytes and macrophages, *N. Engl. J. Med.*, 318, 747, 1988.

257. Mackaness, G. B., The monocyte and cellular immunity, *Semin. Hematol.*, 7, 172, 1970.

258. North, R. J., The concept of the activated macrophage, *J. Immunol.*, 121, 806, 1978.

259. Adams, D. O. and Hamilton, T. A., The cell biology of macrophage activation, *Annu. Rev. Immunol.*, 2, 283, 1984.

260. Nathan, C. F., Prendergast, T. J., Wiebe, M. E., Stanley, E. R., Platzer, E., Remold, H. G., Welte, K., Rubin, B. Y., and Murray, H. W., Activation of human macrophages: comparison of other cytokines with interferon-$\gamma$, *J. Exp. Med.*, 160, 600, 1984.

261. Weiser, W. Y., Van Niel, A., Clark, S. C., David, J. R., and Rewold, H. G., Recombinant human granulocyte/macrophage colony-stimulating factor activates intracellular killing of *Leishmania donovani* by human monocyte-derived macrophages, *J. Exp. Med.*, 166, 1436, 1987.

262. Fels, A. O. S. and Cohn, Z. A., The alveolar macrophage, *J. Appl. Physiol.*, 60, 353, 1986.

263. Fuller, R. W., Morris, P. K., Richmond, R., Sykes, D., Varndell, I. M., Kemeny, D. M., Cole, P. J., Dollery, C. T., and MacDermott, J., Immunoglobulin E-dependent stimulation of human alveolar macrophages: significant of type 1 hypersensitivity, *Clin. Exp. Immunol.*, 65, 416, 1986.

264. Joseph, M., Tonnel, A. B., Torpien, G., Capron, A., Arnoux, B., and Benveniste, J., Involvement of immunoglobulin E in the secretory process of alveolar macrophages from asthmatic patients, *J. Clin. Invest.*, 71, 221, 1983.

265. Spiegelberg, H. L., Structure and function of Fc receptors for IgE on lymphocytes, monocytes and macrophages, *Adv. Immunol.*, 35, 61, 1984.

266. MacDermot, J. and Fuller, R. W., Macrophages, in *Asthma: Basic Mechanisms and Clinical Management*, Barnes, P. J., Rodger, I. W., and Thomson, N. C., Eds., Academic Press, London, 1988, 97.

267. Rankin, J. A., The contribution of alveolar macrophages to hyperreactive airway disease, *J. Allergy Clin. Immunol.*, 83, 722, 1989.

268. Henderson, W. R., Jr., Eicosanoids and lung inflammation, *Am. Rev. Respir. Dis.*, 135, 1176, 1987.

269. Marom, Z., Shelhamer, J. H., and Kaliner, M., The effect of arachidonic acid, monohydroxyeicosatetraenoic acid, and prostaglandins on the release of mucous glycoproteins from human airways *in vitro*, *J. Clin Invest.*, 67, 1695, 1981.

270. Barnes, P. J., Chung, K. F., and Page, C. P., Inflammatory mediators and asthma, *Pharmacol. Rev.*, 40, 49, 1988.

271. Dahlen, S. E., Hedqvist, P., Hammarstrom, S., and Samuelsson, B., Leukotrienes are potent constrictors of human bronchi, *Nature*, 288, 484, 1980.

272. Jones, T. R., Davies, C., and Daniel, E. E., Pharmacological study of the contractile activity of leukotriene C₄ and D₄ on isolated human airway smooth muscle, *Can. J. Physiol. Pharmacol.*, 60, 638, 1982.

273. Court, E. N., Goadby, P., Hendrick, D. J., Kelly, C. A., Kingston, W. P., Stenton, S. C., and Walters, E. H., Platelet-activating factor in bronchoalveolar lavage fluid from asthmatic patients, *Br. J. Clin. Pharmacol.*, 24, 258P, 1987.

274. Bruynzeel, P. L., Koenderman, L., Kok, P. T., Hameling, M. L., and Verhagen, J., Platelet activating factor (PAF-acether) induces leukotriene C₄ formation and luninol dependent chemiluminescence in human eosinophils, *Pharmacol. Res. Commun.*, 18 (Suppl.), 61, 1986.

275. Cuss, F. M., Dixon, C. M. S., and Barnes, P. J., Effects of inhaled platelet activating factor on pulmonary function and bronchial responsiveness in man, *Lancet*, 2, 189, 1986.

276. Rubin, A.-H. E., Smith, L. J., and Patterson, R., The bronchoconstrictor properties of platelet-activating factor in humans, *Am. Rev. Respir. Dis.*, 136, 1145, 1987.

277. Lichtenstein, L. M., Histamine-releasing factors and IgE heterogeneity, *J. Allergy Clin. Immunol.*, 81, 814, 1988.

278. Thueson, D. O., Speck, L. S., Lett-Brown, M. A., and Grant, J. A., Histamine-releasing activity (HRA). 1. Production by mitogen or antigen-stimulated human mononuclear cells, *J. Immunol.*, 123, 626, 1979.

279. Knauer, K. A., Kagey-Sobotka, A., Adkinson, N. F., Jr., and Lichtenstein, L. M., Platelet augmentation of IgE-dependent histamine release from human basophils and mast cells, *Int. Arch. Allergy Appl. Immunol.*, 74, 29, 1984.

280. Bascom, R., Wachs, M., Naclerio, R., Pipkorn, U., Galli, S. J., and Lichtenstein, L. M., Basophil influx occurs after nasal antigen challenge: effects of topical corticosteroid pretreatment, *J. Allergy Clin. Immunol.*, 81, 580, 1988.

281. Melewicz, F. M., Zeiger, R. S., Mellon, M. H., O'Connor, R. D., and Spiegelbreg, H. L., Increased peripheral blood monocytes with Rc receptors for IgE in patients with severe allergic disorders, *J. Immunol.*, 126, 1592, 1981.

282. Kay, A. B., Diaz, P., Carmichael, J., and Grant, I. W., Corticosteroid-resistant chronic asthma and monocyte complement receptors, *Clin. Exp. Immunol.*, 44, 576, 1981.

283. Kishimoto, T., Taga, T., Matsuda, T., et al., Interleukin-6 and its receptor in immune regulation, in *Progress in Immunology*, Vol. 7, Melchers, F., Ed., Springer Verlag, Berlin, 1989, 633.

284. Strieter, R. M., Wiggins, R., Phan, S. H., Wharram, B. L., Showell, H. J., Remick, D. G., Chensue, S. W., and Kunkel, S. L., Monocyte chemotactic protein gene expression by cytokine-treated human fibroblasts and endothelial cells, *Biochem. Biophys. Res. Commun.*, 162, 694, 1989.

285. Gauldie, J., Richards, C., Northermann, W., Fey, G., and Baumann, H., IFNβ-2/BSF2/IL-6 is the monocyte-derived HSF that regulates receptor-specific acute phase gene regulation in hepatocytes, *Ann. N.Y. Acad. Sci.*, 557, 46, 1989.

286. Gauldie, J., Cox, G., and Jordana, M., Myeloid growth factors in the lung, in *Cytokines in the Lung*, Kelley, J., Ed., Marcel Dekker, New York, 1992, 369.

287. Jordana, M., Schulman, J., McSharry, C., Irving, L. B., Newhouse, M. T., Jordana, G., and Gauldie, J., Heterogeneous proliferative characteristics of human adult lung fibroblast lines and clonally derived fibroblasts from control and fibrotic tissue, *Am. Rev. Respir. Dis.*, 137, 579, 1988.

288. Richman, P. I., Tilly, R., Jass, J. R., and Bodmer, W. F., Colonic pericrypt sheath cells: characterisation of cell type with a new monoclonal antibody, *J. Clin. Pathol.*, 40, 593, 1987.

289. Brewster, C. E. P., Howarth, P. H., Djukanovic, R., Wilson, J., Holgate, S. T., and Roche, W. R., Myofibroblasts and sub-epithelial fibrosis in bronchial asthma, *Am. J. Respir. Cell Mol. Biol.*, 3, 507, 1990.

290. Norrby, K., Mast cell histamine, a local mitogen acting via H2-receptors in nearby tissue cells, *Virchows Arch. (B)*, 34, 13, 1980.
291. Roche, W. R., Mast cells and tumors. The specific enhancement of tumor proliferation *in vitro*, *Am. J. Pathol.*, 119, 57, 1985.
292. Pincus, S. A., Ramesh, S. H., and Wyler, D. J., Eosinophils stimulate fibroblast DNA synthesis, *Blood*, 70, 572, 1987.
293. Shimokado, K., Raines, E. W., Madtes, D. K., Barrett, T. B., Benditt, E. P., and Ross, R., A significant part of macrophage-derived growth factor consists of at least two forms of PDGF, *Cell*, 43, 277, 1985.
294. Simonson, M. S., Wann, S., Mene, P., Dubyak, G. R., Kester, M., Nakazato, Y., Sedor, J. R., and Dunn, M. J., Endothelin stimulates phospholipase C2 Na+/H+ exchange, *c-fos* expression, and mitogenesis in rat mesangial cells, *J. Clin. Invest.*, 83, 708, 1989.
295. Skalli, O., Schurch, W., Seemayer, T., Lagace, R., Montandon, D., Pittet, B., and Gabbiani, G., Myofibroblasts from diverse pathologic settings are heterogeneous in their content of actin isoforms and intermediate filament proteins, *Lab. Invest.*, 60, 275, 1989.
296. Barnes, P. J., Asthma as an axon reflex, *Lancet*, 1, 242, 1986.
297. Churchill, L., Friedman, B., Schliemer, R. P., and Proud, D., Production of granulocyte-macrophage colony-stimulating factor by cultured human tracheal epithelial cells, *Immunology*, 75, 189, 1992.
298. Kwon, O. J., Collins, P. D., Au, B., Adcock, M., Yacoub, M., Chung, K. F., and Barnes, P. J., Glucocorticoid inhibition of TNFα-induced IL-8 gene expression in human primary cultured epithelial cells, *Immunology*, 81, 379, 1994.
299. Devalia, J. L., Rusznak, C., Sapsford, R. J., Calderon, M., and Davies, R. J., Nitrogen dioxide ($NO_2$)-induced permeability and synthesis of inflammatory cytokines by human bronchial epithelial cell monolayers *in vitro*, *J. Allergy Clin. Immunol.*, 91, 328, 1993.
300. Tosi, M. F., Stark, J. M., Smith, C. W., Hamedani, A., Gruenert, D. C., and Infeld, M. D., Induction of ICAM-1 expression on human airway epithelial cells by inflammatory cytokines: effects on neutrophil-epithelial cell adhesion, *Am. J. Respir. Cell Mol. Biol.*, 7, 214, 1992.
301. Raulet, D. H., Expression and function of interleukin-2 receptors on immature thymocytes, *Nature*, 314, 101, 1985.
302. Crabtree, G. R., Contingent genetic regulatory events in T lymphocyte activation, *Science*, 243, 355, 1989.
303. Wang, H. M. and Smith, K. A., The interleukin 2 receptor: functional consequences of its bi-molecular structure, *J. Exp. Med.*, 166, 1055, 1987.
304. Crosier, P. S., Granulocyte-macrophage colony stimulating factor (GM-CSF), in *Encyclopedia of Immunology*, Vol. 2, Roitt, J. M., Ed., Academic Press, London, 1992, 630.
305. Beutler, B., Milsark, I. W., and Cerami, A. C., Passive immunization against TNF protects mice from lethal effects of endotoxin, *Science*, 229, 552, 1985.
306. Sherry, B. and Cerami, A., Cachectin/tumor necrosis factor exerts endocrine, paracrine, and autocrine control of inflammatory response, *J. Cell Biol.*, 107, 1269, 1988.
307. Renz, H., Saloga, J., Bradley, K. L., Loader, J. E., Greenstein, J. L., Larsen, G., and Gelfand, E. W., Specific Vβ cell subsets mediate the immediate hypersensitivity response to ragweed allergen, *J. Immunol.*, 151, 1907, 1993.
308. Renz, H., Bradley, K., Larsen, G. L., McCall, C., and Gelfand, D. W., Comparison of the allergenicity of avalbumin and avalbumin peptide 323-339: differential expansion of Vβ-expressing T-cell populations, *J. Immunol.*, 151, 7206, 1994.
309. Busse, W. W., Coffman, R. L., Gelfand, E. W., Kay, A. B., and Rosenwasser, L. J., Mechanisms of persistent airway inflammation in asthma: a role for T cells and T-cell products, *Am. J. Respir. Crit. Care Med.*, 152, 388, 1995.
310. Weller, P. F., The immunobiology of eosinophils, *N. Engl. J. med.*, 324, 1110, 1991.
311. Wardlaw, A. J., Moqbel, R., Cromwell, D., and Kay, A. B., Platelet-activating factor. A potent chemotactic and chemokinetic factor for human eosinophils, *J. Clin. Invest.*, 78, 1701, 1986.

312. Braun, R. K., Hansel, T. T., de Vries, I. J. M., Rihs, S., Blaser, K., Erard, F., and Walker, C., Human peripheral blood eosinophils have the capacity to produce IL-8, *Eur. J. Immunol.*, 23(4), 956, 1993.
313. Bradley, B. L., Azzawi, M., Jacobson, M., Assoufi, B., Collins, J. V., Irani, A.-M., Schwartz, L. B., Durham, S. R., Jeffery, P. K., and Kay, A. B., Eosinophils, T-lymphocytes, mast cells, neutrophils, and macrophages in bronchial biopsy specimens from atopic subjects with asthma: comparison with biopsy specimens from atopic subjects without asthma and normal control subjects, and relationship to bronchial responsiveness, *J. Allergy Clin. Immunol.*, 88, 661, 1991.
314. van Oosterhoust, A. J. M., Ladenius, A. R. C., Savelkoul, H. F. J., van Ark, I., Delsman, K. J., and Nijkamp, F. P., Effect of anti-IL-5 and IL-5 on airway hyperreactivity and eosinophils in guinea pigs, *Am. Rev. Respir. Dis.*, 147, 548, 1993.
315. Nakajima, H., Iwanoto, I., Tomoe, S., Matsumura, R., Tomioka, H., Takatsu, K., and Yoshida, S., CD4+ T-lymphocytes and interleukin-5 mediate antigen-induced eosinophil infiltration into the mouse trachea, *Am. Rev. Respir. Dis.*, 146, 374, 1992.
316. Durham, S. R., Cookson, W. O., Faux, J., Craddock, C. F., and Benson, M. K., Basic mechanisms in allergen-induced late asthmatic responses (Abstract), *Clin. Exp. Allergy*, 19, 117A, 1989.
317. Wardlaw, A. J., Chung, K. F., Moqbel, R., MacDonald, A. J., Hartnell, A., McCusker, M., Collins, J. V., Barnes, P. J., and Kay, A. B., Effects of inhaled PAF in humans on circulating and bronchoalveolar lavage fluid neutrophils. Relationship to bronchoconstriction and changes in airway responsiveness, *Am. Rev. Respir. Dis.*, 141, 386, 1988.

Chapter 4

# FIBROGENIC CYTOKINES IN AIRWAY FIBROSIS

Xun Li and John W. Wilson

## CONTENTS

# I. ASTHMA AND AIRWAY INFLAMMATION

Asthma is characterised by episodic, reversible bronchospasm, wheezing, cough and dyspnoea, associated with endobronchial inflammation and airway hyperreactivity. Despite the wide diversity of precipitating factors and clinical definitions of asthma, the pathological changes observed are those of a well-defined, inflammatory disease process involving the airways.[1-3] The classic features of asthma seen at biopsy or post-mortem include loss of the airway surface epithelium and thickening of the subepithelial collagen layer, bronchial vessel dilatation, congestion and oedema, an intense inflammatory cell infiltrate (most notably with eosinophils, mast cells, and lymphocytes), enlargement of the mass of bronchial smooth muscle and mucus-secreting glands.[1-6] All of these changes contribute to thickening of the airway wall. Such thickening has been postulated as a mechanism by which increased bronchial reactivity to nonspecific stimuli may occur in asthma.[7,8] This hypothesis holds that airway wall thickening gives rise to exaggerated changes in airway calibre with smooth muscle shortening. Effectively, small changes in airway wall thickness that have little effect on baseline airway resistance can markedly increase airway responsiveness to inhaled agonists. This model is supported by several studies.[9,10] Another factor affecting the relationship between smooth muscle shortening and airway narrowing is the elastic recoil of airway and lung parenchyma, which exert an outward force opposing airway narrowing. Uncoupling of the interdependence between the airway smooth muscle and its surrounding cartilage in larger airways (or lung parenchyma surrounding small airways) may contribute to bronchial hyperresponsiveness and the loss of a plateau response to methacholine.[11,12] This uncoupling could be caused by airway wall oedema/inflammatory exudate/adventitial fibrosis in asthma and small airway disease.[12] Airway remodelling, characterised by distension of submucosal vessels,[13] oedema, cellular infiltration, and deposition of collagen in the submucosa[14] within the confines of the muscularis, will further constrain tissue expansion to the luminal side of the muscularis and may consequently act to inhibit full bronchodilatation. Although the characteristics of airway fibrosis and its significance have not been fully addressed, its importance for the pathophysiology of asthma is clear. Fixed airflow obstruction and persisting BHR after steroid treatment may be attributable to fibrotic and other structural changes in the airway wall.[14,15]

# II. SUBEPITHELIAL FIBROSIS
# IN ASTHMATIC AIRWAYS

An apparent increase in thickness of the supporting "basement membrane" has been observed by light microscopy in fatal asthma since the early 1950s.[1,17] Subsequent studies confirmed this "thickened basement membrane" as a consistent finding in asthma, even in mild disease.[18-21] This apparent hyaline, eosinophilic thickening of the bronchial epithelial basement membrane under light microscopy was initially thought to be most likely the result of repetitive injury to the epithelial cell, resulting in basement membrane hypersecretion.[19,22] A recent observation in bronchial biopsies has shown that it is the reticular and not the basal lamina which becomes thickened in atopic asthma.[20] The true basement membrane has been identified by immunostaining with a specific monoclonal antibody to type IV collagen and has been found to be of normal thickness. Immunohistochemical studies have shown this thickened reticular layer to comprise predominantly types I, III, and V collagen (scar-type collagens) present together with fibronectin but not laminin. The term *subepithelial fibrosis* has been introduced to describe these changes.[20] More recently, we have demonstrated scar-type collagen extending deeper into the asthmatic bronchial submucosa in addition to the most superficial 10 µm below the true basement membrane. Typically, sections of the asthmatic airway show a greater percentage area covered with collagen types III and V compared with control airways[14] (Figure 1).

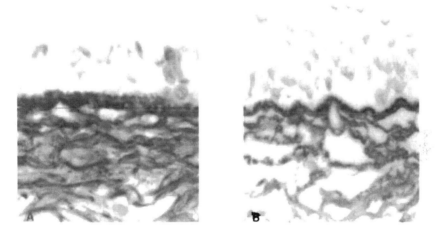

**FIGURE 1** Collagen deposition in the asthmatic bronchial wall. There is a thickened subepithelial collagen layer, and the submucosa shows more immunoreactive collagen type III in asthma (A), compared with control airways (B).

## III. STRUCTURE AND EXTRACELLULAR MATRIX COMPONENT OF THE NORMAL AIRWAY

Extracellular matrix not only serves as scaffolding to stabilise the physical structure of tissues, but also plays a far more active and complex role in regulating the behaviour of the cells it surrounds — influencing their development, migration, proliferation, shape, and metabolic function. The extracellular matrix has a correspondingly complex molecular composition. Unfortunately, our understanding of its nature is still fragmentary. Matrix is made up of two major classes of extracellular macromolecules. They are the collagens and proteoglycans, with collagen being the major constituent.[23]

Collagens are a family of highly characteristic fibrous proteins sharing a common structure, that is, a rigid triple-stranded helical chain. So far, 11 types of collagen molecules encoded by a group of 20 genes[23,24] have been described, each having distinctive structural and metabolic characteristics and different identifiable functions. The predominant are types I, II, III, IV, and V.[23,25] Types I, II, and III are the main types of collagen found in connective tissues.[23,25,26] Type IV collagen is the main constituent of basement membrane and is thought to be a product of cells resting on it, principally epithelial and endothelial cells.[25,26] Type V collagen, the structure of which is still the subject of controversy, is present in laminae and interstitium and smooth muscle.[25-27]

In the normal airway, there are several readily distinguishable layers by light microscopy, namely, surface epithelium, basement membrane, lamina propria, smooth muscle, submucosa, cartilage, and adventitia. Ultrastructurally, the basement membrane of the human airway consists of two distinct layers: a basal lamina and a reticular collagenous lamina (Figure 2).[18,28] The basal lamina (true basement membrane) largely comprises type IV collagen, proteoglycans, laminin, and fibronectin. The reticular collagenous lamina or subepithelial collagen layer predominantly comprises types III and V collagen together with fibronectin.[20] Beneath this is a bed of stromal tissue predominantly comprised of mesenchymal cells, fibroblasts, and smooth muscle cells, embedded in matrix. The matrix substance of normal airways, like other organs, is composed of a wide array of immunologically and biochemically distinct elements: collagens (collagens I, III, V), elastins, proteoglycans, fibronectins, and laminins (Plate 1* and Figure 3). The major components, collagens (types I and III) and elastin, are the primary determinants of the physical properties of bronchioles. In the upper airway there is the additional support to the cartilaginous structures composed predominantly of type II collagen.[29]

## IV. PATHOPHYSIOLOGY OF FIBROSIS

The fibroblast is the effector cell in the fibrotic process. It has four main actions during wound healing: (1) migration to the site of injury, (2) proliferation, (3) production of collagen and matrix proteins, and (4) wound contraction. These actions of fibroblasts are regulated by the soluble products elaborated by activated cells present in chronically inflamed tissues.[30] Jordana and co-workers[31,32] investigated the characteristics of human fibroblast cell lines derived from inflamed airway tissue. These cell lines proliferated at a faster rate and expressed collagen I and III genes at a higher ratio when compared with cell lines from control lung.[31,32] These observations indicate

---

* Plate 1 follows page 80.

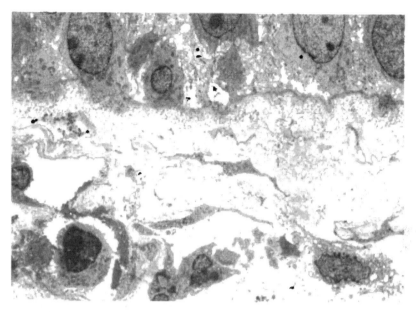

**FIGURE 2** Structure of the subepithelial collagen layer by transmission electron microscopy showing subepithelial collagen, true basement membrane, myofibroblast, epithelial cells, and vessels.

**Subepithelial collagen layer**
**(Collagens I, III, V, fibronectin)**

**True basement membrane**
**(Collagen IV, fibronectin, laminin)**

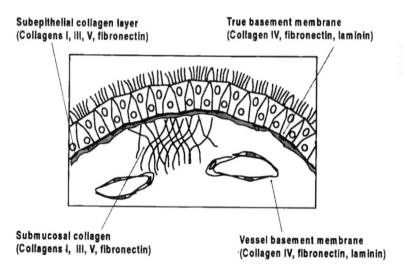

**Submucosal collagen**
**(Collagens I, III, V, fibronectin)**

**Vessel basement membrane**
**(Collagen IV, fibronectin, laminin)**

**FIGURE 3** Distribution of collagen subtypes in the airway submucosa.

that isolated fibroblasts from inflamed airway appear to be activated or to change their phenotype to favour tissue fibrosis.

There are several potential mechanisms for enhanced tissue fibrosis:[33,34] (1) an increase in fibroblast number, as a result of either fibroblast proliferation or recruitment of fibroblasts into the injured tissues, (2) increased collagen biosynthesis by individual fibroblasts, and (3) diminished collagen degradation.

## A. FIBROBLAST PROLIFERATION

Current theories of cell division propose that at least two different classes of signal are required for fibroblast mitosis to occur.[35] These signals are (1) competence factors, which induce cells in G0 phase of the cell cycle to enter G1 and (2) progression factors, which stimulate competence-primed cells to complete G1 and progress to the S phase of the cell cycle. The important competence factors for fibroblasts include platelet-derived growth factor (PDGF), fibroblast growth factor (FGF), and fibronectin. Insulin-like growth factor (IGF) and transforming growth factor-β (TGFβ) are known to be progression factors for fibroblasts. These growth factors will be discussed in the following section.

## B. PRODUCTION OF COLLAGEN

Regulation of collagen production by fibroblasts may occur at every level of the processes of collagen gene expression, including procollagen gene transcription, translation of procollagen mRNA, or posttranslation modification of the procollagen molecule.[36] Again, cytokines and mediators released by activated resident or infiltrating cells play an important role in regulation of expression of collagen genes in both normal and inflamed tissues. One such cytokine fulfilling this role is TGFβ, which is a potent stimulant for the synthesis of procollagen and fibronectin by fibroblasts.[37] In addition to TGFβ, other cytokines such as PDGF(B), IGF-1, interleukin 1 (IL-1), and tumour necrosis factor-α (TNFα) may also influence the production of collagen.

## C. COLLAGEN DEGRADATION

Collagen degradation is a third mechanism responsible for the regulation of collagen homeostasis in injured tissues. Regulation factors include a wide range of enzymes and mediators, including neutral proteases, collagenases, gelatinase,[38] prostaglandin $PGE_2$, and epidermal growth factor (EGF).[39] In addition, TGFβ has also been shown to have an inhibitory action on collagenase secretion by fibroblasts,[40] thereby exhibiting a counterregulatory effect.

The balance between synthesis and degradation of extracellular matrix is essential to maintain tissue integrity following injury and is regulated by cytokines derived from cells present in chronically inflamed tissues.[30] These cytokines include the inflammatory cytokines and growth factors. If this balance is altered when initiating signals override regulatory termination signals, as is seen in repeated injury and chronic inflammation, tissue fibrosis will occur (Figure 4). Understanding the mechanisms of airway wall fibrosis has been greatly enhanced by observations derived from animal models and other human diseases, including idiopathic pulmonary fibrois and ARDS.[36,41-43] There is accumulating evidence to suggest that overexpression of fibrogenic cytokines or growth factors occurs in interstitial pulmonary fibrosis. The

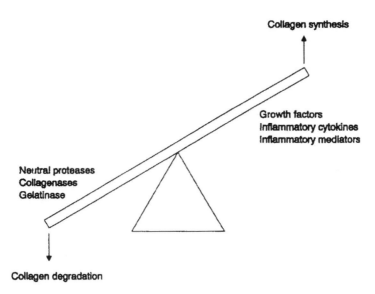

**FIGURE 4**  Balance between synthesis and degradation of extracellular matrix in tissue integrity. Any cause of increased synthesis of collagen or decreased degradation of collagen will result in enhancement of fibrosis.

sequential relationship between pulmonary inflammation with cellular activation and eventual fibrosis with collagen deposition in alveolar spaces has provided information with fundamental bearing on the relationship between airway inflammation and subepithelial fibrosis in asthma.

## V. FIBROGENIC CYTOKINES AND GROWTH FACTORS IMPLICATED IN THE REGULATION OF FIBROSIS

### A. PLATELET-DERIVED GROWTH FACTOR

PDGF is a dimeric molecule of two polypeptide chains, A and B. The AB heterodimer and BB homodymer are capable of binding the PDGFβ ligand, which is the dominant receptor on lung fibroblasts[44] and one of the most important in the fibrotic response.[30] Although initially discovered in platelets, PDGF$_{BB}$ is known to be produced by activated macrophages, endothelial cells, epithelial cells, smooth muscle cells, and fibroblasts.[45,46] PDGF is a highly potent, serum-derived mitogen,[47] particularly for smooth muscle and fibroblasts.[48,49] It is a strong chemoattractant for fibroblasts,[50] stimulates fibroblast contractility,[51] and stimulates fibroblast collagenase production.[52] PDGF may play a role in pathogenesis of fibrotic disorders such as scleroderma, rheumatoid arthritis, and atherosclerosis.[45] PDGF may also act as a secondary stimulus for fibroblast replication, as PDGF production and autostimulation has been shown to occur after priming of fibroblasts with both TNFα[53] and IL-1.[54] Direct evidence for involvement in pulmonary fibrosis comes from the finding of mRNA for PDGF-B in alveolar macrophages from patients with pulmonary fibrosis and sarcoidosis.[55,56] Gene expression has also been found to be increased in alveolar epithelial cells in lung biopsies from patients with fibrotic lung disease, using immunohistochemistry and *in situ* hybridisation techniques.[57] This information suggests that PDGF is capable of acting as a profibrogenic cytokine and is circumstantially present in fibrotic tissues, making it a likely candidate for a link between chronic inflammation and scar formation.

## B. TRANSFORMING GROWTH FACTOR-β

TGFβ is secreted by platelets, macrophages, and activated T-lymphocytes. Receptors have been identified on most cell types.[58] TGFβ was initially recognised by its ability to transform normal rat fibroblasts *in vitro*.[59,60] Subsequent studies have shown this factor to have a broad spectrum of biologic activity including an important role in fibrogenesis. TGFβ is capable of attracting fibroblasts, inducing fibroblast proliferation, stimulating synthesis of collagen and fibronectin by fibroblasts, while also inhibiting collagenase production, thus decreasing degradation of the existing extracellular matrix.[37,61,62] Administration of TGFβ promotes wound repair and fibrosis in animals,[63,64] possibly through its fibroblast-stimulating action. Animal models of pulmonary fibrosis based on the intratracheal instillation of bleomycin have shown the increased expression of mRNA for TGFβ before the onset of histological fibrosis.[65] Biopsies from patients with pulmonary fibrosis have shown increased TGFβ production,[66] while *in situ* hybridisation has revealed high levels of procollagen, fibronectin, and TGFβ mRNA in adjacent macrophages in lung specimens from these patients.[67] These studies provide evidence for the role of TGFβ in pulmonary fibrosis, but have not provided direct information regarding airway changes in these models. Interestingly, following bleomycin exposure, rat lung fibroblasts increase collagen synthesis together with increasing the expression of TGFβ mRNA and TGFβ protein.[68] This work has suggested a possible autocrine loop for fibroblast stimulation in fibrotic disorders, leading to the concept of receptor "upregulation" and a phenotype characterised by more severe and aggressive fibrosis.[69] This most significant finding also links the expression of cytokine mRNA with cytokine product and collagen production, indicating that modulation of gene expression may provide an avenue for future therapy of fibrotic disorders, including airway remodelling. Gauldie and co-workers[69] have suggested that TGFβ has three actions in tissue fibrosis: (1) a direct effect on gene expression of matrix cells to increase collagen synthesis and reduce collagenase production; (2) the induction of fibroblast proliferation, probably indirectly through the actions of PDGF; and (3) the establishment of autostimulatory activation of structural cells, including fibroblasts. The potential involvement of TGFβ in subepithelial fibrosis of asthmatic airways has been suggested, based on expression of the TGFβ gene in eosinophils in inflamed upper airways.[70] Interestingly, immunohistochemical localisation studies in pulmonary fibrosis have shown TFGβ to be found in epithelial cells in patients with active disease,[66] indicating the potential for the epithelium to act as a stimulus for fibrosis. It is therefore curious that other localisation studies[70] have not found such obvious expression, in the presence of subepithelial fibrosis in the upper (nasal) airway. However, a more recent study on both surgical and necropsy specimens from asthmatic patients has not found significant overexpression of TGFβ in asthmatic airways at either the mRNA or protein level when compared with airways from COAD or nonobstructed smoking patients suffering lung cancer.[71] Further studies including healthy controls and more homogeneous asthmatic populations are warranted to confirm this observation.

## C. INSULIN-LIKE GROWTH FACTOR 1

The IGFs are peptides with the capacity to stimulate cell proliferation and differentiation.[72-74] Two main forms of IGFs have been identified: IGF-1 and IGF-2.[73] Although knowledge of the function of IGFs is far from complete, IGF-1 is generally considered as an important postnatal growth factor, whereas IGF-2 is thought to be involved in foetal development and to have a significant role in the development of certain malignant tumours. The liver is the major site of IGF-1 synthesis, contributing to high circulating IGF levels,[75] although synthesis of these factors is known to occur locally in a wide variety of other tissues. In the lung, macrophages and fibroblasts would seem to be an important source of IGF-1.[76] IGF-1 seems likely to play a role in tissue repair after injury based on its ability to enhance division of primed fibroblasts, as well as stimulating collagen production.[77,78] IGF-1 is thought to be an important constituent of progression-type growth factor activity produced by human alveolar macraphages.[79] This progression factor for fibroblasts has been shown to be spontaneously released from alveolar macrophages from patients with fibrosing alveolitis and asbestosis.[80] There is evidence to suggest that IGF-1 production by macrophages may be increased during the process of fibrogenesis. Macrophages at sites of wound repair have been shown to express mRNA for IGF-1.[81] The production of progression-type growth factors by human alveolar macrophages has been demonstrated to be increased in fibrosing conditions, such as pulmonary fibrosis,[82] systemic sclerosis,[83] and asbestosis.[84] These findings imply that IGF-1 may participate in tissue remodelling following chronic inflammation or injury.

## D. TUMOUR NECROSIS FACTOR

The term *tumour necrosis factor* describes two distinct peptides, TNFα and TNFβ. TNFα is produced predominantly by monocytes and macrophages,[85] while TNFβ (lymphotoxin) is produced predominantly by lymphocytes.[86,87] Both molecules bind to the same receptors (TNFα p55 and TNFα p75 receptors) and target cells and have similar biologic activities.[88,89] TNFα is a multifunctional cytokine and is generally considered to be a proinflammatory cytokine that acts together with IL-1 to orchestrate local inflammation. This proinflammatory action is most likely mediated by (1) activating neutrophils, lymphocytes, and monocytes, (2) inducing endothelial cells to express

leukocyte adhesion molecules, and (3) inciting production of secondary cytokines and other inflammatory mediators. All of these actions would be likely
to indirectly initiate local tissue-remodelling processes, including a biphasic
effect on growth of airway smooth muscle.[90] At the same time, TNFs have
direct actions on fibroblast proliferation and collagen synthesis. TNFα can
directly stimulate fibroblast replication.[91,92] TNFα has been reported to be able
to modulate fibroblast extracellular matrix degradation,[93] inhibit fibroblast
collagen production, and increase collagenase production.[94,95] TNFα can also
induce the synthesis of another potent fibroblast growth factor — TGFβ.[95]
TNF may be an important cytokine in the development of pulmonary fibrosis.
TNFα mRNA from whole lung was found to be increased in bleomycin-
induced pulmonary fibrosis in a rat model, while antiserum to TNFα was able
to prevent the development of pulmonary fibrosis.[97] The importance of TNF
in silica-induced pulmonary fibrosis has also been demonstrated in mice.[98]
The relationship of TNFα to other growth factors is not yet established;
however, in the rat–bleomycin model, TNFα appeared early, while TGFβ
mRNA and proteins were subsequently expressed during a phase of collagen
production.[99] TNFα might therefore be acting to prime fibroblasts for stimulation by other factors.

Recent evidence suggests that the production of TNFα is increased in
asthmatic airways. Significantly elevated levels of TNFα derived from cultured
asthmatic bronchoalveolar lavage (BAL) cells has been reported in both
stable[100] and allergen-challenged states.[101] Elevated levels of TNFα have been
found in BAL from symptomatic asthmatic subjects.[102] mRNA for TNFα was
found to be increased in stable, atopic asthmatic subjects when compared with
controls.[103] Bradding and co-workers[104] have shown a sevenfold increase in
TNFα within mast cells in biopsies from the airways of patients with mild
asthma. Thus, TNFα is likely to act as an important signal to activate fibroblast
and initiate tissue remodelling in chronic asthmatic airways.

## E. GRANULOCYTE/MACROPHAGE
## COLONY-STIMULATING FACTOR

Granylocyte/macrophage colony-stimulating factor (GM-CSF) is a glycoprotein of 127 amino acids encoded by a gene on chromosome 5, produced
by a range of cells resident within the airway, including T-lymphocytes,
macrophages, epithelium, fibroblasts, eosinophils, and mast cells.[105-113] It acts
to prime, activate, and induce replication of constituent airway cells in asthma,
including eosinophils, mast cells, and fibroblasts.[114-117] Gauldie et al.[69] have
raised the prospect that GM-CSF may be influential in airway fibrosis, as well
as in the perpetuation of inflammation. Fibroblasts actively produce GM-CSF
capable of supporting eosinophils,[107] and subcutaneous administration of
GM-CSF by infusion pump may induce a fibroblast proliferate response.[117]
GM-CSF-derived fibroblast proliferation led to an accumulation of alpha-
actin-positive myofibroblasts, such as those seen below the subepithelial collagen layer in asthma.[118] The ability of GM-CSF to induce fibroblast phenotype

differentiation may be inferred from its ability to induce fibroblast colony formation from bone marrow stromal cells in anchorage-independent growth conditions.[119] Hence, GM-CSF, although considered to be predominantly proinflammatory in nature, may be relatively influential in regulating fibroblast replication and activity within the bronchial submucosa.

## F. INTERLEUKIN 1

IL-1 is produced predominantly by monocytes and macrophages but may be liberated by other cell types. IL-1 comprises two gene products, IL-1$\alpha$ and IL-1$\beta$, which are chemically distinct but have similar biologic activities and bind the same membrane receptor.[120] In addition to its action as a signal for lymphocyte activation, IL-1 stimulates fibroblast proliferation, probably through indirect means by the induction of the PDGF-A gene.[54,121] IL-1 also increases synthesis of extracellular matrix components such as fibronectin and types I, III, and IV collagen.[122,123] Increased IL-1 produced by alveolar macrophages has been found in patients with the fibrosing pulmonary disorder of sarcoidosis.[124] Furthermore, this increased activity has been shown to correlate with the degree of alveolitis, suggesting that IL-1 may initiate and maintain inflammation in the lung in a form that has pulmonary fibrosis as a sequel.[125] There is evidence that IL-1 may participate in the development of other forms of pulmonary fibrosis. It has been demonstrated that alveolar macrophages release increased amounts of IL-1 after exposure to silica,[126] asbestos fibres,[127] and bleomycin[128] in animal models. IL-1 may also act indirectly, through T-lymphocyte activation, with the secondary release of other fibrogenic cytokines, including TNF$\beta$, TFG$\beta$, and PGDF.[16]

## G. INTERFERONS

The interferons (IFNs) are a heterogenous group of molecules with a range of antiviral, antiproliferative, and immunomodulatory functions.[129,130] IFNs have the capacity to inhibit many aspects of the fibrotic response while also acting as proinflammatory cytokines through the induction of macrophage activation and class I and II MHC antigen expression. IFNs inhibit fibroblast chemotaxis,[131] and proliferation.[131-133] Accordingly, IFN$\gamma$, secreted by stimulated T-lymphocytes, plays dual roles in the pathogenesis of fibrosis in inflammatory disorders. It may act early in fibrogenesis to promote macrophage activation and secretion of fibrogenic cytokines, including TGF$\beta$, PDGF, IGF-I, and TNF$\beta$, and later in a regulatory role to inhibit collagen synthesis.[134] Indeed, a recent study in patients with sarcoidosis has shown that higher serum levels of IFN$\gamma$ are associated with a more favourable outcome and responsiveness to corticosteroids on clinical assessment.[135] In contrast, Moseley and coworkers[136] have demonstrated that BAL cells from patients with pulmonary sarcoidosis spontaneously release IFN$\gamma$ *in vitro*. However, this release of IFN$\gamma$ was associated with the simultaneous elaboration of growth factor activity for fibroblasts *in vitro* and focal abnormalities seen on chest X-rays.[136] This paradoxical role of INF$\gamma$ in the development of lung fibrosis associated with sarcoidosis may act to maintain the dynamic balance between pro- and anti-fibrogenic cytokines in collagen homeostasis. It is noteworthy that local T-lymphocyte activation and mast cell infiltration are both associated with sarcoidosis[137-140] and bronchial asthma.[6,29,141-143]

## H. FIBROBLAST GROWTH FACTORS

Originally purified from pituitary extracts, FGFs are mitogenic for fibroblasts, endothelial cells, epithelial cells, and other cells of mesenchymal origin. They are described as acidic FGF (aFGF) and basic FGF (bFGF), depending upon their isoelectric point. bFGF was first described by Gospodarowicz[144] who extracted it from bovine brain. A second factor, also isolated from brain, had an acidic isoelectric point and was also capable of stimulating 3T3 cell proliferation.[145] Further characterisation of FGFs has shown at least five other polypeptides with amino acid sequence homology and mitogenic activity.[146]

Basic fibroblast growth factor is a 146 amino acid protein with an isoelectric point of 9.6.[147] The gene for bFGF on chromosome 4 codes for both the 155 amino acid protein and a number of forms of higher molecular weight. The source of bFGF is unclear, although it is produced *in vitro* by fibroblasts, endothelial cells, glial cells, and smooth muscle cells.[148-154] Both bFGF and aFGF undergo heparin binding, a factor which may alter biologic potency.[155] Several associated FGFs have also been described, predominantly in developing tissues rather than in the adult state, or in tumours.[146] A family of FGF receptors has been identified and cloned.[156] At least one member of the FGF receptor family (FGFR-3) can be activated by both aFGF and bFGF. bFGF has been shown to bind to heparin-like molecules in basement membranes,[157] suggesting a "storage" form, which may be more stable and protected from denaturation. Also, the biologic activity of aFGF is enhanced by the addition of heparan sulphate proteoglycans.[158] Such an effect may be due to conformational changes in the molecule brought about by this interaction.

Other than inducing fibroblast proliferation, FGFs are powerful inducers of angiogenesis.[159] Studies on cultured endothelial cells have shown that bFGF may induce penetration of basement membranes *in vitro*.[160] The FGFs, therefore, have the capacity to induce wound healing in animal models[161] and induce angiogenesis. Although true neovascularisation has not been shown to occur in asthma, the increased vascularity seen in the distal airway may be attributable to bFGF.[13] bFGF has been localised to epithelial cells of the trachea and bronchi,[162] suggesting a local effect on fibroblasts in the region of the basement membrane. Possibly, bFGF may act as a factor responsible for the laying down of subepithelial collagen beneath the epithelium and in the deep submucosa in asthma, as has been recently described.[14,20]

## VI. AIRWAY INFLAMMATION AND FIBROSIS

The finding that there is more type III and V collagen in the subepithelial region of the asthmatic airway implies a site-directed insult by the inflammatory response to the injured epithelium.[16] Indeed, epithelial denudation of the trachea in graft experiments leads to an intense fibrotic reaction, which may be abrogated by re-epithelialisation.[163] Other structures, including bronchial capillary endothelium, may also be contributory to fibrosis. Capillary leakage, the hallmark of ARDS, which has fibrosis as a sequel, has been clearly demonstrated in models of pulmonary fibrosis before the onset of overt scar formation.[164-167] It is well established that bronchial capillary leakage and oedema are features of asthma.[168] Possibly, mast cells (which produce the vasoactive mediators $LTC_4$, $PGD_2$, and tryptase) may provide the link between vascular leakage and fibrosis.[169] However, bleomycin has been shown to induce pulmonary fibrosis in congenitally mast cell-deficient mice.[170]

Since collagen types III and V are cross-linked interstitial collagen, whereas type IV collagen is epithelial cell derived,[26,171] expansion of the subepithelial collagen layer is most likely to originate from fibroblasts rather than from the epithelium. Indeed, a study combining electron microscopic and immunohistochemical methods has shown that there is an increased number of myofibroblasts in lower levels of reticular collagen in bronchial biopsies from atopic asthmatic subjects. There was a close correlation between actin-negative myofibroblast numbers and thickness of the collagen layer.[118] This observation suggests proliferation of myofibroblasts under the influence of mitogens produced by inflammatory cells in the asthmatic airway may be responsible for the characteristic subepithelial fibrosis. This hypothesis is supported by evidence indicating that the thickness of the basement membrane estimated by light microscopy correlates with the degree of submucosal mast cell infiltration in bronchial biopsies[172] and numbers of eosinophils in BAL from asthmatic asthma.[173] Haslam reported increased numbers of mast cells and eosinophils in BAL from patients with pulmonary fibrosis, although lung biopsies did not provide correlative evidence for their role in causing alveolar damage.[174,175] BAL fluid from such patients significantly stimulated the replication of fibroblasts *in vitro* through the action of unidentified factors.[176]

Eosinophils contain major basic protein, eosinophil cationic protein, and eosinophil peroxidase, all of which may cause tissue injury.[177] There are several important observations suggesting that eosinophils may play a role in the stimulation of collagen production. Asthmatic subjects frequently have an eosinophilia in blood and bronchial lavage, increased numbers of eosinophils can be demonstrated beneath the epithelial basement membrane, and IL-5, a supporting cytokine for eosinophils, as well as its mRNA, can be found in asthmatic airways.[178,179] In other eosinophilic disorders, excessive eosinophilia may be associated with collagen deposition and tissue fibrosis. These include the hypereosinophilic syndrome, in which endomyocardial fibrosis is a known complication,[180] and cryptogenic fibrosing alveolitis, in which an elevated eosinophil count in BAL is frequently associated with a more likely progression to lung fibrosis.[181] There is increasing recognition that tissue-dwelling eosinophils and fibroblasts may interact. It has been demonstrated that eosinophil-conditioned media can stimulate human lung fibroblasts to proliferate *in vitro*[182] and eosinophil cationic protein can stimulate fibroblasts in culture to synthesise hyaluronan and proteoglycans.[183] The discovery that human blood eosinophils produce both the mRNA for TGFβ and its protein product provides molecular evidence for their fibroblast-stimulating potential.[184] Furthermore, Ohno and co-workers[70] found that eosinophils were the major cell type expressing mRNA for TGFβ in human nasal polyp biopsy tissue. Histopathologically, nasal polyposis and asthma, both respiratory tract inflammatory disorders related by atopy, share a number of common features, including fibroblast proliferation, an inflammatory cell infiltrate, especially with eosinophils, and a thickened basement membrane.[3,185] This work implies that eosinophils may be a potent local source of this fibrogenic cytokine, through which they link chronic airway inflammation and fibrosis.

Mast cells, considered for some time to play a central role in the pathogenesis of asthma,[186] are another potential candidate for a link between asthmatic airway inflammation and fibrosis. Mast cells have been demonstrated in increased numbers and activation status within the mucosa and bronchial lavage from asthmatic patients.[6,142,143] There are several lines of evidence implicating mast cells with the induction of fibrosis. First, mast cell hyperplasia has been described in a variety of conditions characterised by inflammation and fibrosis.[187] These include systemic sclerosis,[188] sarcoidosis, hypersensitivity pneumonitis, and idiopathic pulmonary fibrosis.[140,189] Mast cells have been described in animal models of pulmonary fibrosis resulting from exposure to asbestos,[190] bleomycin,[191] and ionizing radiation.[192] Second, mast cells have been shown to be capable of stimulating fibroblast proliferation and collagen synthesis. Mouse mast cells in culture induce multiplication of fibroblasts and increase collagen accumulation in the extracellular matrix.[193] Histamine, a major preformed mediator of human mast cells, has been shown to stimulate the growth of fibroblasts *in vitro* and *in vivo*.[194,195] Recent studies by Tomlinson and co-workers[196] showed that the mast cell granule contents stimulates, while heparin inhibits, proliferation of human airway fibroblasts *in vitro*. In addition to mediator production, murine mast cells have the ability to produce fibrogenic cytokines such as TGFβ.[197] Third, a correlation between numbers of mast cells and degree of fibrosis has been recently described in human lung biopsy specimens from fibrotic lung disorders.[140] Aldenborg et al.[192] have shown that numbers of mast cells, as well as histamine content, strongly correlate with exposure to radiation in fibrotic regions of the lung in radiation-induced pulmonary fibrosis. Mast cell numbers are also increased, albeit to a lesser extent, in lung regions exposed to irradiation but without fibrosis. Finally, ultrastructural studies provide evidence of mast cell activation in the form of piecemeal degranulation present in the same irradiated animal model.[192] Such mast cells bear close resemblance to the activated cells described in asthmatic airways by Djukanovic and co-workers.[169] These observations bring forth the notion of a major role for the mast cell in fibrosis.

Other types of cells may also participate in the progression of fibrosis in asthmatic airways. Monocyte/macrophages, the predominant cells in bronchial lavage, are capable of the synthesis and release a wide range of growth factors and mediators, such as PDGF, TGFβ, FGF, IL-1β, IL-1α, and TNFα, which are known regulators of fibroblast proliferation and collagen synthesis.[30] Indeed, there are increased numbers of macrophages in lung biopsy specimens from patients with lung fibrotic disorders.[198] Products of tissue injury, including collagen and elastin peptide fragments, may be chemotactic for macrophages and lymphocytes. Furthermore, it is likely that the production of growth factors by macrophages may be secondarily enhanced in inflammatory disorders.

Recent evidence suggests that T-lymphocytes may also play a role in the pathogenesis of fibrosis by releasing cytokines. They may act on fibroblast possible subclass effects (Th, Ts, Th1, Th2), either directly (IFNγ) or indirectly (IL-2, IL-3, IL-5, GM-CSF), by enhancing the activation of macrophages, eosinophils, or mast cells. Thus, while T-lymphocytes very likely orchestrate the allergic inflammatory response in asthma, they are capable of modulating fibrogenic cytokine release by other cells and driving the repair processes manifest as subepithelial fibrosis and submucosal collagen deposition.[14,16] Pulmonary fibrosis, sarcoidosis, and asthmatic inflammation are all characterised by infiltration with activated T-lymphocytes.[29,137,138,141,199-201] Taking all this evidence together, a working hypothesis to explain the pathogenesis of airway fibrosis in asthma can be described and is schematically represented in Figure 5.

Genetic and/or environmental factors favour the proliferation of allergen-specific T cell clones which produce and release IL-3, IL-4, IL-5, and GM-CSF. These cytokines induce principal immunological events, including the release of IgE from B cells, activation and degranulation of mast cells and migration, and increased survival and activation of eosinophils in the airway. The end result is chronic airway inflammation with eosinophilia. The persistence of inflammation and injury leads to an imbalance between stimulatory and inhibitory mechanisms in favour of fibrosis. This enhanced stimulation is most likely mediated by persistently activated eosinophils, mast cells, and macrophages that are present in chronically inflamed tissues. Since the reported association between EBV and pulmonary fibrosis,[202] several studies have provided evidence proposing the expression of viral genes in mesenchymal and epithelial cells of the lung. Such gene activation could act permissively, resulting in extracellular matrix production, presumably by initiating expression of genes for synthesis of collagen,[203,204] as well as by directly inducing the expression of fibrogenic cytokines (TNFα and TGFβ).[205,206] Following acute bronchiolitis, Macek and co-workers[207] have found that there was a persistent and/or latent adenoviral infection in the lungs of children with subsequent chronic airway obstruction, compared with those without chronic airflow obstruction. These observations are reminiscent of viral–gene incorporation theories invoked to explain the presence of persistent airway inflammation in asthma and may also shed new light on the pathogenesis of tissue fibrosis.

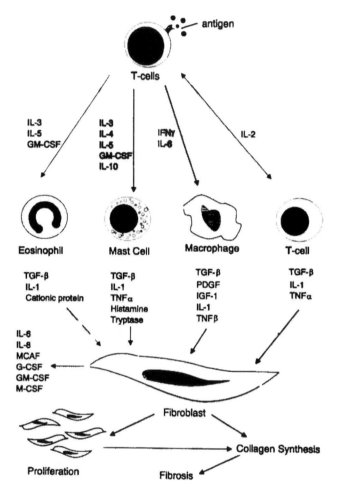

**FIGURE 5**  Hypothetical pathogenesis of airway fibrosis in asthma. The dependence of the fibroblast on growth factors produced by inflammatory cells in the asthmatic airway.

## VII. SIGNIFICANCE OF AIRWAY FIBROSIS IN ASTHMA

To date, the pathophysiological significance of subepithelial fibrosis is not clear. It has been postulated that it may be contributory to irreversible airway obstruction with incomplete responsiveness to $\beta_2$-agonists and persisting BHR after steroid treatment.[14-16] Evidence exists to show that asthmatic airways are more rigid and less distensible than controls.[208] Airway rigidity with loss of normal conducting ability may be seen as analogous to the functional deficit seen in myocardial fibrosis or collagenous colitis.[209,210] Treatment of asthma with $\beta$-agonists alone has little or no effect on airway inflammation and may result in poorer control of disease.[211,212] Normally, $FEV_1$ annually decreases with age, but this decline is accelerated in some individuals with asthma.[211,213] A recent study has shown that long-term inhaled corticosteroid therapy (BDP 800 μg for 2 years) reduced the accelerated decline in $FEV_1$ in one group of patients with asthma.[214] Whether this effect was due to reduced airway inflammation and collagen deposition or to changes in other components of the airway is not certain. In one long-term, uncontrolled study in which inflammation was suppressed with inhaled corticosteroids over 10 years, there was no apparent change in the thickness of sub-basement membrane collagen seen by light microscopy.[15] Similarly, a small, uncontrolled study of six patients by Jeffery and co-workers[21] using budesonide 400 μg per day for 4 weeks found no change in subepithelial collagen. A longer, 3-month placebo-controlled study using 1200 μg budesonide daily also found no effect on subepithelial collagen.[215] Trigg and co-workers,[216] however, have recently reevaluated these findings in a controlled study using beclomethesone dipropionate 500 μg twice daily for 4 months. There was a significant reduction in deposition of type III collagen in the sub-basement membrane region, indicating that inhaled steroids are capable of reversing this facet of airway remodelling in asthma. Further studies to elucidate the relationship between this pathological remodelling and physiological impairment of the airway in asthma are needed.

## ACKNOWLEDGMENTS

The authors wish to acknowledge the assistance of Ms. Barbara Welton with the preparation of the manuscript.

## REFERENCES

1. Dunnill, M. S., The pathology of asthma, with special changes in the bronchial mucosa, *J. Clin. Pathol.*, 13, 27, 1960.
2. Hogg, J. C., James, A. L., and Pare, P. D., Evidence for inflammation in asthma, *Am. Rev. Respir. Dis.*, 143(3), S39, 1991.
3. Jeffery, P. K., Pathology of asthma, *Br. Med. Bull.*, 48, 23, 1992a.
4. Beasley, R., Roche, W. R., Roberts, J. A., and Holgate, S. T., Cellular events in the bronchi in mild asthma and after bronchial provocation, *Am. rev. Respir. Dis.*, 139, 806, 1989.
5. Bradley, B. L., Azzawi, M., Jacobson, M., Assoufi, B., Collins, J. V., Irani, A. M., Schwartz, L. B., Durham, S. R., Jeffrey, P. K., and Kay, A. B., Eosinophils, T-lymphocytes, mast cells, neutrophils, and macrophages in bronchial biopsy specimens from atopic subjects with asthma: comparison with biopsy specimens from atopic subjects without asthma and normal control subjects and relationship to bronchial hyperresponsiveness, *J. Allergy Clin. Immunol.*, 88, 661, 1991.
6. Djukanovic, R., Lai, C. K., Wilson, J. W., Britten, K. M., Wilson, S. J., Roche, W. R., Howarth, P. H., and Holgate, S. T., Bronchial mucosal manifestations of atopy: a comparison of markers of inflammation between atopic asthmatics, atopic nonasthmatics and healthy controls, *Eur. Respir. J.*, 5, 538, 1992.

7. Moreno, R. H., Hogg, J. C., and Paré, P. D., Mechanics of airway narrowing, *Am. Rev. Respir. Dis.*, 133, 1171, 1986.

8. Wiggs, B. R., Moreno, R., Hogg, J. C., Hilliam, C., and Pare, P. D., A model of the mechanics of airway narrowing, *J. Appl. Physiol.*, 69, 849, 1990.

9. Stephens, N. L. and Van Nickerk, W., Isometric and isotonic contractions in airway smooth muscle, *Can. J. Physiol. Pharmacol.*, 55, 833, 977.

10. James, A. L., Pare, P. D., and Hogg, J. C., The mechanics of airway narrowing in asthma, *Am. Rev. Respir. Dis.*, 139, 242, 1989.

11. Ding, D. J., Martin, J. G., and Macklem, P. T., Effects of lung volume on maximal methacholine-induced bronchoconstriction in normal humans, *J. Appl. Physiol.*, 62, 1324, 1987.

12. Macklem, P. T., Factors determining bronchial smooth muscle shortening, *Am. Rev. Respir. Dis.*, 143 (Suppl.), 47, 1991.

13. Kuwano, K., Bosken, C. H., Paré, P. D., Bai, T. R., Wiggs, B. R., and Hogg, J. C., Small airways dimensions in asthma and in chronic obstructive pulmonary disease, *Am. Rev. Respir. Dis.*, 148, 1220, 1993.

14. Wilson, J. W. and Li, X., The measurement of airway collagen in asthmatic airways, *Am. Rev. Respir. Crit. Care Med.*, 149, A959, 1994.

15. Lundgren, R., Soderberg, M., Horstedt, P., and Stenling, R., Morphological studies on bronchial mucosal biopsies from asthmatics before and after ten years treatment with inhaled steroids, *Eur. Respir. J.*, 1, 883, 1988.

16. Holgate, S. T. et al., The T cell and the airway's fibrotic response in asthma, *Chest*, 103 (Suppl.), 125S, 1993.

17. Houston, J. C. S., de Navasquez, S., and Trounce, J. R., A clinical and pathological study of fatal cases of status asthmatics, *Thorax*, 8, 207, 1953.

18. McCarter, J. H., Vazquez, J. J., and Durham, N. C., The bronchial basement membrane in asthma, *Arch. Pathol.*, 82, 328, 1966.

19. Pierce, G. B. and Nakane, P. K., Basement membranes: synthesis and deposition in response to cellular injury, *Lab. Invest.*, 21, 27, 1969.

20. Roche, W. R., Beasley, R., Williams, J. H., and Holgate, S. T., Subepithelial fibrosis in the bronchi of asthmatics, *Lancet*, 1, 520, 1989.

21. Jeffery, P. K., Godfrey, R. W., Ädelroth, E., Nelson, F., Rogers, A., and Johansson, S. A., Effects of treatment on airway inflammation and thickness of basement membrane reticular collagen in asthma: a quantitative light and electron microscopic study, *Am. Rev. Respir. Dis.*, 145, 890, 1992.

22. Thurlbeck, W. M. and Hogg, J. C., Pathology of asthma, in *Allergy: Principle and Practice*, 3rd ed., Middleton, E., Reed, C. E., Ellis, E. F., Adkinson, N. F., and Yunginger, J. W., Eds., C.V. Mosby, St. Louis, MO, 1988, 1008–1017.

23. Alberts, B., Bray, D., Lewis, J., Raff, M., Roberts, K., and Watson, J. D., *Molecular Biology of the Cell*, Garland Publishing, New York, 1983, 692.

24. Cheah, K. S., Collagen genes and inherited connective tissue disease, *Biochem. J.*, 229, 287, 1985.

25. Leeson, T. S., Leeson, C. R., and Paparo, A. A., Connective tissue property, in *Text/Atlas of Histology*, Wonsiewicz, M., Ed., W.B. Saunders, Philadelphia, 1988, 126–158.

26. Martinez-Hernandez, A. and Amenta, P. S., The basement membrane in pathology, *Lab. Invest.*, 48, 656, 1983.

27. Laurent, G. J., Lung collagen: more than scaffolding, *Thorax*, 41, 418, 1986.

28. Jeffery, P. K., Microscopy anatomy, in *Respiratory Medicine*, Brewis, R. A. L., Gibson, G. J., and Geddes, D. M., Eds., Bailliere Tindall, London, 1990, chap. 1.3.

29. Campa, J. S., Harrison, N. K., and Laurent, G. J., Regulation of matrix production in the airways, in *T-lymphocyte and Inflammation Cell Research in Asthma*, Jolles, G., Karlsson, J.-A., and Taylor, J., Eds., Academic Press, New York, 1993, 221–239.

30. Shaw, R. J., The role of lung macrophages at the interface between chronic inflammation and fibrosis, *Respir. Med.*, 85, 267, 1991.

31. Jordana, M., Shulman, J., McSharry, C., Irving, L. B., Newhouse, M. T., Jordana, G., and Gauldie, J., Heterogeneous proliferative characteristics of human adult lung fibroblast lines and clonally derived fibroblasts from control and fibrotic tissue, *Am. Rev. Respir. Dis.*, 137, 579, 1988.

32. Jordana, M., Vancheri, C., Ohtoshi, T., Harnish, D., Gauldie, J., Dolovich, J., and Denburg, J., Hemopoietic function of the microenvironment in chronic airway inflammation, *Agents Actions Suppl.*, 28, 85, 1989.

33. Harrison, N. K., Argent, A. C., McAnulty, R. J., Black, C. M., Corrin, B., and Laurent, G. J., Collagen synthesis and degradation by systemic sclerosis lung fibroblasts: respones to TGF-β, *Chest*, 99, S71, 1991.

34. Laurent, G. J., Regulation of lung collagen production during wound healing, *Chest*, 99, 67, 1991.

35. McIntosh, J. R. and Koonce, M. P., Mitosis, *Science*, 246, 622, 1989.

36. Sheppard, M. N. and Harrison, N. K., Lung injury, inflammatory mediators, and fibroblast activation in fibrosing alveolitis, *Thorax*, 47, 1064, 1992.

37. Ignotz, R. A. and Massague, J., Transforming growth factor-B stimulates expression of fibronectin and collagen and their incorporation into the extracellular matrix, *J. Biol. Chem.*, 261, 4337, 1986.

38. Sakamoto, S. and Sakamoto, M., Degradative processes of connective tissue protein with special emphasis on collagenolysis and bone resorption, *Mol. Aspects Med.*, 10, 299, 1988.

39. Baum, B. J., Moss, J., Breul, S. D., Berg, R. A., and Crystal, R. G., Effect of cyclic AMP on the intracellular degradation of newly synthesized collagen, *J. Biol. Chem.*, 255, 2843, 1980.

40. Sporn, M. B., Roberts, A. B., Wakefield, L. M., and de Crombrugghe, B., Some recent advances in the chemistry and biology of transforming growth factor-beta, *J. Cell Biol.*, 105, 1039, 1987.

41. Rinaldo, J. E. and Rogers, R. M., Adult respiratory distress syndrome, *N. Engl. J. Med.*, 315, 578, 1986.

42. Scadding, J. G., Fibrosing alveoltitis, *Br. Med. J.*, 2, 686, 1964.

43. Turner-Warwick, M., *Immunology of the Lung*, Arnold, London, 1978, 165.

44. Siegbahn, A., Hammacher, A., Westermark, B., and Heldin, C. H., Differential effects of various isoforms of platelet-derived growth factor on chemotaxis of fibroblasts, monocytes and granulocytes, *J. Clin. Invest.* 85, 916, 1990.

45. Ross, R., Platelet-derived growth factor, *Lancet*, 1(8648), 1179, 1989.

46. Fabisiak, J. P. and Kelley, J., Platelet-derived growth factor, in *Cytokines of the Lung*, Kelley, J., Ed., Marcel Dekker, New York, 1992, 3–40.

47. Seppa, H., Grotendorst, G., Seppa, S., Schiffman, E., and Martin, G. R., The platelet-derived growth factor is chemotactic to fibroblasts, *J. Cell Biol.*, 92, 584, 1982.

48. Larrson, O., Latham, C., Zickert, P., and Zetterberg, A., Cell cycle regulation of human diploid fibroblasts: possible mechanisms of platelet-derived growth factor, *J. Cell Physiol.*, 139, 477, 1989.

49. Marinelli, W. A., Polunovsky, V. A., Harmon, K. R., and Bitterman, P. B., Role of platelet-derived growth factor in pulmonary fibrosis, *Am. J. Respir. Cell Mol. Biol.*, 5, 503, 1991.

50. Deuel, T. F. and Huang, J. S., Platelet-derived growth factor structure, function and roles in normal and transformed cells, *J. Clin. Invest.*, 74, 669, 1984.

51. Clark, R. A., Folkvord, J. M., Hart, C. E., Murray, M. J., and McPherson, J. M., Platelet isoforms of platelet derived growth factor stimulate fibroblasts to contract collagen matrices, *J. Clin. Invest.*, 84, 1036, 1989.

52. Bauer, E. A., Cooper, T. W., Huang, J. S., Altman, J., and Deuel, T. F., Stimulation of *in vitro* human skin collagenase expression by platelet-derived growth factor, *Proc. Natl. Acad. Sci. U.S.A.*, 82, 4132, 1985.

53. Paulsson, Y., Austgulen, R., Hofsli, E., Heldin, C.-H., Westermark, V., and Nissen-Meyer, J., Tumor necrosis factor-induced expression of platelet-derived growth factor-A-chain messenger RNA in fibroblasts, *Exp. Cell Res.*, 1810, 490, 1989.

54. Raines, E. W., Dower, S. K., and Ross, R., Interleukin-1 mitogenic activity for fibroblasts and smooth muscle cells is due to PDGF-AA, *Science*, 243, 393, 1989.

55. Nagaoka, I., Trapnell, B. C., and Crystal, R. G., Regulation of insulin-like growth factor 1 gene expression in the human macrophage-like cell line U937, *J. Clin. Invest.*, 85, 448, 1990.

56. Shaw, R. J., Benedict, S. H., Clark, R. A. F., and King, T. E., Jr., Pathogenesis of pulmonary fibrosis in interstitial lung disease: alveolar macrophage PDGF(B) gene activation and upregulation by interferon gamma, *Am. Rev. Respir. Dis.*, 143, 167, 1991.

57. Antoniades, H. N., Bravo, M. A., Avila, R. E., Galanopoulos, T., and Selman, M., Platelet-derived growth factor in idiopathic pulmonary fibrosis, *J. Clin. Invest.*, 86, 1055, 1990.

58. Sporn, M. B. and Roberts, A. B., Peptide growth factors and inflammation, tissue repair and cancer, *J. Clin. Invest.*, 78, 329, 1986.

59. Moses, H. L., Branum, E. L., Proper, J. A., and Robinson, R. A., Transforming growth factor production by chemically transformed cells, *Cancer Res.*, 41, 2842, 1981.

60. Roberts, A. B., Anzano, M. A., Lamb, L. C., Smith, J. M., and Sporn, M. B., New class of transforming growth factors potentiated by epidermal growth factor, *Proc. Natl. Acad. Sci. U.S.A.*, 78, 5339, 1981.

61. Postlethwaite, A. E., Keski-Oja, J., Moses, H. I., and Kang, A. H., Stimulation of the chemotactic migration of human fibroblasts by transforming growth factor b, *J. Exp. Med.*, 165, 251, 1987.

62. Overall, C. M., Wrana, J. L., and Sodek, J., Independent regulation of collagenase, 72-kDa progelatinase and metalloproteinase inhibitor expression in human fibroblasts by transforming growth factor-beta, *J. Biol. Chem.*, 264, 1860, 1989.

63. Sporn, M. B., Roberts, A. B., Shull, J. H., Smith, J. M., Ward, J. M., and Sodek, J., Polypeptide transforming growth factors isolated from bovine sources and used for wound healing *in vivo*, *Science*, 219, 1329, 1983.

64. Roberts, A. B., Sporn, M. B., Assoian, R. K., Smith, J. M., Roche, N. S., Wakefield, L. M., Heine, U. I., Liotta, L. A., Falanga, V., Kehrl, J. H., et al., Transforming growth factor type b: rapid induction of fibrosis and angiogenesis in vivo and stimulation of collagen formation in vitro, *Proc. Natl. Acad. Sci. U.S.A.*, 83, 4167, 1986.

65. Hoyt, D. G. and Lazo, J. S., Alterations in pulmonary mRNA encoding procollagens, fibronectin and transforming growth factor-precede bleomycin-induced pulmonary fibrosis in mice, *J. Pharmacol. Exp. Ther.*, 246, 765, 1988.

66. Khalil, N., O'Conner, R. N., Unruh, H. W., Warren, P. W., Flanders, K. C., Kemp, A., Bereznay, O. H., and Greenberg, A. H., Increased production and immunohistochemical localization of transforming growth factor-β in idiopathic pulmonary fibrosis, *Am. J. Respir. Cell Mol. Biol.*, 5, 155, 1991.

67. Broekelmann, T. J., Limper, A. H., Colby, T. V., and McDonald, J. A., Transforming growth factor β1 is present at sites of extracellular matrix gene expression in human pulmonary fibrosis, *Proc. Natl. Acad. Sci. U.S.A.*, 88, 6642, 1991.

68. Breen, E., Shull, S., Burne, S., Absher, M., Kelley, J., Phan, S., and Kutroneo, K. R., Bleomycin regulation of transforming growth factor β mRNA in rat lung fibroblasts, *Am. J. Respir. Cell Mol. Biol.*, 6, 146, 1992.

69. Gauldie, J., Jordana, M., and Cox, G., Cytokines and pulmonary fibrosis, *Thorax*, 48, 931, 1993.

70. Ohno, I., Lea, R. G., Flanders, K. C., Clark, D. A., Banwatt, D., Dolovich, J., Denburg, J., Harley, C. B., Gauldie, J., and Jordana, M., Eosinophils in chronically inflamed human upper airway tissue express transforming growth factor beta 1 gene (TGF beta 1), *J. Clin. Invest.*, 89(5), 1662, 1992.

71. Aubert, J. D., Dalal, B. L., Bai, T. R., Robert, C. R., Hayashi, S., and Hogg, J., Transforming growth factor $b_1$ gene expression in human airways, *Thorax*, 49, 225, 1994.

72. Van Wyk, J. J., The somatomedins: biological actions and physiologic control mechanisms, in *Hormonal Proteins and Peptides*, Vol. 7, Li, C. H., Ed., Academic Press, New York, 1984.

73. Humbel, R. E., Insulin-like growth factors I and II, *Eur. J. Biochem.*, 190, 445, 1990.
74. Hepler, J. E. and Lund, P. K., Molecular biology of the insulin-like growth factors, *Mol. Neurobiol.*, 2, 93, 1990.
75. Scott, C. D., Martin, J. L., and Baxter, R. C., Production of insulin-like growth factor 1 and its binding protein by adult rat hepatocytes in primary culture, *Endocrinology,* 116, 1094, 1985.
76. Stiles, A. D. and D'Ercole, A. J., The insulin-like growth factors and the lung, *Am. J. Respir. Cell Mol. Biol.*, 3(2), 93, 1989.
77. Stiles, A. D. and Moats-Staats, B. M., Production and action of insulin-like growth factor 1/somatomedin C in primary cultures of fetal lung fibroblasts, *Am. J. Respir. Cell Mol. Biol.*, 1, 21, 1989.
78. Goldstein, R. H., Poliks, C. F., Pilch, P. F., Smith, B. D., and Fine, A., Stimulation of collagen formation by insulin and insulin-like growth factor 1 in cultures of human lung fibroblasts, *Endocrinology,* 124, 964, 1989.
79. Rom, W. N., Bassett, P., Fells, G. A., Nukiwa, T., Trapnell, B. C., and Crystal, R. G., Alveolar macrophages release an insulin-like growth factor I-type molecule, *J. Clin. Invest.*, 82, 1658, 1988.
80. Bitterman, P. B., Rennard, S. I., Hunninghake, G. W., and Crystal, R. G., Human alveolar macrophage growth factor for fibroblasts: regulation and partial characterisation, *J. Clin. Invest.*, 70, 806, 1982.
81. Rappolee, D. A., Mark, D., Banda, M. J., and Werb, Z., Wound macrophages express TGF-alpha and other growth factors in vivo: analysis by mRNA phenotyping, *Science*, 241, 708, 1988.
82. Bitterman, P. B., Adelberg, S., and Crystal, R. G., Mechanisms of pulmonary fibrosis: spontaneous release of the alveolar macrophage-derived growth factor in the interstitial lung disorders, *J. Clin. Invest.*, 72, 1801, 1983.
83. Rossi, G. A., Bitterman, P. B., Rennard, S. I., Ferrans, V. J., and Crystal, R. G., Evidence for chronic inflammation as a component of the interstitial lung disease associated with progressive systemic sclerosis, *Am. Rev. Respir. Dis.*, 131, 612, 1985.
84. Rom, W. N., Bitterman, P. B., Rennard, S. I., Cantin, A., and Crystal, R. G., Characterization of the lower respiratory tract inflammation of nonsmoking individuals with interstitial lung disease associated with chronic inhalation of inorganic dusts, *Am. Rev. Respir. Dis.*, 136, 1429, 1987.
85. Beutler, B., Greenwald, D., Hulmes, J. D., et al., Identity of TNF and the macrophage-secreted factor cachectin, *Nature*, 316, 552, 1984.
86. Pennica, D., Nedwin, G. E., Hayflick, J. S., Seeburg, P. H., Derynck, R., Palladino, M. A., Kohr, W. J., Aggarwal, B. B., and Goeddel, D. V., Human tumour necrosis factor. Precursor structure, expression, and homology to lymphotoxin, *Nature*, 312, 724, 1985.
87. Turner, M., Londer, M., and Feldmann, M., Human T-cells from autoimmune and normal individuals can produce tumor necrosis factor, *Eur. J. Immunol.*, 17, 1807, 1987.
88. Old, L. J., Tumour necrosis factor (TNF), *Science*, 230, 630, 1985.
89. Le, J. and Vilcek, J., TNF and IL-1: cytokines with multiple overlapping biological activities, *Lab. Invest.*, 56, 234, 1987.
90. Stewart, A. G., Tomlinson, P. R., Fernandes, D. J., Wilson, J. W., and Harris, T., Tumor necrosis factor α modulates mitogenic responses of human cultured airway smooth muscle, *Am. J. Respir. Cell Mol. Biol.*, 12, 110, 1995.
91. Kohase, M., May, L. T., Tamm, I., Vilcek, J., and Sehgal, P. B., A cytokine network in human diploid fibroblasts: interactions of interferons, tumor necrosis factor, platelet derived growth factor, and interleukin-1, *Mol. Cell Biol.*, 7, 273, 1987.
92. Vilcek, J., Palombella, V. J., Henriksen-DeStefano, D., Svenson, C., Feinman, R., Hirai, M., and Tsujimoto, M., Fibroblast growth enhancing ability of tumor necrosis factor and its relationship to other polypeptide growth factors, *J. Exp. Med.*, 163, 632, 1986.
93. Ito, A., Sato, T., Iga, T., and Mori, Y., Tumour necrosis factor bifunctionally regulates matrix metalloproteinases and tissue inhibitor of metalloproteinases (TIMP) production by human fibroblasts, *FEBS Lett.*, 269, 93, 1990.

94. Solis-Herruzo, J. A., Brenner, D. A., and Chojkier, M., Tumor necrosis factor alpha inhibits collagen gene transcription and collagen synthesis in cultured human fibroblasts, *J. Biol. Chem.*, 263, 5841, 1988.
95. Scharffetter, K., Heckmann, M., Hatamochi, A., Maunch, C., Stein, B., Reithmuller, G., Ziegler-Heitbrock, H. W., and Krieg, T., Synergistic effect of tumor necrosis factor-alpha and interferon-gamma on collagen synthesis of human skin fibroblasts in vitro, *Exp. Cell Res.*, 181, 409, 1989.
96. Tracey, K. J., Vlassara, H., and Cerami, A., Cachectin/TNF, *Lancet*, 1, 1122, 1989.
97. Piguet, P. F., Collart, M. A., Frau, G. E., Kapanci, Y., and Vassalli, P., Tumour necrosis factor/cachectin play a key role in bleomycin-induced pneumopathy and fibrosis, *J. Exp. Med.*, 170, 655, 1989.
98. Piguet, P. F., Collart, M. A., Frau, G. E., Sappino, A. P., and Vassalli, P., Requirement of tumour necrosis factor for development of silica-induced pulmonary fibrosis, *Nature*, 344, 245, 1990.
99. Phan, S. H. and Kunkel, S. L., Lung cytokine production in bleomycin-induced pulmonary fibrosis, *Exp. Lung Res.*, 18, 29, 1992.
100. Cembrzynska-Nowak, M., Szklarz, E., Inglot, A. D., and Teodorcyzk-Injeyan, J. A., Elevated release of tumour necrosis factor-alpha and interferon-gamma by bronchoalveolar leukocytes from patients with bronchial asthma, *Am. Rev. Respir. Dis.*, 147, 291, 1993.
101. Gosset, P., Tsicopoulos, A., Wallaert, B., Vannimenus, C., Joseph, M., Tonnel, A.-B., and Capron, A., Increased secretion of tumour necrosis factor-a and interleukin-6 by alveolar macrophages consecutive to the development of the late asthmatic reaction, *J. Allergy Clin. Immunol.*, 88, 561, 1991.
102. Broide, D. H., Lotz, D., Cuomo, A. J., Coburn, D. A., Federman, E. C., and Wasserman, S. I., Cytokines in symptomatic asthma airways, *J. Allergy Clin. Immunol.*, 89, 958, 1992.
103. Ying, S., Robinson, D. S., Varney, V., Meng, Q., Tsicopoulos, A., Moqbel, R., Durham, S. R., Kay, A. B., and Hamid, Q., TNF-a mRNA expression in allergic inflammation, *Clin. Exp. Allergy*, 21, 745, 1991.
104. Bradding, P., Roberts, J. A., Britten, K. M., Montefort, S., Djukanovic, R., Mueller, R., Heusser, C. H., Howarth, P. H., and Holgate, S. T., Interleukin-4, -5, and -6 and tumor necrosis facor-a in normal and asthmatic airways: evidence for the human mast cell as a source of these cytokines, *Am. J. Respir. Cell Mol. Biol.*, 10, 471, 1994.
105. Yamato, K., El-Hajjaoui, Z., Kuo, J. F., and Koeffler, K. P., Granulocyte-macrophage colony stimulating factor: signals for its mRNA accumulation, *Blood*, 74, 1314, 1989.
106. Wodnar-Filipowicz, A., Heusser, C. H., and Moroni, C., Production of the hemopoietic growth factors GM-CSF and interleukin-3 by mast cells in response to IgE receptors-mediated activation, *Nature*, 339, 150, 1989.
107. Vancheri, C., Gauldie, J., Bienenstock, J., Cox, G., Scicchitano, R., Stanisz, A., and Jordana, M., Human lung fibroblast-derived granulocyte-macrophage colony stimulating factor (GM-CSF) mediates eosinophil survival in vitro, *Am. J. Respir. Cell Mol. Biol.*, 1, 289, 1989.
108. Lee, M. T., Kaushansky, K., Ralph, P., and Ladner, M. B., Differential expression of M-CSF, G-CSF and GM-CSF by human monocytes, *J. Leukocyte Biol.*, 47, 275, 1990.
109. Cromwell, O., Hamid, Q., Corrigan, C. J., Barkans, J., Meng, Q., Collins, P. D., and Kay, A. B., Expression and generation of IL-6, IL-8 and GM-CSF by human bronchial epithelial cells and enhancement by IL-1β and TNF-α, *Immunology*, 77, 330, 1992.
110. Zucali, J. R., Dinarello, C. A., Oblon, D. J., Gross, M. A., Anderson, L., and Weiner, R. S., Interleukin 1 stimulates fibroblasts to produce granulocyte-macrophage colony-stimulating activity and prostaglandin E2, *J. Clin. Invest.*, 77, 1857, 1986.
111. Howell, C. J., Pujol, J.-L., Crea, A. E. G., Davidson, R., Gearing, A. J. H., Godard, P. H., and Lee, T. H., Identification of an alveolar-macrophage-derived activity in bronchial asthma that enhances LTD4, generation by human eosinophils stimulated by ionophore (A23187) as granulocyte-macrophage colony-stimulating factor (GM-CSF), *Am. Rev. Respir. Dis.*, 140, 1340, 1989.

112. Clark, S. C. and Kamen, R., The human hematopoietic colony-stimulating factors, *Science,* 236, 1229, 1987.

113. Moqbel, R., Hamid, Q., Sun, Y., Barkans, J., Hartnell, A., Tsicopoulos, A., Wardlaw, A. J., and Kay, A. B., Expression of mRNA for the granulocyte/macrophage colony-stimulating factor (GM-CSF) in activated human eosinophils, *J. Exp. Med.,* 174, 749, 1991.

114. Silberstein, D. S., Eosinophils, in *Encyclopedia of Immunology,* Vol. 1, Roitt, J. M., Ed., Academic Press, London, 1992, 512–514.

115. Owen, W. F., Jr., Rothenberg, M. E., Silberstein, D. S., Gasson, J. C., Stevens, R. L., Austen, K. F., and Soberman, R. J., Regulation of human eosinophil viability, density and function by granulocyte/macrophage colony-stimulating factor in the presence of 3T3 fibroblasts, *J. Exp. Med.,* 166, 129, 1987.

116. Siraganian, R. P., Mast cells, in *Encyclopedia of Immunology,* Vol. 2, Roitt, J. M., Ed., Academic Press, London, 1992, 1035–1038.

117. Rubbia-Brandt, L., Sappino, A., and Gabbiani, G., Locally applied GM-CSF induces the accumulation of alpha smooth muscle actin containing fibroblasts, *Virchows Arch. (B),* 60, 73, 1991.

118. Brewster, C. E. P., Howarth, P. H., Djukanovic, R., Wilson, J., Holgate, S. T., and Roche, W. R., Myofibroblasts and subepithelial fibrosis in bronchial asthma, *Am. J. Respir. Cell Mol. Biol.,* 3, 507, 1990.

119. Dedhar, S., Gaboury, L., Galloway, P., and Eaves, C., Human granulocyte-macrophage colony-stimulating factor is growth factor active on a variety of cell types of non-hemopoietic origin, *Proc. Natl. Acad. Sci. U.S.A.,* 85, 9253, 1988.

120. March, C. J., Mosley, B., and Larsen, A., Coloning, sequence and expression of two distinct human interleukin 1 complementary DNAs, *Nature,* 64, 641, 1985.

121. Schmidt, J. A., Mizel, S. B., Cohen, D., and Green, I., Interleukin 1, a potential regulator of fibroblast proliferation, *J. Immunol.,* 128, 2177, 1982.

122. Krane, S., Dayer, J. M., Simon, L., and Byrne, S., Mononuclear cell-conditioned medium containing mononuclear cell factor (MCF), homologous with interleukin-1, stimulates collagen and fibronectin synthesis by adherent rheumatoid synovial cells: effects of prostaglandin E2 and indomethacin, *Collagen Relat. Res.,* 5, 99, 1985.

123. Dinarello, C. and Savage, N., Interleukin-1 and its receptor, *Crit. Rev. Immunol.,* 9, 1, 1989.

124. Hunninghake, G. W., Release of IL-1 by alveolar macrophages of patients with active pulmonary sarcoidosis, *Am. Rev. Respir. Dis.,* 129, 569, 1984.

125. Yamaguchi, E., Okazaki, N., Tsuneta, Y., Abe, S., Terai, T., and Kawakami, Y., Ineterleukins in pulmonary sarcoidosis. Dissociative correlation of lung interleukins 1 and 2 with the intensity of alveolitis, *Am. Rev. Respir. Dis.,* 138, 645, 1988.

126. Schmidt, J. A., Oliver, C. N., Lepe-Zuniga, J. L., Green, I., and Gery, I., Silica-stimulated monocyte release of fibroblast proliferation factors identical to interleukin 1. A potential role for interleukin 1 in the pathogenesis of silicosis, *J. Clin. Invest.,* 73, 1462, 1984.

127. Hartmann, D. P., Georgian, M. M., Oghiso, Y., and Kagan, E., Enhanced interleukin activity following asbestos inhalation, *Clin. Exp. Immunol.,* 55, 643, 1984.

128. Jordana, M., Richard, C., Irving, L. B., and Gauldie, J., Spontaneous in vitro release of alveolar-macrophage cytokines after the intratracheal instillation of bleomycin in rats. Characterization and kinetic studies, *Am. Rev. Respir. Dis.,* 137, 1135, 1988.

129. Kelley, J., Cytokines of the lung, *Am. Rev. Respir. Dis.,* 141, 756, 1990.

130. Barnes, P. J., Inflammation, in *Bronchial Asthma: Mechanisms and Therapeutics,* 3rd ed., Weiss, E. B. and Stein, M., Little Brown, Boston, 1993, 80–94.

131. Adelmann-Grill, B. C., Hein, R., Wach, F., and Krieg, T., Inhibition of fibroblast chemotaxis by recombinant human interferon gamma and interferon alpha, *J. Cell. Physiol.,* 130, 270, 1987.

132. Oleszak, E., Inhibition of mitogenic activity of PDGF, EGF, and FGF by interferon-gamma, *Exp. Cell Res.,* 179, 575, 1988.

133. Elias, J. A., Jiminez, S. A., and Freundlich, B., Recombinant gamma, alpha and beta interferon regulation of human lung fibroblast proliferation, *Am. Rev. Respir. Dis.,* 135, 62, 1987.

134. Kovacs, E. J., Fibrogenic cytokines: the role of immune mediators in the development of scar tissue, *Immunol. Today,* 12, 17, 1991.

135. Prior, C. and Haslam, P. L., Increased levels of serum interferon-gamma in pulmonary sarcoidosis and relationship with response to corticosteroid therapy, *Am. Rev. Respir. Dis.,* 143, 53, 1991.

136. Moseley, P. L., Hemkin, C., Monick, M., Nugent, K., and Hunninghake, G. W., Interferon and growth factor activity for human lung fibroblasts release from bronchoalveolar cells from patients with active sarcoidosis, *Chest,* 89(5), 657, 1986.

137. Du Bois, R. M., Recent advances in the immunology of interstitial lung disease, *Clin. Exp. Allergy,* 21, 9, 1991.

138. O'Connor, C. M. and FitzGerald, M. X., Speculations on sarcoidosis, *Resp. Med.,* 86, 277, 1992.

139. Bjermer, L., Engstrom-Laurent, A., Thunell, M., and Hallgren, R., Hyaluronic acid in bronchoalveolar lavage fluid in patients with sarcoidosis: relationship to lavage mast cell, *Thorax,* 42, 933, 1987.

140. Pesci, A., Bertorelli, G., Gobrielli, M., and Olivieri, D., Mast cells in fibrotic lung disorders, *Chest,* 103(4), 989, 1993.

141. Azzawi, M., Bradley, B., Jeffery, P. K., Frew, A. J., Wardlaw, A. J., Knowles, G., Assoufi, B., Collins, J. V., Durham, S., and Kay, A. B., Identification of activated T lymphocytes and eosinophils in bronchial biopsies in stable atopic asthma, *Am. Rev. Respir. Dis.,* 142, 1407, 1990.

142. Wardlaw, A. J., Dunnett, S., Gleich, G. J., Collins, J. V., and Kay, A. B., Eosinophils and mast cells in bronchoalveolar lavage in mild asthma: relationship to bronchial hyperreactivity, *Am. Rev. Respir. Dis.,* 136, 379, 1988.

143. Kirby, J. G., Hargreave, F. E., Gleich, G. J., and O'Bryne, P. M., Bronchoalveolar cell profiles of asthmatic and non-asthmatic subjects, *Am. Rev. Respir. Dis.,* 136, 379, 1987.

144. Gospodarowicz, D., Purification of a fibroblast growth factor from bovine pituitary, *J. Biol. Chem.,* 250, 2515, 1975.

145. Maciag, T., Cerundolo, J., Ilsley, S., Kelley, P. R., and Forand, R., An endothelial cell growth factor from bovine hypothalamus: identification and partial characterization, *Proc. Natl. Acad. Sci. U.S.A.,* 76, 5674, 1979.

146. Moscatelli, D., Fibroblast growth factors, in *Cytokines of the Lung,* Vol. 61, Kelley, J., Ed., Marcel Dekker, New York, 1993, 41–76.

147. Esch, F., Baird, A., Ling, N., Ueno, N., Hill, F., Denoroy, L., Klepper, R., Gospodarowicz, D., Bohlen, P., and Guillemin, R., Primary structure of bovine pituitary basic fibroblast growth factor (FGF) and comparison with the amino-terminal sequence of bovine brain acidic FGF, *Proc. Natl. Acad. Sci. U.S.A.,* 82, 6507, 1985.

148. Connolly, D. T., Stoddard, B. L., Harakas, N. K., and Feder, J., Human fibroblast-derived growth factor is a mitogen and chemoattractant for endothelial cells, *Biochem. Biophys. Res. Commun.,* 144, 705, 1987.

149. Gospodarowicz, D., Ferrara, N., Haaparanta, T., and Neufeld, G., Basic fibroblast growth factor: expression in cultured bovine vascular smooth muscle cells, *Eur. J. Cell. Biol.,* 46, 144, 1988.

150. Hatten, M. E., Lynch, M., Rydel, R. E., Sanchez, J., Joseph-Silverstein, J., Moscatelli, D., and Rifkin, D. B., In vitro neurite extension by granule neurons is dependent upon astroglial-derived fibroblast growth factor, *Dev. Biol.,* 125, 280, 1988.

151. Moscatelli, D., Presta, M., Joseph-Silverstein, J., and Rifkin, D. B., Both normal and tumor cells produce basic fibroblast growth factor, *J. Cell. Physiol.,* 129, 273, 1986.

152. Schweigerer, L., Neufeld, G., Friedman, J., Abraham, J. A., Fiddes, J. C., and Gospodarowicz, D., Capillary endothelial cells express basic fibroblast growth factor, a mitogen that promotes their own growth, *Nature,* 325, 257, 1987.

153. Vlodavsky, I., Folkman, J., Sullivan, R., Fridman, R., Ishai-Michaeli, R., Sasse, J., and Klagsbrun, M., Endothelial cell-derived basic fibroblast growth factor: synthesis and deposition into subendothelial extracellular matrix, *Proc. Natl. Acad. Sci. U.S.A.,* 84, 2292, 1987.

154. Weich, H. A., Iberg, N., Klagsbrun, M., and Folkman, J., Expression of acidic and basic fibroblast growth factors in human and bovine vascular smooth muscle cells, *Growth Factors*, 2, 313, 1990.
155. Harper, J. W. and Lobb, R. R., Reductive methylation of lysine residues in acidic fibroblast growth factor: effect on mitogenic activity and heparin affinity, *Biochemistry*, 27, 671, 1988.
156. Lee, P. L., Johnson, D. E., Cousens, L. S., Fried, V. A., and Williams, L. T., Purification and complementary DNA cloning of a receptor for basic fibroblast growth factor, *Science*, 245, 57, 1989.
157. Jeanny, J.-C., Fayein, N., Moenner, M., Chevallier, B., Barritault, D., and Courtois, Y., Specific fixation of bovine brain and retinal acidic and basic fibroblast growth factors to mouse embryonic eye basement membranes, *Exp. Cell Res.*, 171, 63, 1987.
158. Gordon, P. B., Choi, H. U., Conn, G., Ahmed, A., Ehrmann, B., Rosenberg, L., and Hatcher, V. B., Extracellular matrix heparan sulfate proteoglycans modulate the mitogenic capacity of acidic fibroblast growth factor, *J. Cell. Physiol.*, 140, 584, 1989.
159. Folkman, J. and Klagsbrun, M., Angiogenic factors, *Science*, 235, 442, 1987.
160. Mignantti, P., Tsuboi, R., Robbins, E., and Rifkin, D. B., In vitro angiogenesis on the human amniotic membrane: requirement for basic fibroblast growth factor-induced proteinases, *J. Cell Biol.*, 108, 671, 1989.
161. Tsuboi, R., Sato, Y., and Rifkin, D. B., Correlation of cell migration, cell invasion, receptor number, proteinase production, and basic fibroblast growth factor levels in endothelial cells, *J. Cell Biol.*, 110, 511, 1990.
162. Cordon-Cardo, C., Vlodavsky, I., Haimovitz-Friedman, A., Hicklin, D., and Fuks, Z., Expression of basic fibroblast growth factor in normal tissues, *Lab. Invest.*, 63, 832, 1990.
163. Terzaghi, M., Nettesheim, P., and Williams, M. L., Repopulation of denuded tracheal grafts with normal, preneoplastic and neoplastic epithelial cell populations, *Cancer Res.*, 38, 4546, 1978.
164. Corrin, B., Dewar, A., Rodriguez-Rogin, R., and Turner-Warwick, M., Fine structural changes in cryptogenic fibrosing alveolitis and asbestosis, *J. Pathol.*, 147, 107, 1985.
165. Wangensteen, D., Yankovich, R., Hoidal, J., and Niewochner, D., Bleomycin induced changes in pulmonary microvascular albumin permeability and extravascular space, *Am. Rev. Respir. Dis.*, 127, 204, 1983.
166. Adamson, I. Y. R. and Bowden, D. H., Endothelial injury and repair in radiation-induced pulmonary fibrosis, *Am. J. Pathol.*, 112, 224, 1983.
167. Hay, J. G., Haslam, P. L., Staple, L. H., and Laurent, G. J., Role of iron and oxygen in bleomycin-induced pulmonary edema, *Adv. Microcirc.*, 13, 239, 1987.
168. Widdicombe, J., New perspectives on basic mechanisms in lung disease. 4. Why are the airways so vascular?, *Thorax*, 48, 290, 1993.
169. Djukanovic, R., Wilson, J. W., Britten, K. M., Wilson, S. J., Walls, A. F., Roche, W. R., Howarth, P. H., and Holgate, S. T., Quantitation of mast cells and eosinophils in the bronchial mucosa of symptomatic atopic asthmatics and healthy control subjects using immunohistochemistry, *Am. Rev. Respir. Dis.*, 142, 863, 1990.
170. Mori, H., Kawada, K., Zhang, P., Uesugi, Y., Sakamoto, O., and Koda, A., Bleomycin-induced pulmonary fibrosis in genetically mast cell-deficient WBB6F1-W/Wv mice and mechanism of the suppressive effect of tranilast, an antiallergic drug inhibiting mediator release from mast cells, on fibrosis, *Int. Arch. Allergy Appl. Immunol.*, 95, 195, 1991.
171. Kefalides, N. A., Alper, R., and Clark, C. C., Biochemistry and metabolism of basement membranes, *Int. Rev. Cytol.*, 61, 167, 1979.
172. Foresi, A., Bertorelli, G., Pesci, A., Chetta, A., and Olivieri, D., Inflammatory markers in bronchoalveolar lavage and in bronchial biopsy in asthma during remission, *Chest*, 98, 528, 1990.
173. Olivieri, D. and Foresi, A., Correlation between cell content of bronchoalveolar lavage and histologic findings in asthma, *Respiration*, 5, 182, 1992.

174. Haslam, P., Turton, C. W. G., Heard, B., Lukoszek, A., Collins, J. V., Salsbury, A. J., and Turner-Warwick, M., Bronchoalveolar lavage in pulmonary fibrosis: comparison of cells obtained with lung biopsy and clinical features, *Thorax*, 35, 9, 1980.

175. Allan, J. N., Davies, W. B., and Pacht, E. R., Diagnostic significance of increased bronchoalveolar lavage fluid eosinohphils, *Am. Rev. Respir. Dis.*, 42, 642, 1991.

176. Cantin, A. M., Boileau, R., and Begin, R., Increased procollagen III aminoterminal peptide-related antigens and fibroblast growth signals in the lungs of patiens with idiopathic pulmonary fibrosis, *Am. Rev. Respir. Dis.*, 137, 572, 1988.

177. Hoidal, J. R., The eosinophil and acute lung injury, *Am. Rev. Respir. Dis.*, 142, 1245, 1990.

178. Hamid, Q., Azzawi, M., Ying, S., Moqbel, R., Wardlaw, A. J., Corrigan, C. J, Bradley, B., Durham, S. R., Collins, J. V., Jeffrey, P. K., and Kay, A. B., Expression of mRNA for interleukin-5 in mucosal bronchial biopsies from asthmatics, *J. Clin. Invest.*, 87, 1541, 1991.

179. Robinson, D. S., Durham, S. R., and Kay, A. B., Cytokines in asthma, *Thorax*, 48, 845, 1993.

180. Spry, C. J. F., Davies, J., Tai, P. C., Olsen, E. J. G., Oakley, C. M., and Goodwin, J. F., Clinical features of fifteen patients with hypereosinophilic syndrome, *Q. J. Med.*, 205, 1, 1983.

181. Turner-Warwick, M. and Haslam, P. L., The value of serial bronchoalveolar lavages in assessing the clinical progress of patients with cryptogenic fibrosing alveolitis, *Am. Rev. Respir. Dis.*, 135, 26, 1987.

182. Shock, A., Rabe, K. F., Dent, G., Chambers, R. C., Gray, A. J., Chung, K. F., Barnes, P. J., and Laurent, G. J., Eosinophils adhere to and stimulate replication of lung fibroblasts in vitro, *Clin. Exp. Immunol.*, 86, 185, 1991.

183. Sarnstrand, B., Hernnas, J., Peterson, C., Venge, P., and Malmstrom, A., Eosinophil cationic protein stimulates synthesis of hyaluron and proteoglycan in fibroblast cultures, *Am. Rev. Respir. Dis.*, 139, A209, 1989.

184. Wong, D. T., Weller, P. F., Galli, S. J., Elovic, A., Rand, T. H., Gallagher, G. T., Chiang, T., Chou, M. Y., Matossian, K., McBride, J., et al., Human eosinophils express transforming growth factor $\alpha$, *J. Exp. Med.*, 172, 673, 1990.

185. Cauna, N., Hinderer, K. H., Manzetti, G. W., and Swanson, E. W., Fine structure of nasal polyps, *Ann. Otol.*, 81, 41, 1972.

186. Holgate, S. T. and Church, M. K., The mast cell, *Br. Med. Bull.*, 48, 40, 1991.

187. Bienenstock, J., Tomioka, M., Stead, R., Ernst, P., Jordana, M., Gauldie, J., Dolovich, J., and Denburg, J., Mast cell involvement in various inflammatory processes, *Am. Rev. Respir. Dis.*, 135(6 Pt. 2), S5, 1987.

188. Hawkins, R. A., Claman, H. N., Clark, R. A., and Steigerwald, J. C., Increased dermal mast cell proliferation in progressive systemic sclerosis: a link in chronic fibrosis?, *Ann. Intern. Med.*, 102, 182, 1985.

189. Kawanami, O., Ferrans, V. J., Fulmer, J. D., and Crystal, R. G., Ultrastructure of pulmonary mast cells in patients with fibrotic lung disorders, *Lab. Invest.*, 40, 717, 1979.

190. Keith, I., Day, R., Lemaire, S., and Lemaire, I., Asbestos-induced fibrosis in rats: increase in lung mast cells and autacoid contents, *Exp. Lung Res.*, 13, 311, 1987.

191. Tomioka, M., Goto, T., Lee, T. D. G., Bienenstock, J., and Befus, D., Isolation and characterization of lung mast cells from rats with bleomycin-induced pulmonary fibrosis, *Immunology*, 66, 439, 1989.

192. Aldenborg, F., Nilsson, K., Jarlshammar, B., Bjermer, L., and Enerback, L., Mast cells and biogenic amines in radiation-induced pulmonary fibrosis, *Am. J. Respir. Cell Mol. Biol.*, 8, 112, 1993.

193. Dayton, E. T., Caufield, J. P., Hein, A., Austen, K. F., and Stevens, R. L., Regulation of the growth rate of mouse fibroblasts by IL-3-activated mouse bone marrow-derived mast cells, *J. Immunol.*, 142, 4307, 1989.

194. Jordana, M., Befus, A. D., Newhouse, M. T., Bienenstock, J., and Gauldie, J., Effect of histamine on proliferation of normal human adult lung fibroblasts, *Thorax*, 43, 552, 1988.

195. Norrby, K., Mast cell histamine: a local mitogen acting via H2-receptors in nearby tissue cells, *Virchows Arch.*, 34, 13, 1980.

196. Tomlinson, P. R., Wilson, J. W., and Stewart, A. G., Proliferative responses of human airway subepithelial fibroblasts obtained from non-asthmatic patients, *Proc. Aust. Physiol. Pharmacol. Soc.*, 24, 18P, 1993.

197. Tsai, M., Gordon, J. R., and Galli, S. J., Mast cells constitutively express transforming growth factor-beta mRNA, *FASEB J.*, 4, A1944, 1990.

198. Campbell, D. A., Poulter, L. W., and du Bois, R. M., Phenotypic analysis of alveolar macrophages in normal subjects and in patients with interstitial lung disease, *Thorax*, 41, 429, 1986.

199. Haslam, P. L., Evaluation of alveolitis by studies of lung biopsies, *Lung*, 168 (Suppl.), 984, 1990.

200. Kradin, R. L., Divertie, M. B., and Colvin, R. B., Usual interstitial pneumonitis is a T-cell alveolitis, *Immunol. Immunopathol.*, 40, 224, 1986.

201. Wilson, J. W., Djukanovic, R., Howarth, P. H., and Holgate, S. T., Lymphocyte activation in bronchoalveolar lavage and peripheral blood in atopic asthma, *Am. Rev. Respir. Dis.*, 145, 958, 1992.

202. Vergnon, J. M., De The, G., Weynants, P., Vincent, M., Mornex, J. F., and Brune, J., Fibrosing alveolitis and Epstein-Barr virus: an association?, *Lancet*, 2, 768, 1984.

203. Matsui, R., Goldstein, R. H., Mihal, K., Brody, J. S., Steele, M. P., and Fine, A., Type I collagen formation in rat type II alveolar cells immortalised by viral gene products, *Thorax*, 49, 201, 1994.

204. Jimenez, S. A., New insights into the pathogenesis of interstitial pulmonary fibrosis, *Thorax*, 49, 193, 1994.

205. Buonaguro, L., Barillari, G., Chang, H. K., Bohan, V. A., Kao, V., Morgan, R., Gallo, R. C., and Ensoli, B., Effects of the human immunodeficiency virus type I Tat protein on the expression of inflammatory cytokines, *J. Virol.*, 66, 7159, 1992.

206. Cupp, C., Taylor, J. P., Khalili, K., and Amini, S., Evidence for stimulation of the transforming growth factor-$\beta 1$ promoter by HIV-I Tat in cells derived from CNS, *Oncogene*, 8, 2231, 1993.

207. Macek, V., Sorli, J., Kopriva, S., and Marin, J., Persistent adenoviral infection and chronic airway obstruction in children, *Am. J. Respir. Crit. Care Med.*, 150, 7, 1994.

208. Wilson, J. W., Li, X., and Pain, M. C. F., The lack of distensibility of asthmatic airways, *Am. Rev. Respir. Dis.*, 148, 806, 1993.

209. Rams, H., Rogers, A. J., and Ghandur-Mnaymnch, L., Collagenous colitis, *Ann. Intern. Med.*, 106, 108, 1987.

210. Hwang, W. S., Kelly, J. K., Shaffer, E. A., and Hershfield, N. B., Collagenous colitis: a disease of the pericryptal fibroblast sheath?, *J. Pathol.*, 149, 33, 1986.

211. Peat, J. K., Woolcock, A. J., and Cullen, K., Rate of decline of lung function in subjects with asthma, *Eur. J. Respir. Dis.*, 70, 171, 1987.

212. Reed, C. E., New therapeutic approaches in asthma, *J. Allergy Clin. Immunol.*, 27, 537, 1986.

213. Woolcock, A. J., Worldwide differences in asthma prevalence and mortality, Why is asthma mortality so low in the USA?, *Chest*, 90(5 Suppl.), 40S, 1986.

214. Dompeling, E., van Schayck, C. P., van Grunsven, P. M., van Herwaarden, C. L. A., Akkermans, R., Molema, J., Folgering, H., and van Weel, C., Slowing the deterioration of asthma and chronic obstructive pulmonary disease observed during bronchodilator therapy by adding inhaled corticosteroids: a 4-year prospective study, *Ann. Intern. Med.*, 118, 770, 1993.

215. Laitinen, L. A., Laitinen, A., and Haahtela, T., A comparative study of the effects of an inhaled corticosteroid, budesonide, and a $b_2$-agonist, terbutaline, on airway inflammation in newly diagnosed asthma: a randomized, double-blind, parallel-group controlled trial, *J. Allergy Clin. Immunol.*, 90, 32, 1992.

216. Trigg, C. J., Manolitsas, N. D., Wang, J., Calderon, M. A., McAulay, A., Jordan, S. E., Herdman, M. J., Jhalli, N., Duddle, J. M., Hamilton, S. A., Devalia, J. L., and Davies, R. J., Placebo-controlled immunopathologic study of four months of inhaled corticosteroids in asthma, *Am. J. Respir. Crit. Care Med.*, 150, 17, 1994.

217. Swain, S. L., Huston, G., Tonkonogy, S., and Weinberg, A., Transforming growth factor-β and IL-4 cause helper T cell precursors to develop into distinct effector helper cells that differ in lymphokine secretion pattern and cell surface phenotype, *J. Immunol.*, 147, 2991, 1991.

218. Daynes, R. A., Dowell, T., and Araneo, B. A., Platelet-derived growth factor is a potent biologic response modifier of T cells, *J. Exp. Med.* 174, 1323, 1991.

219. Hackett, R. J., Davis, L. S., and Lipsky, P. E., Comparative effects of tumor necrosis factor-alpha and IL-1-beta on mitogen-induced T cell activation, *J. Immunol.*, 140, 2639, 1988.

220. Philip, R. and Epstein, L. B., TNF as immunomodulator and mediator of monocyte cytotoxicity induced by itself, *Nature*, 323, 86, 1986.

221. Silberstein, D. S. and Davis, J. R., Tumour necrosis factor enhances eosinophil toxicity to *Schistosoma mansoni* larvae, *Proc. Natl. Acad. Sci. U.S.A.*, 83, 1055, 1986.

222. Ulich, T. R., del Castillo, J., Ni, R. X., Bikhazi, N., and Calvin, L., Mechanisms of TNF-induced lymphopenia, neutropenia, and biphasic neutrophilia: a study of lymphocyte recirculation and hematologic interactions of TNF with endogenous mediators of leukocyte trafficking, *J. Leukocyte Biol.*, 45, 155, 1989.

223. Thorton, S. C., Pot, S. B., Walsh, B. J., Penny, R., and Breit, S. N., Interaction of immune and connective tissue cells: I. The effect of lymphokines and monokines on fibroblast growth, *J. Leukocyte Biol.*, 47, 312, 1990.

224. Oppenheim, J. J., Kovacs, F. J., Matsushima, K., and Durum, S. K., There is more than one interleukin 1, *Immunol. Today*, 7, 45, 1986.

225. Greenbaum, L. A., Horowitz, J. B., Woods, A., Pasqualini, T., Reich, E.-P., and Bottomly, K., Autocrine growth of CD4+ T cells. Differential effects of IL-1 on helper and inflammatory T cells, *J. Immunol.*, 140, 1555, 1988.

226. Pober, J. S., Gimbrone, M. A., Lapierre, L. A., Mendrick, D. L., Fiers, W., Rothlein, R., and Springer, T. A., Overlapping patterns of activating of human endothelial cells by interleukin 1, tumor necrosis factor, and immune interferon, *J. Immunol.*, 137, 1893, 1986.

227. Murray, H. W., Interferon-gamma, the activated macrophage, and host defence against microbial challenge, *Ann. Intern. Med.*, 108, 595, 1988.

228. Trinchieri, G. and Perussia, B., Immune interferon: a pleiotropic lymphokine with multiple effects, *Immunol. Today*, 6, 131, 1985.

229. Pestka, S. and Langer, J., Interferons and their actions, *Annu. Rev. Biochem.*, 56, 727, 1987.

Chapter 5

# EPITHELIAL FUNCTION AND AIRWAY RESPONSIVENESS

Roy G. Goldie and Janet M. H. Preuss

## CONTENTS

0-8493-7813-3/97/$0.00+$.50
© 1997 by CRC Press, Inc.

# I. INTRODUCTION

Until relatively recent times, the physical barrier role played by the airway epithelium to protect underlying structures was considered to be the major function of this tissue. However, it has become apparent that the airway epithelium is a very complex and highly specialised structure, containing numerous cell types and subserving an array of functions critical to homeostasis in the respiratory tract. The secretion of fluids and mucus, the synthesis of many biologically active substances, and the metabolism of various endogenous and exogenous substances are but a few of these (Figure 1). This chapter will focus on the potential modulatory influences of the airway epithelium on airway smooth muscle responsiveness to chemical stimuli, including various proinflammatory mediators relevant to the pathogenesis of asthma.

There is a basal release from the airway epithelium of both relaxant and spasmogenic substances which might diffuse to the underlying airway smooth muscle to directly influence tone. However, various chemical stimuli can also initiate the synthesis and release of substances from the epithelium, which might subsequently alter the state of airway smooth muscle contraction. Both of these cases will be dealt with in this review. Importantly, the airway epithelium can influence the concentration of mediators within submucosal biophases in a variety of ways, each of which will also be addressed. First, however, it is necessary to recognise the structural and functional heterogeneity of the airway epithelium.

## II. AIRWAY EPITHELIAL CELL TYPES

The mammalian airway epithelium is a remarkably diverse and complicated layer, consisting of at least 11 major cell types, although the function of many of them remains uncertain.[1,2] These include ciliated cells, goblet, brush and K cells (including neuroepithelial body cells), basal and Clara cells, and globule leukocytes (derived from subepithelial mast cells). There are both inter- and intraspecies differences in the composition of the epithelium of the airways and a striking diversity in both the epithelial architecture and the relative distribution of the various cells in different regions.[1,3,4]

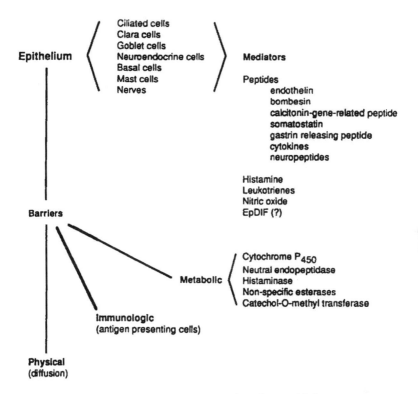

FIGURE 1 The functional roles of the airway epithelium.

The significant morphological differences in the various epithelial cell types are reflected in important differences in their functional characteristics and in the response to injury. Thus, whereas ciliated cells primarily promote the flow of mucus,[3] secretory cells, including goblet serous cells and Clara cells, play a key role in the generation and maintenance of the mucociliary system. Cytochrome $P_{450}$–metabolising isozymes are present only in Clara cells, which possess the highest rate of cytochrome $P_{450}$–mediated metabolism of any cell type.[5,6] Several inflammatory cells, including lymphocytes[1,3] and mast cells,[7] have been localised to the airway epithelium. In particular in asthma, the bronchial epithelium contains appreciable numbers of eosinophils which have significant capacity to release powerful proinflammatory mediators.[8]

The bronchial epithelium is also well innervated. For example, peripheral branches of peptide-containing sensory nerves are readily detected.[9,10] The materials released from these nerves include tachykinins, such as substance P (SP), which have been implicated in neurogenic airway inflammation.[11] Intraepithelial axons are observed associated with all cell types, but in particular basal cells,[12] brush cells,[13] K cells,[14] and neuroepithelial bodies.[15]

Neuroendocrine cells are in low density, scattered throughout the respiratory tract, with increasing numbers detected with decreasing airway size.[16]

Importantly, pulmonary neuroendocrine cells (PNEC) contain a number of substances with potentially important biologic activities in the airways. For example, PNECs contain 5-hydroxytryptamine, bombesin, calcitonin gene-related peptide, somatostatin, and endothelin, as well as gastrin-releasing peptide, katacalcin, and calcitonin.[16] Rather than secreting their contents into the airway lumen, mediator release from these cells is polarised such that products are directed towards cells beneath the epithelial basement membrane, including nerves, blood vessels, and airway smooth muscle.[17-19] Neuroepithelial bodies are clusters of neuroendocrine cells and are often seen in close apposition to nerves. In such cases, they may act as intrapulmonary chemoreceptors.[15,20] It is also noteworthy that the numbers of PNECs increase in various respiratory disorders, including cystic fibrosis, emphysema, chronic bronchitis, bronchopulmonary dysplasia, and asthma.[16]

Clearly then, the airway epithelium is a complex, multifunctional cellular network which plays a critical role in the normal physiology and regulation of homeostasis in the respiratory tract. In the following section, the impact of epithelium-derived substances on airway wall function will be examined.

## III. EPITHELIUM-DERIVED MEDIATORS

The airway epithelium is capable of generating, releasing, and metabolising a diverse array of biologically active substances. No attempt will be made here to exhaustively describe all of these. Rather, this section will focus on those substances which are most likely to impact on airway smooth muscle tone.

### A. OXIDATIVE METABOLITES OF ARACHIDONIC ACID
### 1. Cyclooxygenase Products

The first report concerning the potential modulatory influence of the epithelium on the level of tone in airway smooth muscle was published by Orehek et al.[21] in 1975. They demonstrated that scraping the mucosal surface of the guinea pig trachea stimulated the release of prostaglandins (PGs). It was hypothesised that the local release of PGs played an important role in the regulation of airway smooth muscle tone.[21] Support for this concept was provided by the study of O'Byrne and colleagues,[22] which demonstrated that $PGF_{2\alpha}$ enhanced the responsiveness of the pulmonary airways of the dog.

Certainly, cyclooxygenase and lipoxygenase products of arachidonic acid metabolism can be produced by the airway epithelium,[23] and these can influence the activity of various neighbouring cells. The major arachidonic acid metabolites released from primary tracheal epithelial cultures from humans and animal species are $PGE_2$ and $PGF_{2\alpha}$.[21,24-27] Furthermore, mechanical disruption of the guinea pig tracheal epithelium results in the release of both $PGE_2$ and $PGF_{2\alpha}$. Importantly, inhibition of cyclooxygenase with indomethacin in guinea pig tracheal preparations increased the contractile response to histamine and 5-HT.[21,28] Arachidonic acid which relaxes guinea pig[29,30] and canine[31] airway smooth muscle with an intact epithelium, caused contraction in epithelium-denuded preparations,[29] consistent with the view that the epithelium can release inhibitory PGs under conditions of significant basal tone. Interestingly, $PGE_2$ and $PGF_{2\alpha}$ caused contraction in guinea pig trachea in the absence of basal tone and may be responsible for "intrinsic" airway smooth muscle tone.[32,33]

Various mediators have also been shown to promote the generation and release of epithelium-derived PGs. For example, SP causes relaxation of precontracted rat trachea, a response which is epithelium-dependent and indomethacin-sensitive.[34,35] Furthermore, $PGE_2$ release from canine tracheal epithelium has been reported in response to bradykinin,[36] leukotriene $C_4$ ($LTC_4$), and $LTD_4$.[37] $PGE_2$ release has also been detected in epithelial cultures from canine,[31,38] rabbit, and rat[39] airways in response to bradykinin and the calcium ionophore A23187.

## 2. Lipoxygenase Products

There are numerous cellular sources of the LTs, including a variety of inflammatory cells such as eosinophils, mast cells, macrophages, basophils, neutrophils, and monocytes. The qualitative and quantitative nature of the release of the LTs depends on the cell type and also the stimulus.[40-42]

The LTs have been implicated in the pathogenesis of a variety of disorders. Asthma is a disease for which there is the most convincing evidence that the LTs, particularly the peptidoleukotrienes, play a key role. Thus, the LTs mimic many of the features of the disease. For example, the peptidoleukotrienes are very potent bronchoconstrictor agonists in human airways *in vitro* and *in vivo*, being more than 1000-fold as potent as histamine or cholinoceptor agonists.[43-48] In addition, they potently stimulate mucus secretion from human airways *in vitro*[49,50] and increase microvascular permeability,[51-53] actions which are consistent with the mucus plugging and oedema seen characteristically in asthma.[54]

The predominant lipoxygenase pathway in human epithelium appears to be via 15-lipoxygenase.[26,55,56] In contrast, 12-lipoxygenase predominates in bovine epithelium[57] and 12-lipoxygenase in canine and sheep cells. Low levels of 5-lipoxygenase, which catalyses the synthesis of the sulphidopeptidoleukotrienes $LTC_4$, $LTD_4$, and $LTE_4$, as well as the potent chemotactic factor $LTB_4$, were also detected in canine and sheep epithelial cells.[26,56,58,59]

It was recently reported that platelet-activating factor (PAF) stimulated the release of 15-HETE from cultured human bronchial epithelial cells in sufficient quantities to elicit airway smooth muscle contraction[60] and of $LTC_4$ and $LTD_4$ from rabbit tracheal explants.[61] Similar rabbit explants also released 5-, 12-, and 15-HETEs in response to arachidonic acid.[62] Whereas the 12-HETEs are the primary metabolites from rabbit epithelium, the 15-HETEs predominate from human bronchial epithelial cultures in response to arachidonic acid, PAF, bradykinin, and acetylcholine.[23,26,60] Exposure to ozone also stimulated the release of cyclooxygenase and lipoxygenase products from cultured bovine tracheal epithelial cells.[25]

Interestingly, epithelium-derived prostanoids and LTs may cause the slow decline in cholinergic nerve-mediated airway smooth muscle contraction in both ferrets and dogs.[63-65] The release of the chemoattractant $LTB_4$ from freshly isolated canine airway epithelial cells has also been demonstrated.[59] More-recent studies have indicated that the airway epithelium is also able to release various nonlipoxygenase products, which are chemotactic for several respiratory cell types. For example, bovine and human bronchial epithelial cells in culture release fibronectin, which is chemotactic for lung fibroblasts.[66] Supernatants from cultured bovine bronchial epithelial cells possess chemotactic activity for T helper lymphocytes and B-lymphocytes.[67] In addition, bronchial epithelial cells, which are capable of directed migration, release substances such as fibronectin, which are chemotactic for epithelial cells.[68]

## B. HISTAMINE

In the airways, the major site of histamine storage is in mast cells found predominantly in the mucosa and submucosa near blood vessels and glands, although some are located in the airway epithelium.[69,70] Histamine-induced effects may be mediated via activation of $H_1$, $H_2$, or $H_3$ receptors. Histamine elicits $H_1$-mediated bronchospasm in most species, including humans.[71] Histamine-induced increased microvascular permeability in airways is also mediated via $H_1$ receptor activation causing endothelial cell contraction and intercellular gap formation,[72,73] a process which can promote mucosal oedema.[74,75] Furthermore, it has been suggested that histamine-induced stimulation of epithelial $H_1$ receptors alters ion and fluid transport and affects the viscosity of the mucus.

Histamine $H_2$ receptor–mediated events include bronchial dilation, stimulation of suppressor T cells, and increases in mucus secretion.[75] $H_2$ receptors are present in airway smooth muscle of the rat, rabbit, cat, and sheep, where they mediate airway smooth muscle relaxation, but these receptors do not appear to be present in airway smooth muscle from the pig, goat, calf, horse, or human. $H_2$ histamine receptors have been detected in human bronchial epithelium,[78] activation of which has been demonstrated to stimulate airway mucus secretion.[79]

$H_3$ receptor activation has been linked to inhibition of cholinergic neurotransmission in human[80] and guinea pig[81] airways, inhibition of excitatory nonadrenergic, noncholinergic (e-NANC) neural bronchoconstriction in the guinea pig,[82] as well as to inhibition of neurogenic airway microvascular leakage.[83] In addition, $H_3$ receptors on mast cells can be activated to reduce histamine release.[84]

## C. CYTOKINES

Airway epithelial cells express and produce several cytokines, including granulocyte/macrophage colony-stimulating factor (GM-CSF), interleukin (IL)-1α, IL-1β, IL-6, and IL-8.[85-88] Exposure of human bronchial epithelial cell cultures to toluene diisocyanate resulted in a marked increase in the release of IL-1β and IL-6.[86] In guinea pig isolated trachea, IL-1 reduced the relaxant effect of isoprenaline,[89] although this is not always observed.[90] Interestingly, cultured bronchial epithelial cells from asthmatic individuals released more GM-CSF than cells from nonasthmatic individuals, and they also expressed increased levels of mRNA for GM-CSF.[91] Furthermore, the production of proinflammatory cytokines by the human airway epithelial cells is increased following infection with respiratory syncytial virus,[92,93] a virus commonly associated with exacerbations of asthma in young children.[94]

## D. ENDOTHELIN

It is well established that the endogenous peptide endothelin-1 (ET-1) is synthesised in vascular endothelial cells.[95] However, it is also now established that the bronchial epithelium is a major site of synthesis and release of this peptide.[96,97] ET-1 is a potent spasmogen in human bronchial smooth muscle,[98,99] accelerates the growth of airway smooth muscle cells in culture[100,101] and stimulates mucus gland secretion.[102] These activities suggest a role for ET-1 in asthma, since elevated airway tone, airway smooth muscle hyperplasia, and hypersecretion of mucus are characteristic features of this disease.[103] Immunoreactive ET has also been shown to be released from human bronchial,[104] canine,[105] and guinea pig[106] tracheal epithelial cells. In addition, ET-like immunoreactivity can be demonstrated in bronchiolar epithelial cells *in vivo* in rats, and mice, as well as in mucus, serous, and Clara cells with very little observed in basal or ciliated cells.[107] Importantly, levels of ET-like immunoreactive material are significantly elevated in the bronchial epithelium[97] and bronchoalveolar lavage fluid of asthmatic individuals,[108] a finding which may be of particular relevance to putative pathophysiological actions of this peptide.

In this regard, we have recently reported that low concentrations of ET-1 caused marked potentiation of cholinergic nerve-mediated contraction of murine airway smooth muscle, an effect involving activation of postganglionic, neuronal $ET_B$ receptors.[109] This indicates that ET-1 can have a marked amplifier action on this important bronchoconstrictor mechanism. ET-3 had a similar effect in rabbit bronchus, where receptors for ET-1 were identified on parasympathetic ganglion cells.[110] It is interesting to note that, whereas the bronchial epithelium is a significant site of ET synthesis, epithelial cells contain relatively few receptors for ET-1.[98,111,112] Studies using cultured feline tracheal epithelial cells suggest that such receptors mediate the production of a variety of arachidonic acid metabolites, including $PGE_2$ and $PGF_{2\alpha}$, 5-HETE, and 12-HETE.[113]

Epithelium-derived ET-1 may have a physiological role in tissue repair and regeneration, as well as in the maintenance of airway smooth muscle tone. However, in inflammatory airway diseases such as asthma, where ET-1 is produced in greater than usual amounts, pathological airway responses may result, including airway smooth muscle hyperplasia, mucus gland hyperplasia and hypersecretion, and excessive airway smooth muscle contraction.

### E. TACHYKININS

SP, neurokinin A (NKA), and neurokinin B (NKB; also known as neuro-kinin K) belong to the family of sensory neuropeptides known as the tachy-kinins. In the pulmonary system, the tachykinins are contained in capsaicin-sensitive peripheral unmyelinated branches of primary afferent neurons, also known as "sensory C-fibres." The airway epithelium, blood vessels associated with several ganglia and mucus glands, and airway smooth muscle from many species all have SP- and NKA-containing neurones.[10,50]

The tachykinins are potent bronchoconstrictors of isolated airway prepa-rations from several species including humans in which bronchospasm appears to be via an NK2 receptor.[114-116] SP induces mucus secretion in animal and human airways *in vitro*[117-119] and may be also responsible for e-NANC bron-choconstriction.[120-122] Exogenous neurokinins increase microvascular perme-ability in rat and guinea pig airways and may also mediate neurogenic leak-age.[11,123] The ability of the tachykinins to modulate responses of inflammatory cells suggests that they have a role as immunomodulators.[124,125]

In asthma, SP may play a role via an axon reflex, excessively activated as a result of epithelial damage which exposes sensory afferent nerves. Stimula-tion of these nerve fibres by proinflammatory substances such as bradykinin or LTs released from inflammatory cells might in turn release neuronal tachy-kinins to exert effects including bronchospasm, mucus secretion, microvascu-lar leakage, and cough.[117,124,126,127]

The tachykinins are effective substrates for neutral endopeptidase (NEP), which is present in abundance in airway epithelium and which modulates responses to the tachykinins. SP-induced bronchospasm in guinea pigs may also be modulated by angiotensin-converting enzyme.[128]

### F. NITRIC OXIDE

Current evidence suggests that nitric oxide (NO) is a primary mediator of inhibitory NANC (i-NANC) neurotransmission in animal[129-131] and human[132,133] airways. The airway epithelium contains NO synthase (NOS),[134] raising the possibility that this source of NO may have a modulatory influence on airway smooth muscle tone. This concept is supported by data showing that ET-1 can cause relaxation of precontracted isolated guinea pig trachea, a response which was apparently mediated by epithelium-derived NO,[135] and that NOS inhibition results in airway hyperresponsiveness to histamine in the guinea pig.[136]

A form of NOS can be induced in the lung by endotoxin[137] and by cytokines including TNFα.[138] Interestingly, levels of the inducible form of this enzyme were significantly elevated in the bronchial epithelium in asthma[138] and raised levels of NO can be detected in the expired air.[139] However, rather than subserving a beneficial airway dilator function, NO in asthma may be associ-ated with tissue damage,[140] but in expired air may also be a useful marker of bronchial inflammation.[139,141]

# IV. THE EPITHELIUM IN DEFENCE
# OF THE AIRWAY WALL

## A. BARRIER FUNCTIONS

The airway epithelium serves as an effective barrier between the underlying tissues of the airway wall and the external environment. This barrier is created in physical, immunologic, and metabolic terms. In each case, the result can be modulation of the presentation of biologically active molecules to the internal milieu and, thus, modification of responses of tissue elements including the microvasculature, nerves, and airway smooth muscle to these penetrating substances.

## 1. Physical Barriers
### a. Intercellular Junctions

Intercellular junctions, which connect the apical surfaces of individual cells, form critical elements of the physical barrier system in the airway epithelium.[1,142] These junctions protect the airways from noxious inhaled substances and also prevent the uncontrolled leakage of water and solutes into the airway lumen. The tight junction complexes which consist of a proximal, continuous zonula occludens provide the barrier function. In addition, intermediate, continuous zonula adherens exist which subserve cell adhesion and recognition functions, whereas desmosomes are involved in maintaining the structural integrity of the epithelium.[142-145] In addition, gap junctions exist which are involved in cell–cell communication,[146-148] permitting the nonspecific intercellular exchange of small molecules and ions, apparently via passive diffusion.

### b. Secretion of Mucus

Cells in the airway epithelium secrete a diverse array of materials, including mucus, water, and electrolytes,[149,150] as part of the complex of defence mechanisms to protect the lungs from harmful substances inhaled from the external environment. The epithelium presents the first barrier to allergens by providing a blanket of mucus over the airway surface which traps allergens for transport back to the pharynx by the beating cilia. The mucus contains proteolytic enzymes which also degrade allergens.[151] In healthy airways, the production of mucus is limited to provide an adequate system for airway lubrication and the entrapment of inhaled foreign particles. However, the amount, composition, and viscosity of mucus may be altered in airway diseases, including viral infections, asthma, bronchitis, and cystic fibrosis.[1,152,153] In the larger airways, submucosal glands provide the bulk of the material secreted to the airway surface.[1,3,6] However, epithelial serous, goblet, and Clara cells also contribute significantly to airway mucus production.[154,155]

## 2. Immunologic Barrier

It is also well established that the epithelium can play an active role in preventing antigen access to submucosal tissues. The epithelium is at the interface between the immune system and the external environment. The efficient identification, clearance, and disposal of inspired pathogenic antigens is critical to the maintenance of immunologic homeostasis in the respiratory tree.[151] Allergens which have escaped mucociliary clearance and resident macrophages may bind to airway epithelial cells via specific receptors. Adhesion molecules present in the epithelium are then responsible for the attachment of lymphocytes to these antigen-presenting cells, thereby directing inflammatory cells to the site to allow clearance and/or detoxification of the allergen and the initiation of tissue repair.[156]

In humans and animal species, airway epithelial cells have been shown to express class I and class II major histocompatibility complex (MHC) antigens. Since these are necessary for accessory cell function in antigen presentation,[157-159] the epithelium plays a role in regulating the immune response subsequent to inhalation of antigens.[158] Of particular interest is the finding that a complex network of dendritic cells, located in the airway epithelium, is involved in the trapping of inhaled antigen and in its presentation to T-lymphocytes as part of the local immune response in airways.[160-163]

## 3. Metabolic Barrier

The epithelium has a capacity to metabolise a broad spectrum of substances. For example, the airway epithelium is a rich source of neutral endopeptidase (NEP).[164,165] This enzyme is a membrane-bound neutral metalloendopeptidase, also known as enkephalinase.[166] NEP, which is localised at the surface of airway epithelial cells, can cleave many peptide substances,[167] including the tachykinins, bradykinin,[168] vasoactive intestinal peptide (VIP),[169] and endothelin.[170] Inhibitors of NEP, such as thiorphan or phosphoramidon, potentiate the effects of SP on mucus gland secretion *in vitro*,[118] ciliary beat frequency,[171] and airway smooth muscle contraction.[165,172,173] In potentiating the actions of bradykinin,[174] endothelin,[170] atrial natriuretic peptides,[175] and VIP,[176,177] the effect of NEP inhibitors in epithelium-containing airway smooth muscle preparations mimics to a large extent the effects of epithelium removal, suggesting that the epithelium can act as a significant site of peptide metabolism.

Furthermore, recent evidence suggests that histaminase present in guinea pig tracheal epithelium contributes to the inhibitory effect of the epithelium on histamine-induced contraction.[178] Metabolism of histamine can also occur in human bronchial epithelium via histamine N-methyltransferase, inhibition of which caused enhanced contractile responses to histamine.[179] In isolated guinea pig tracheal strips, the epithelium may be a major site of extraneuronal uptake and *O*-methylation of catecholamines, such as isoprenaline.[180] The guinea pig tracheal epithelium may also be a site for the uptake and degradation of adenosine.[180,181]

The Clara cell (nonciliated bronchiolar secretory cell) is highly metabolically active and possesses a variety of enzymes including acid and alkaline phosphatases, nonspecific esterase, hydroxylases, transferases, peroxidases, and catalase, in addition to cytochrome $P_{450}$ monoxygenase.[1,182,183] A primary function of the Clara cell is to metabolise xenobiotic cytotoxic agents that enter the respiratory tract via the air or blood. This is achieved via cytochrome $P_{450}$—mediated metabolism, a pathway which is more active in the Clara cell than in any other pulmonary cell type.[3,184-186]

## V. FUNCTIONAL CONSEQUENCES OF EPITHELIAL DISRUPTION

Clearly then, if the integrity of epithelial structure is significantly compromised, for example, via the disruption of intercellular tight junctions, the potential exists for perturbations of responsiveness of underlying tissues to inhaled chemical stimuli. A signal feature of asthma is damage to or desquamation of the epithelium.[8,164,187,188] Importantly, a correlation between the extent of damage and the degree of airway hyperresponsiveness to airway smooth muscle spasmogens has been reported,[187] although a study by Lozewicz and co-workers[189] comparing airway biopsies from nonasthmatic and stable asthmatic subjects did not confirm such a relationship.

Epithelial damage may result in increased permeability and easier access of allergens, pollutants, and inflammatory and contractile agents to intra- and subepithelial nerves, inflammatory cells, and vascular and airway smooth muscle. Epithelial damage with associated bronchial hyperresponsiveness is observed in patients with farmer's lung[190] and viral infections.[191] Aerosol administration of substances that cause bronchial epithelial damage, including ozone, nitrogen dioxide, and toluene diisocyanate,[192-194] results in bronchial hyperresponsiveness. In experimental animals exposure of the airways to inflammatory stimuli, such as cigarette smoke, which increase epithelium permeability, increased the responsiveness of the airways to spasmogens.[195-197] Experiments in humans have provided conflicting data, with some suggesting increased permeability in asthma,[198] while others failed to observe this.[199,200]

The precise mechanism(s) responsible for asthma-associated airway epithelial damage have not been completely elucidated. However, a significant contribution from the cytotoxic products of eosinophils, notably major basic protein (MBP), has been proposed.[201] In asthma, eosinophils are recruited into the airways and can be detected in the epithelial layer.[70,187] Currently, it is believed that eosinophils play a critical role in the pathogenesis of asthma, and a correlation between eosinophil number and the changes in pulmonary function has been reported.[202] MBP can induce airway epithelial damage that is histologically similar to that observed in asthma.[54,188,201,203] Perhaps importantly, this damage has been associated with increased responsiveness of isolated airway tissues.[204,205]

Neutrophil numbers are also elevated in the bronchoalveolar lavage fluid in asthma, temporally associated with the late-phase asthmatic response to antigen, and this may also be associated with epithelial damage.[206] A link between increased epithelial permeability, enhanced microvascular permeability, submucosal oedema and desquamation, and damage to the epithelium has not been evaluated fully.

## A. AIRWAY SMOOTH MUSCLE TONE

Ten years after the novel observations of Orehek et al.,[21] experiments in canine bronchus demonstrated the modulatory influence of mechanical removal of the epithelium on contractile responses to several agonists and also on relaxant responses to isoproterenol.[207] These studies suggested that the airway epithelium exerted an inhibitory influence on neighbouring smooth muscle cells. Subsequently, various groups have confirmed the modulatory effects of the epithelium on isolated tissue responsiveness to spasmogenic and relaxant agonists (for reviews, see Referencs 208 through 210) (Table 1).

### TABLE 1
**Examples of Studies Reporting Increased Responsiveness
of Isolated Airway Smooth Muscle Preparations to
Spasmogens and Relaxants Following Epithelium Removal**

| Agonist | Species | Tissue | Ref. |
|---|---|---|---|
| Acetylcholine | Guinea pig | Trachea | 211, 212 |
| | Canine | Bronchus | 207, 213 |
| | Bovine | Trachea | 214 |
| | Human | Bronchus | 215 |
| Methacholine | Guinea pig | Trachea | 212, 216 |
| | Canine | Bronchus | 217 |
| | Human | Trachea | 218 |
| Bethanechol | Rabbit | Bronchus | 219 |
| Histamine | Guinea pig | Trachea | 211, 216, 220 |
| | Canine | Bronchus | 213, 217 |
| | Bovine | Bronchus | 214 |
| | Human | Bronchus | 215 |
| 5-HT | Guinea pig | Trachea | 211 |
| | Canine | Bronchus | 213 |
| | Bovine | Bronchus | 214 |
| Adenosine | Guinea pig | Trachea | 181, 211 |
| Leukotriene $C_4/D_4$ | Guinea pig | Trachea | 224, 225 |
| Isoprenaline | Guinea pig | Trachea | 176, 180 |
| | Bovine | Bronchi | 214 |
| Sodium nitroprusside | Guinea pig | Trachea | 180 |
| PAF | Guinea pig | Trachea | 226, 227 |
| Substance P | Guinea pig | Trachea | 173, 221 |
| VIP | Guinea pig | Trachea | 176 |
| Endothelin | Guinea pig | Trachea | 170 |
| | Rabbit | Trachea | 222 |
| | Human | Bronchus | 223 |

Several mechanisms may be involved in this epithelium-dependent modulatory effect, with their contributions varying depending on the bronchoactive substance involved. These mechanisms include the epithelium acting as

1. A diffusion barrier
2. A site of metabolism
3. A source of inhibitory and/or contractile substances

This section will focus on the influence and possible reasons for epithelium-dependent modulation of airway smooth muscle responsiveness to various mediators. Many studies involved determining the effects of mechanical removal of the epithelium on responsiveness of isolated airway smooth muscle.

### 1. Histamine

Several studies showed that epithelium removal caused twofold to eightfold increases in histamine potency in guinea pig tracheal smooth muscle preparations.[216,220,228] In some cases, maximum contraction was also increased,[28,216,229,230] but in others no effect was observed.[211,220] Interestingly, the influence of epithelial ablation on airway smooth muscle responsiveness to histamine in the guinea pig, was age-dependent, with the greatest increases in histamine potency seen during the early stages of animal maturation.[228] Epithelial ablation also increased responsiveness to histamine in guinea pig isolated bronchus.[230] Epithelium removal in canine bronchus also produced significant increases in airway sensitivity and maximum response to histamine.[207,231] In guinea pig trachea, responsiveness to histamine after epithelial ablation was greater in preparations previously sensitised to ovalbumin than in tissues from nonsensitised controls.[232] Importantly, human bronchial sensitivity to histamine was also significantly increased following epithelium removal[233,234] (Figure 2), although epithelium ablation in bronchial preparations from human asthmatic lung failed to result in increased sensitivity to histamine.[234]

Having demonstrated that histamine caused a greater release of $PGE_2$ from epithelium-intact compared with epithelium-free guinea pig trachea, Braunstein and colleagues[28] concluded that the modulatory influence of the epithelium was in large part attributable to the release of relaxant $PGE_2$, although such release could not be confirmed in a separate study.[235] The epithelium contains histaminase and thus may act as a site of metabolism to modulate histamine-induced responses in guinea pig trachea.[178] Güc et al.[236] postulated the existence of a non-$H_1$-/non-$H_2$-histamine receptor which mediated the release of a nonprostanoid epithelium-derived inhibitory factor.

### 2. Muscarinic Cholinoceptor Agonists

As for histamine, mechanical ablation of the epithelium has been shown to significantly increase the potencies of acetylcholine, methacholine, and bethanechol by twofold to sevenfold in airways from the rat,[228] guinea

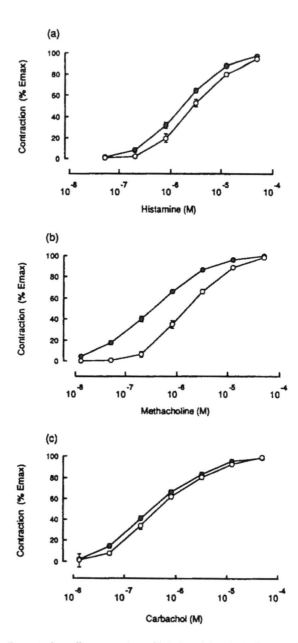

**FIGURE 2** Concentration–effect curves to (a) histamine, (b) methacholine, and (c) carbachol in bronchial preparations with an intact epithelium (O) or with the epithelium removed (●), isolated from nondiseased human lung. Vertical bars represent means ± s.e.m. of responses from 12-20 bronchial preparations. (Reproduced with permission from Fernandes et al. (1990). *Eur. J. Pharmacol.*, 187, 331-336.)

pig,[173,211,212,216,220,229,237] rabbit,[218,238] dog,[207,239] pig,[240] cow,[215] and human[215,234] (see Table 1). In contrast, the spasmogenic effects of carbachol were not increased in epithelium-denuded airway preparations.[211,212,216,228,234] The reasons for this difference are not well defined, but do not seem to relate to muscarinic receptor subtype selectivities.[237] Although seemingly unlikely, it is possible that the epithelium is more permeable to carbachol than to related agonists and is thus less affected by removal of this tissue.

It has also been proposed that the epithelium-dependent augmentation of acetylcholine-induced contractions of canine trachea *in situ*, induced by eosinophil MBP, was mediated by an epithelium-derived contractile factor,[205] perhaps ET-1.

### 3. Potassium Ions

Airway smooth muscle sensitivity to $K^+$ was not significantly altered by epithelium removal in bovine,[214] canine,[241] rabbit,[218] rat,[228] or guinea pig[211,216,220,229] airways. However, it has been suggested that mechanical stripping of the epithelium can induce the release of tryptase from mast cells, which causes potentiation of several spasmogens including $K^+$.[242,243]

### 4. Leukotrienes

There is general agreement that epithelium removal increases isolated airway sensitivity to LTs. However, the mechanisms underlying this effect remain the subject of controversy, with some evidence for the involvement of both prostanoid and nonprostanoid inhibitory mediators. In addition, species differences complicate any attempt to arrive at a unifying explanation for all the data. Thus, guinea pig tracheal sensitivity to the spasmogenic effects of $LTC_4$ and $LTD_4$ was increased twofold to fourfold after epithelium removal, whereas $LTD_4$-induced responses were unaltered.[224] Interestingly, indomethacin mimicked the effect of epithelium removal on sensitivity to $LTC_4$, suggesting that the contractile effect of this substance was modulated by a smooth muscle inhibitory prostanoid derived from the epithelium. In contrast, indomethacin did not increase responsiveness to $LTD_4$, perhaps because that to $LTD_4$ was influenced by a nonprostanoid substance.[224] However, these data are at odds with a report from Hisayama et al.[225] who showed that epithelium removal shifted the concentration–effect curve to $LTD_4$ to the left by 6.3-fold and that this was inhibited by the cyclooxygenase inhibitor flurbiprofen.

Prié and colleagues[230] confirmed that responsiveness to all three peptidoleukotrienes was increased following epithelial denudation of guinea pig tracheal and bronchial preparations. Furthermore, $LTD_4$ and histamine stimulated the release of $PGE_2$ and 6-keto-$PGF_{1\alpha}$. However, this release was not reduced by removal of the epithelium.[230] In contrast, no effect of $LTD_4$ on release of $PGE_2$, $PGF_{2\alpha}$, and 6-keto-$PGF_{1\alpha}$ from guinea pig trachea was observed in either the presence or absence of the epithelium,[235] suggesting that the modulatory effect of the epithelium involved the release of a nonprostanoid inhibitory factor(s).

Epithelium removal also produced a threefold increase in sensitivity to $LTD_4$ in human bronchus via an indomethacin-sensitive mechanism, but had no influence on the responsiveness to $LTC_4$ or $LTE_4$.[244] This suggested that an epithelium-derived inhibitory cyclooxygenase product, perhaps $PGE_2$, modulated $LTD_4$-induced responses in human airways. However, in the same study it was noted that, whereas epithelium removal potentiated sensitivity of isolated guinea pig trachea to $LTC_4$ and $LTD_4$, a threefold decrease in sensitivity to $LTE_4$ was seen which was abolished by lipoxygenase inhibitors. Thus, the inhibitory effect of epithelium removal on responses to $LTE_4$ might have involved an $LTE_4$-induced release of a smooth muscle excitatory product of 5-lipoxygenase.[46]

### 5. Platelet-Activating Factor

Brunelleschi and co-workers[226] showed that PAF induced epithelium-dependent relaxation in precontracted guinea pig trachea. In addition, PAF stimulated the release of $PGE_2$,[226] which was abolished by epithelium removal and markedly decreased in the presence of indomethacin. Thus, PAF may have caused relaxation of guinea pig isolated trachea following the synthesis and release of epithelium-derived $PGE_2$.

### 6. Bradykinin

Bradykinin is a potent bronchoconstrictor in asthmatics, but has little direct spasmogenic activity in airway smooth muscle from all animal species, except guinea pigs and ferrets.[245] In ferrets, bradykinin-induced tracheal contraction was not influenced by the epithelium,[168] whereas, in guinea pigs, this peptide was a relaxant agonist in epithelium-intact trachea and a spasmogen following epithelium removal.[246-248] In the presence of indomethacin, bradykinin contracted guinea-pig trachea whether or not the epithelium was intact.[247,248] A similar picture was observed with $PGE_2$, such that relaxation was observed in epithelium-intact guinea pig tracheal preparations and relaxation in epithelium-denuded tissue.[247] The ability of bradykinin to increase $PGE_2$ production in this tissue was also dramatically reduced by epithelium removal. Accordingly, it was suggested that the epithelium-dependent relaxation of guinea pig trachea in response to bradykinin, was mediated by $PGE_2$.

Medium from canine epithelial cell culture stimulated with bradykinin inhibited neurogenic contractions of canine bronchial preparations, and this was apparently due to bradykinin-induced production of an epithelium-derived product of cyclooxygenase.[38] This inhibitor was probably $PGE_2$, since it is generated by canine airway epithelium[31,249,250] and is known to inhibit neurogenic contractions in the dog airway.[251] These data are consistent with the hypothesis that bradykinin may indirectly modulate cholinergic neurotransmission in canine airways via the release of $PGE_2$ from the epithelium.

### 7. Tachykinins

The epithelium has a major modulatory influence on the responsiveness of guinea pig trachea to the tachykinins, primarily by providing NEP for peptide metabolism and perhaps by releasing an inhibitory substance(s). Thus, removing the epithelium increased the potency of SP by 20- to 150-fold and significantly increased the maximum response.[172,173,221,252] Inhibitors of NEP, such as phosphoramidon, mimicked the effects of epithelium removal.[165,172,173,253,254]

In the presence of the cyclooxygenase inhibitor indomethacin, removal of guinea pig tracheal epithelium still caused a 150-fold increase in sensitivity to SP. In the presence of phosphoramidon, this was dramatically reduced to 18-fold, suggesting that the residual potency increase was due to the effect of a nonprostanoid inhibitory substance.[173]

Epithelium removal enhanced responsiveness to SP[254] and to stimulation of intramural noncholinergic nerve endings in guinea pig bronchial preparation.[253] Epithelium removal also increased the potency of SP in ferret tracheal[165] and human bronchial preparations, where the increase was only about eightfold.[116]

Phosphoramidon and epithelium removal have both been shown to potentiate responsiveness of human bronchial smooth muscle to SP.[116,255] Naline and colleagues[116] also found that epithelium removal increased sensitivity to NKA. Although inhibition of NEP abolished the effect of epithelium removal on sensitivity to SP, epithelium removal still increased the sensitivity to NKA in the presence of phosphoramidon,[116] suggesting that, for NKA, another inhibitory mechanism was also involved. In contrast, in rat trachea SP caused relaxation which was markedly inhibited after removal of the epithelium, indicating that in this tissue SP induced the release of an epithelium-derived smooth muscle relaxant.[34]

### 8. Endothelin

The spasmogenic effect of ET-1 in guinea pig isolated tracheal smooth muscle[98,170] was enhanced by removing the epithelium.[170] Inhibitors of epithelium-derived PG production, angiotensin-converting enzyme, endopeptidase, or aminopeptidase had little effect on the potentiating influence of epithelium removal.[170] The ETs are good substrates for NEP.[256,257] Since the potentiating effect of epithelium removal was abolished by phosphoramidon, increased responsiveness of denuded guinea pig trachea to ET-1 was probably due to removal of a major site of metabolism, i.e., epithelial NEP.[170]

### 9. Antigen

Antigen-induced contraction in human and guinea pig airway preparations is mediated exclusively via the release of histamine and LTs.[258] The epithelium exerts a significant modulatory effect on the actions of these two mediators. Not surprisingly then, it has been shown that removal of the epithelium increased the sensitivity to ovalbumin of tracheal smooth muscle isolated from actively sensitised guinea pigs by sixfold to eightfold.[259,260] While it is possible that epithelium-derived substances influenced antigen-induced mediator release from mast cells, the relatively small changes observed with epithelial ablation are unlikely to be due to loss of inhibitory prostanoids, since in the presence of indomethacin, denudation produced a 300-fold increase in sensitivity to ovalbumin. Furthermore, superfusion cascade studies provided no direct evidence for the release of an inhibitory factor from the guinea pig tracheal epithelium.[260] However, the loss of the protective epithelial diffusion barrier may enhance responses to antigen, given the size of this molecule.

### 10. Nerve-Induced Responses

In guinea pig trachea, neuronal release of [$^3$H]-acetylcholine, in response to electrical field stimulation (EFS), was significantly increased following epithelium removal.[261] However, conflicting data have been reported concerning the influence of the epithelium on cholinergic nerve-induced contractile responses of various isolated airway smooth muscle preparations. For example, epithelium removal has been shown to have no effect[211] or to slightly potentiate[229] responses to EFS. In addition, in bovine trachea, epithelium removal had little effect on EFS-induced responses,[214] but did reverse the fade-in responses usually seen in dog bronchus.[207] Similar data were reported in ferret trachea,[262] in which the release of both prostanoid and nonprostanoid inhibitory factors from the epithelium was postulated in response to vagus nerve stimulation.[262] These data contrast sharply with results in porcine bronchial smooth muscle preparations in which epithelium removal inhibited the frequency–response relationship.[31]

Removal of epithelium resulted in a small potentiation of e-NANC responses in guinea pig trachea.[253] This appeared to be due to loss of epithelial NEP, as phosphoramidon abolished the effect.[253]

The inhibitory effects of the epithelium on membrane potential, neurotransmission, and the level of tone in canine trachea and bronchus precontracted via EFS in the presence of indomethacin has also been observed.[65] Hyperpolarisation of the smooth muscle membrane was also observed following addition of isolated and dispersed epithelial cells, an effect which was not altered by indomethacin.[65]

### 11. Relaxant Agonists

Several studies have examined the influence of epithelium removal on *in vitro* airway smooth muscle responses to β-adrenoceptor agonists such as isoprenaline and salbutamol. The results have sometimes been contradictory. For example, studies examining the relaxant effects of isoprenaline in guinea pig trachea[220,263] have shown that epithelial stripping had no significant influence on potency, but caused a reduction in maximal relaxant response (Emax). Similar data were reported for canine[207,264] and porcine airways.[240] In canine bronchial preparations, the attenuating effect of epithelial stripping on maximal relaxant responses to isoprenaline increased with decreasing airway diameter, suggesting an increasingly important modulatory role for this tissue down the respiratory tract.[239] Epithelium removal caused no change, or a small decrease in isoprenaline potency was observed in bovine tracheal preparations[214] and human bronchus.[233] In contrast, the guinea pig tracheal epithelium has been described as a potential extraneuronal uptake compartment for catecholamines, since epithelium removal increased isoprenaline potency.[176,180] Epithelium removal also had little effect upon responsiveness to the noncatecholamine β-agonists terbutaline[263] and salbutamol[180] or on the non-β-adrenoceptor relaxants theophylline and enprophylline[263] and nitroglycerine, although a small decrease in relaxant Emax for forskolin was seen in guinea pig trachea.[220]

Epithelium denudation also caused significant potentiation of the relaxant responses to exogenously applied VIP,[176] a peptide which, with NO, may be a neurotransmitter in the i-NANC nervous system.[129,130,132] Similar potentiation of VIP-induced relaxation of human bronchial preparations has been reported.[265] Atrial natriuretic peptide (ANP) causes airway smooth muscle relaxation,[266,267] which was markedly potentiated in epithelium-denuded preparations[175] (Figure 3). The neutral endopeptidase inhibitor phosphoramidon largely mimicked the potentiation observed with epithelium stripping for both VIP[177] and ANP,[175] further evidence that the airway epithelium has a significant capacity to act as a metabolic sink for various peptide substances. Interestingly, a tetrodotoxin-resistant i-NANC component of relaxation to EFS was reported in epithelium-intact guinea pig trachea, raising the possibility of the release of an epithelium-derived inhibitory factor.[177]

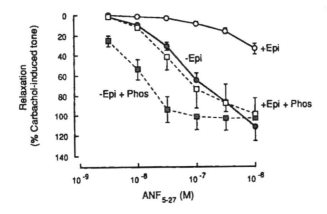

**FIGURE 3** Concentration-dependent relaxation to $ANF_{5-27}$ in epithelium-intact (+Epi, open symbols) and epithelium-denuded (–Epi, filled symbols) guinea pig tracheal preparations precontracted with carbachol $EC_{50}$ in the absence (circles; n = 10) or presence of 1 µM phosphoramidon (Phos; squares; n = 8). Each data point represents the mean ± s.e.m. of n preparations. (Reproduced with permission from Fernandes et al. (1992). *Eur. J. Pharmacol.*, 212, 187-194.)

## B. MUCOUS GLANDS

The influence of the epithelium on mucus secretion in feline tracheal submucosal glands has been assessed using [³H]-glucosamine-labelled mucus glycoconjugate.[268] The release of mucus was decreased in the presence of isolated epithelium to the level observed in tracheal explants. The epithelium-derived mediator of this effect was neither a cyclooxygenase nor a lipoxygenase product of arachidonic acid metabolism. These intriguing findings suggest that an epithelium-derived, nonprostanoid inhibitory factor can modulate secretory function in a fashion similar to that reported for modulation of tone in airway smooth muscle.

## C. INFLAMMATORY CELLS

The epithelium may also markedly influence the recruitment of inflammatory cells into the airways,[144] which in turn can affect epithelial function. For example, epithelial ion transport and mucus secretion may be influenced via the local release of inflammatory cell-derived mediators.[269,270]

The airway epithelium can alter inflammatory cell migration and direction via the release of chemotactic substances and as a result of the expression of epithelial adhesion molecules. Evidence for the release of various substances that are chemotactic for neutrophils, monocytes, lymphocytes, eosinophils, basophils, and mast cells has been obtained.[144] These factors include $LTB_4$[21] and cytokines such as GM-CSF and G-CSF,[87,271,272] in addition to several, as yet, unidentified materials.[144]

Neutrophil adherence to bovine bronchial epithelium was increased by exposure to cigarette smoke, lipopolysaccharide, or phorbol ester and was associated with epithelial cell cytotoxicity.[66] Furthermore, human parainfluenza virus type 2 markedly increased adherence of neutrophils to human tracheal epithelial cells. This response apparently involved adhesion molecule-1 (ICAM-1) and ICAM-1-independent mechanisms.[273] Mast cells also selectively adhered to canine epithelial cells, to surface epithelial or submucosal glands, but not to basal membrane or connective tissue.[274] Interestingly, ICAM-1 expression was increased in airway epithelium *in vitro* and *in vivo* in a monkey model of airway hyperreactivity following antigen inhalation accompanied by increased epithelial eosinophils.[275]

## VI. EPITHELIUM-DERIVED INHIBITORY FACTOR

It is clear that the epithelium of the airways of many animal species, as well as of humans, can produce and release $PGE_2$ in response to various chemical stimuli and that this substance may be considered to be an epithelium-derived inhibitory or relaxant factor (EpDIF or EpDRF). An epithelium-derived spasmogenic factor that augmented contractile responses to endogenous acetylcholine either prejunctionally or postjunctionally has also been postulated.[31] A cyclooxygenase-derived constrictor substance from a hamster lung epithelial cell line was also recently described.[33] However, the possibility that the epithelium can also release a nonprostanoid EpDIF was suggested as early as 1985, when Flavahan et al.[207] and Barnes and co-workers[214] described epithelium-dependent enhancement of histamine-induced airway contraction *in vitro*. This putative factor has been the focus of a great deal of research aimed at its isolation, identification, and pharmacological and biochemical characterisation. As was initially the case with endothelium-derived inhibitory factor (EDRF), now generally believed to be NO, EpDIF has proved to be an elusive target. Indeed, the very existence of a nonprostanoid EpDIF remains a matter of continuing controversy. Some of the evidence for and against a nonprostanoid EpDIF is presented in the following section.

The consistent feature of experiments reporting changes in airway smooth muscle responses *in vitro* to spasmogens after ablation of the epithelium is that concentration–effect curves are significantly shifted to the left, i.e., agonist potency is increased. In addition, in many cases significant increases in maximal response to agonists were detected. If removal of the epithelium were simply destroying a barrier to agonist diffusion, an increase in response rate for agents that are not subject to degradation would be expected. However, it is unlikely to alter the sensitivity or magnitude of equilibrium responses to such agents. Furthermore, in isolated airway preparations in which airway smooth muscle tension changes are assessed in a bathing medium, agonists have access to the submucosa from all sides, reducing the effectiveness of the epithelium as a barrier to the diffusion of agonist to airway smooth muscle. It is also difficult to see how changes in airway smooth muscle responses resulting from stimulation of intramural cholinergic nerves might result from the loss of an external diffusion barrier.[207,262]

It is also clear that the effects of epithelium removal are selective, in that the responses to some, but not all, bioactive agents are affected. For example, it is well established that contractile responses of airway preparations to carbachol are not significantly altered by epithelial denudation, whereas the potencies of methacholine and bethanechol are increased.[220,237] This would seem to be more consistent with the selective stimulation of EpDIF release than with differences in agonist permeation rates or metabolism.

Further indirect evidence for a nonprostanoid EpDIF was obtained from experiments utilising perfused whole trachea from guinea pigs.[276] Although convincing data for the production and transfer of an EpDIF capable of relaxing airway smooth muscle were lacking, Munakata and co-workers[277] elegantly demonstrated epithelium-dependent airway smooth muscle relaxation in response to osmotic stimuli in a perfused tracheal preparation, consistent with the release of a nonprostanoid EpDIF. Holroyde[211] and Undem et al.[260] tried unsuccessfully to detect such a mediator in superfusion cascade systems involving a potential EpDIF donor preparation and a recipient airway assay preparation. However, Vanhoutte[278] was able to provide limited preliminary evidence for the release and transfer of an effective epithelium-derived relaxant of canine airway smooth muscle.

Other groups also described the transfer of epithelium-dependent relaxant activity in response to various agonists in superfusion/perfusion bioassay preparations. However, these involved both vascular and non-vascular smooth muscle.[279,281,282] In these systems, a coaxial assembly was used in which an

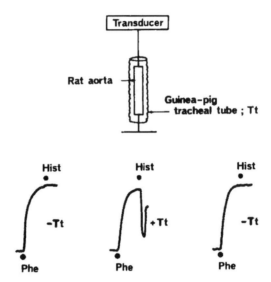

**FIGURE 4** A diagrammatic representation of a coaxial assembly for the bioassay of EpDIF released from epithelium-intact guinea pig tracheal tube tissue (Tt). EpDIF released in response to histamine (Hist) is detected by the assay tissue, i.e., phenylephrine (Phe) contracted, endothelium-denuded rat aorta strip, which relaxes while suspended within the lumen of the tracheal tube. Removal of the EpDIF donor tissue (–Tt) results in no response to histamine.

endothelium-denuded vascular smooth muscle preparation (e.g., rat aorta) was suspended in the long axis for tension measurement within an epithelium-intact guinea pig tracheal tube preparation, which was acting as an EpDIF donor (Figure 4). Agonists, such as histamine and methacholine which do not contract such vessels but which might release EpDIF from the airway, were applied and vascular relaxation responses measured.[208,234,281,283] While strong relaxations were detected (Figure 5), these studies did not provide evidence for an EpDIF which was active in airway smooth muscle. Indeed, relaxations were not seen in coaxial assemblies that used airway smooth muscle as the assay tissue.[283] This raises the possibility that at least two nonprostanoid inhibitory factors can be derived from the epithelium. The first, which is detectable in coaxial bioassay systems, is selective for vascular smooth muscle and may modulate the activity of ingested chemical stimuli at airway smooth muscle by increasing the volume of the airway microvascular sink for their removal.[283,284] This substance is not NO,[234,285] but is capable of causing significant increases in intracellular guanosine 3',5'-cyclic monophosphate (cGMP) in rat aorta in coaxial bioassay assemblies.[286] The data from this study suggested that EpDIF might induce vasorelaxation via stimulation of the membrane-bound form of guanylate cyclase, as occurs in response to ANP. The second might be selective for airway smooth muscle.[234,278] However, the identities of these putative substances remain unknown. Certainly, the vasoactive

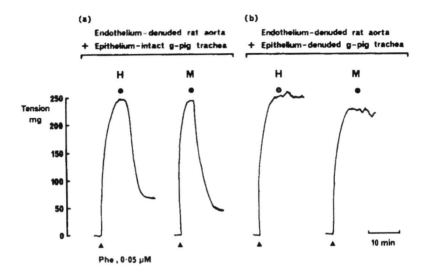

**FIGURE 5**  Responses to histamine (H, 100 μM) and methacholine (M, 25 μM) in endothelium-denuded rat aorta (a) mounted coaxially within the epithelium-intact guinea pig trachea or (b) mounted coaxially within epithelium-denuded guinea pig trachea. All preparations were pre-contracted with phenylephrine (Phe, 0.05 μM; ▲). Indomethacin (5 μM) was present throughout all experiments. (Reproduced with permission from Fernandes et al. (1989). *Br. J. Pharmacol.,* 96, 117-124.)

EpDIF and ANP are not identical, since ANP also causes relaxation of airway smooth muscle.[175,266]

Care must be taken when interpreting the data from coaxial bioassay studies of this kind. For example, Gunn and Piper[287] have suggested that a component of the airway epithelium-dependent vascular relaxations in coaxial assemblies may be related to luminal hypoxia resulting from the epithelial uptake of oxygen and exacerbated by airway tube constriction. However, not all airway smooth muscle spasmogens induce relaxation of rat aorta in coaxial bioassay experiments.[234] Other pharmacological and biochemical evidence is also at odds with the concept of a significant role for hypoxia in these systems.[286,288]

The relative importance of EpDIFs vs. the diffusion barrier function of the epithelium has also been the subject of intense investigation during the last 4 to 5 years. Iriarte et al.[289] showed that in guinea pig tracheal strip preparations, epithelium removal had a marked effect on responses to mucosally applied acetylcholine or histamine, whereas no effect occurred on adventitial application. This would again suggest a significant diffusion barrier role for the epithelium in guinea pig trachea. However, conflicting evidence has been reported in studies employing guinea pig or rat perfused tracheal tubes. Some studies have demonstrated a much greater influence of the epithelium on the potency of luminally (mucosal side) applied agonists than on serosally (adventitial side) applied agonists, suggesting a substantial diffusion barrier role for the epithelium.[212,290] In contrast, others found minimal differences.[291] Despite these discrepancies between studies, a growing body of evidence indicates that the airway epithelium does have a powerful influence as a diffusion barrier against mucosally applied spasmogens in perfused airway preparations. This has been demonstrated for hydrophillic charged agonists such as acetylcholine in porcine,[292,293] canine,[294] bovine, and human bronchial tube preparations,[295] where epithelium removal increased potency by 30- to 100-fold. These data suggest that the diffusion barrier role played by the airway epithelium is of considerably greater importance with respect to the modulation of the spasmogenic potency of some agents than is the influence of putative EpDIFs. However, it remains possible that the lesser potencies of luminally applied than of serosally applied spasmogens are in part due to EpDIF release preceding contraction on luminal administration, whereas serosal application would allow contraction to occur largely in the absence of EpDIF release.

## VII. PATHOLOGICAL SIGNIFICANCE

The pathophysiological significance of epithelial damage in asthma and other respiratory diseases also remains a subject of controversy. In 1984 Hogg and Eggleston[296] suggested that the basic defect in asthma was the inability of the epithelium to control the osmolarity of fluid lining the bronchial mucosa, although in the same year O'Byrne et al.[200] showed that while asthmatic subjects were markedly more sensitive to inhaled histamine, the permeabilities of their bronchial epithelia were within the normal range. It was subsequently demonstrated that epithelial damage in the airways was often present in asthmatic subjects with airway hyperresponsiveness to inhaled histamine.[188]

The increased exposure of nerve fibres in asthmatic airways as a result of epithelial damage[188,297] may well permit enhanced access of inhaled stimulants, including allergens, to submucosal target tissues, as well as to the release of proinflammatory substances such as LTs and bradykinin which may cause direct or reflex bronchoconstriction via vagal or local pathways. Perhaps more importantly, stimulation of sensory nerve C-fibres may result in the establishment of an axon reflex involving antidromic conduction and release of proinflammatory sensory neuropeptides, including the tachykinins, which may result in numerous deleterious effects including neurogenic inflammation, enhanced mucus secretion, and bronchoconstriction.[117] In addition, loss of NEP as a result of damage to epithelial cells will enhance the effects of endogenously released tachykinins. Overall, these events have the potential to create a significantly amplified inflammatory response in the affected region of the airways. Although there is widespread support for the notion that damage or dysfunction to the epithelium contributes significantly to the airway hyperreactivity to spasmogens that is a feature of asthma,[8] it is important to note that such damage is not always observed in this disease, even where hyperresponsiveness is apparent.[189]

Despite the relative uncertainty about the precise mechanisms, and their relative importance, whereby the epithelium is involved in the pathogenesis of respiratory disorders, there is unequivocal agreement that by virtue of its location and biologic characteristics, it plays a central role in the complex inflammatory processes which are characteristic of airway diseases, such as asthma. In fact, it has been suggested that injury to the epithelial cell is the initial event during airway inflammation.[298]

## VIII. CONCLUSIONS

It is now universally recognised that the mammalian airway epithelium does not act only as a barrier to solute diffusion or particle penetration, but is a complex, multifunctional, and extremely dynamic cellular layer consisting of several different specialised cell types. Its strategic location makes it the first line in defence of the submucosa from inhaled stimuli. In addition, its diverse biologic activities ensure that the epithelium plays a critical role in the homeostatic control of the pulmonary system. Certainly, the epithelium appears to be a key player in the initiation (perhaps as a result of epithelial cell injury), progression, and regulation of the airway inflammatory process. While various mechanisms have been postulated to explain its powerful influence on airway function, it seems likely that the various barrier functions of the epithelium are the most important components of its modulatory activity.

## ACKNOWLEDGMENTS

RGG is a Principal Reseach Fellow with the National Health and Medical Research Council (Australia).

## REFERENCES

1. Breeze, R. G. and Wheeldon, E. B. (1977). The cells of the pulmonary airways. *Am. Rev. Respir. Dis.*, 116, 705–777.
2. Jeffery, P. K. (1983). Morphologic features of airway surface epithelial cells and glands. *Am. Rev. Respir. Dis.*, 128, S14–S20.
3. Breeze, R. G. and Turk, M. (1984). Cellular structure, function and organization in the lower respiratory tract. *Environ. Health Perspect.*, 55, 3–24.
4. Harkema, J. R., Mariassy, A., St. George, J., Hyde, D. M., and Plopper, C. G. (1991). Epithelial cells of the conducting airways: a species comparison, in *The Airway Epithelium*, pp. 3–39, S. G. Farmer and D. W. P. Hay, Eds., Marcel Dekker, New York.
5. Devereux, T. R., Serabjit-Singh, C. J., Slaughter, S. R., Wolf, C. R., Philpot, R. M., and Fouts, J. R. (1981). Identification of cytochrome $P_{450}$ isozymes in nonciliated bronchial epithelial (Clara) and alveolar type II cells isolated from rabbit lung. *Exp. Lung Res.*, 2, 221–230.

6. Penney, D. P. (1988). The ultrastructure of epithelial cells of the distal lung, in *International Review of Cytology*, Vol. 111, pp. 231–269. (Eds. G. H. Bourne, K. W. Keon, and M. Friedlander). Academic Press, New York.

7. Irani, A. A., Schechter, N. M., Craig, S. S., DeBlois, G., and Schwartz, L. B. (1986). Two types of human mast cells that have distinct neutral protease compositions. *Proc. Natl. Acad. Sci. U.S.A.*, 83, 4464–4468.

8. Jeffery, P. K., Wardlaw, A. J., Nelson, F. C., Collins, J. V., and Kay, A. B. (1989). Bronchial biopsies in asthma. An ultrastructural, quantitative study and correlation with hyperreactivity. *Am. Rev. Respir. Dis.*, 140, 1745–1753.

9. Wharton, J., Polak, J. M., Bloom, S. R., Will, J. A., Brown, M. R., and Pearse, A. G. E. (1979). Substance P-like immunoreactive nerves in mammalian lung. *Invest. Cell Pathol.*, 2, 3–10.

10. Lundberg, J. M., Hokfelt, T., Martling, C.-R., Saria, A., and Cuello, C. (1984). Sensory substance P-immunoreactive nerves in the lower respiratory tract of various mammals including man. *Cell Tissue Res.*, 235, 251–261.

11. McDonald, D. M. (1987). Neurogenic inflammation in the respiratory tract: actions of sensory nerve mediators on blood vessels and epithelium of the airway mucosa. *Am. Rev. Respir. Dis.*, 136, S65–S72.

12. Jeffrey, P. and Reid., L. (1973). Intraepithelial nerves in normal rat airways: a quantitative electron microscopic study. *J. Anat.*, 114, 35–45.

13. Luciano, L., Reale, E., and Ruska, H. (1968). Uber eine 'chemorezeptive' Sinneszelle in der Treachea der Ratte. *Z. Zellforsch. Mikrosk. Anat.* 85, 350.

14. Hung, K.-S., Hertweck, M. D., Hardy, J. D., and Loosli, C. G. (1973). Ultrastructure of nerves and associated cells in bronchiolar epithelium of the mouse lung. *J. Ultrastruct. Res.*, 43, 426.

15. Lauweryns, J. M., Cokelaere, M., and Theunynck, P. (1972). Neuroepithelial bodies in the respiratory mucosa of various mammals: a light optical, histochemical and ultrastructural investigation. *Z. Zellforsch. Mikrosk. Anat.*, 135, 569.

16. Johnson, D. E. (1991). Pulmonary neuroendocrine cells, in *The Airway Epithelium: Physiology, Pathophysiology and Pharmacology*, pp. 335–397. (Eds. S. G. Farmer and D. W. P. Hay). Marcel Dekker, New York.

17. Becker, K. L. (1984). Historical perspective on the pulmonary endocrine cell, in *The Endocrine Cell in Health and Disease*, pp. 156–161. (Eds. K. L. Becker and A. F. Gazdar). Saunders, Philadelphia.

18. DiAugustine, R. P. and Sonstegard, K. S. (1984). Neuroendocrine-like (small granule) epithelial cells in the lung. *Environ. Health Perspect.*, 55, 271–295.

19. Hoyt, R. F., Jr., Sorokin, S. P., and Feldman, H. (1982). Small granule (neuro)endocrine cells in the intracardiac lobe of a hamster lung. *Exp. Lung Res.*, 3, 273–298.

20. Lauweryns, J. M., and Van Lommel, A. (1987). Ultrastructure of nerve endings and synaptic junctions in rabbit intrapulmonary neuroepithelial bodies. A single and serial section analysis. *J. Anat.*, 151, 65–83.

21. Orehek, J., Douglas, J. S., and Bouhuys, A. (1975). Contractile responses of the guinea-pig trachea *in vitro*: modification by the prostaglandin synthesis inhibiting drugs. *J. Pharmacol. Exp. Ther.*, 194, 554–564.

22. O'Byrne, P. M., Aizawa, H., Bethel, R. A., Chung, K. F., Nadel, J. A., and Holtzman, M. J. (1984). Prostaglandin $F_{2\alpha}$ increases responsiveness of pulmonary airways in dogs. *Prostaglandins*, 28, 537–543.

23. Holtzman, M. J. (1991). Epithelial cell regulation of arachidonic acid oxygenation, in *The Airway Epithelium*, pp. 65–115. S. G. Farmer and D. W. P. Hay, Eds.. Marcel Dekker, New York.

24. Churchill, L., Chilton, F. H., Resau, J. H., Bascom, R., Hubbard, W. C., and Proud, D. (1989). Cyclooxygenase metabolism of endogenous arachidonic acid by cultured human tracheal epithelial cells. *Am. Rev. Respir. Dis.*, 140, 449–459.

25. Leikauf, G. D., Driscoll, K. E., and Wey, H.E . (1988). Ozone-induced augmentation of eicosanoid metabolism in epithelial cells from bovine trachea. *Am. Rev. Respir. Dis.*, 137, 435–442.
26. Salari, H. and Chan-Yeung, M. (1989). Release of 15-hydroxyeicosatetraenoic acid (15-HETE) and prostaglandin $E_2$ ($PGE_2$) by cultured human bronchial epithelial cells. *Am. J. Respir. Cell Mol. Biol.*, 1, 245–250.
27. Widdicombe, J. H., Ueki, I. F., Emery, D., Margolskee, D., Yergey, J., and Nadel, J. A. (1989). Release of cyclooxygenase products from primary cultures of tracheal epithelia of dog and human. *Am. J. Physiol.*, 256, L351–L355.
28. Braunstein, G., Labat, C., Brunelleschi, S., Benveniste, J., Marsac, J., and Brink, C. (1988). Evidence that the histamine sensitivity and responsiveness of guinea-pig isolated trachea are modulated by epithelial prostaglandin $E_2$. *Br. J. Pharmacol.*, 95, 300–308.
29. Farmer, S. G., Hay, D. W. P., Raeburn, D., and Fedan, J. S. (1987). Relaxation of guinea-pig tracheal smooth muscle to arachidonate is converted to contraction following epithelium removal. *Br. J. Pharmacol.*, 92, 231–236.
30. Tschirhart, E., Frossard, N., Bertrand, C., and Landry, Y. (1987). Arachidonic acid metabolites and airway epithelium-dependent relaxant factor. *J. Pharmacol. Exp. Ther.*, 243, 310–316.
31. Stuart-Smith, K. and Vanhoutte, P. M. (1988). Airway epithelium modulates the responsiveness of porcine bronchial smooth muscle. *J. Appl. Physiol.*, 65, 721–727.
32. Coleman, R. A. and Kennedy, I. (1980). Contractile and relaxant actions of prostaglandins on guinea-pig isolated trachea. *Br. J. Pharmacol.*, 68, 533–539
33. Wilkens, J. A., Becker, A., Wilkens, H., Emura, M., Riebe-Imre, M., Plein, K., Schöber, S., Tsikas, D., Gutzki, F. M., and Frölich, J. C. (1992). Bioassay of a tracheal smooth muscle-constricting factor released by respiratory epithelial cells. *Am. J. Physiol.*, 263, L137–L141.
34. Frossard, N. and Müller, F. (1986). Epithelial modulation of tracheal smooth muscle responses to antigenic stimulation. *J. Appl. Physiol.*, 61, 1449–1456.
35. DeVillier, P., Acker, G. M., Advenier, C., Marsac, J., Regoli, D., and Frossard, N. (1992). Activation of an epithelial neurokinin NK-1 receptor induces relaxation of rat trachea through release of prostaglandin $E_2$. *J. Pharmacol. Exp. Ther.*, 263, 767–772.
36. Leikauf, G. D., Ueki, I. F., Nadel, J. A., and Widdicombe, J. H. (1985). Bradykinin stimulates Cl secretion and prostaglandin $E_2$ release by canine tracheal epithelium. *Am. J. Physiol.*, 248, F48–F55.
37. Leikauf, G. D., Ueki, I. F., Widdicombe, J. H., and Nadel, J. A. (1986). Alterations of chloride secretion across canine tracheal epithelium by lipoxygenase products of arachidonic acid. *Am. J. Physiol.*, 250, F47–F53.
38. Barnett, K., Jacoby, D. B., Nadel, J. A., and Lazarus, S. C. (1988) The effects of epithelial cell supernatant on contractions of isolated canine tracheal smooth muscle. *Am. Rev. Respir. Dis.*, 138, 780–783.
39. Xu, G. L., Sivarajah, K., Wu, R., Nettesheim, P., and Eling, T. (1986). Biosynthesis of prostaglandins by isolated and cultured airway epithelial cells. *Exp. Lung Res.*, 10, 101–114.
40. Borgeat, P. and Samuelsson, B. (1979). Arachidonic acid metabolism in polymorphonuclear leukocytes: effects of ionophore A23187. *Proc. Natl. Acad. Sci. U.S.A.*, 76, 2148–2170.
41. Fels, A. O. S., Pawlowski, N. A., Cramer, E. B., King, T. K. C., Cohn, Z. A., and Scott, W. A. (1982). Human alveolar macrophages produce leukotriene $B_4$. *Proc. Natl. Acad. Sci. U.S.A.*, 79, 7866–7870.
42. Peters, S. P., Schleimer, R. P., Naclerio, R. M., MacGlashan, D. W., Togias, A. G., Proud, D., Freeland, H. S., Fox, C., Adkinson, N. J., and Lichtenstein, L. M. (1987). The pathophysiology of human mast cells: *in vitro* and *in vivo* function. *Am. Rev. Respir. Dis.*, 135, 1196–1200.

43. Adelroth, E., Morris, M. M., Hargreave, F. E., and O'Byrne, P. M. (1986). Airways responsiveness to leukotrienes $C_4$ and $D_4$ and to methacholine in patients with asthma and normal control. *N. Engl. J. Med.*, 315, 480–484.

44. Barnes, N. C., Piper, P. J., and Costello, J. F. (1984). Comparative effects of inhaled leukotriene $C_4$, leukotriene $D_4$, and histamine in normal human subjects. *Thorax*, 39, 500–504.

45. Bisgaard, H., Groth, S., and Madsen, F. (1985). Bronchial hyperreactivity of leukotriene $D_4$ and histamine in exogenous asthma. *Br. Med. J.*, 290, 1468–1471.

46. Buckner, C. K., Krell, R. D., Laravuso, R. B., Coursin, D. B., Bernstein, P. R., and Will, J. A. (1986). Pharmacological evidence that human intralobar airways do not contain different receptors that mediate contractions to leukotriene $C_4$ and leukotriene $D_4$. *J. Pharmacol. Exp. Ther.*, 237, 558–562.

47. Davidson, A. E., Lee, T. H., Scanlon, P. D., Solway, J., McFadden, E. R., Ingram, R. H., Corey, E. J., Austen, K. F., and Drazen, J. M. (1987). Bronchoconstrictor effects of leukotriene $E_4$ in normal and asthmatic subjects. *Am. Rev. Respir. Dis.*, 135, 333–337.

48. Griffin, M., Weiss, J. W., and Leitch, A. G. (1983). Effects of leukotriene D on the airways in asthma. *N. Engl. J. Med.*, 308, 436–439.

49. Coles, S. J., Neill, K. H., Reid, L. M., Austen, K. F., Nu, Y., Corey, E. J., and Lewis, R. A. (1983). Effects of leukotrienes $C_4$ and $D_4$ on glycoprotein and lysozyme secretion by human bronchial mucosa. *Prostaglandins*, 25, 155–170.

50. Marom, Z., Schelhamer, J. H., Bach, M. K., Morton, D. R., and Kaliner, M. A. (1982). Slow reacting substances, leukotrienes $C_4$ and $D_4$ increase the release of mucus from human airways *in vitro*. *Am. Rev. Respir. Dis.*, 126, 449–451.

51. Dahlén, S.-E., Björk, J., Hedqvist, P., Arfors, K.-E., Hammarström, S., Lindgren, J. A., and Samuelsson, B. (1981). Leukotrienes promote plasma leakage and leukocyte adhesion in postcapillary venules: *in vivo* effects with relevance to the acute inflammatory response. *Proc. Natl. Acad. Sci. U.S.A.*, 78, 3887–3891.

52. Evans, T. W., Rogers, D. F., Aursudkij, B., Chung, K. F., and Barnes, P. J. (1989). Regional and time-dependent effects of inflammatory mediators on microvascular permeability in the guinea-pig. *Clin. Sci.*, 76, 479–485.

53. Hua, X. Y., Dahlén, S. E., Lundberg, J. M., Hammerström, S., and Hedqvist, P. (1985). Leukotrienes $C_4$ and $E_4$ cause widespread and extensive plasma extravasation in the guinea pig. *Naunyn-Schmiedebergs Arch. Pharmacol.*, 330, 136–141.

54. Dunnill, M. S. (1960). The pathology of asthma with specific reference to changes in the bronchial mucosa. *J. Clin. Pathol.*, 13, 27–33.

55. Henke, D., Danilowicz, R. M., Curtis, J. F., Boucher, R. C., and Eling, T. E. (1988). Metabolism of arachidonic acid by human nasal and bronchial epithelial cells. *Arch. Biochem. Biophys.*, 267, 426–436.

56. Holtzman, M. J., Hansbrough, J. R., Rosen, G. D., and Turk, J. (1988). Uptake, release, and novel species-dependent oxygenation of arachidonic acid in human and animal airway epithelial cells. *Biochim. Biophys. Acta*, 963, 401–413.

57. Hansbrough, J. R., Atlas, A. B., Turk, J., and Holtzman, M. J. (1989). Arachidonate 12-lipoxygenase and cyclooxygenase: PGE isomerase are predominant pathways for oxygenation in bovine tracheal epithelial cells. *Am. J. Respir. Cell Mol. Biol.*, 1, 237–244.

58. Eling, T. E., Danilowicz, R. M., Henke, D. C., Sivarajah, K., Yankaskas, J. R., and Boucher, R. C. (1986). Arachidonic acid metabolism by canine tracheal epithelial cells. *J. Biol. Chem.*, 261, 12841–12849.

59. Holtzman, M. J., Aizawa, H., Nadel, J. A., and Goetzl, E. J. (1983). Selective generation of leukotriene $B_4$ by tracheal epithelial cells from dogs. *Biochem. Biophys. Res. Commun.*, 114, 1071–1076.

60. Salari, H. and Schellenberg, R. R. (1991). Stimulation of human airway epithelial cells by platelet activating factor (PAF) and arachidonic acid produces 15-hydroxyeicosatetraenoic acid (15-HETE) capable of contracting bronchial smooth muscle. *Pulm. Pharmacol.*, 4, 1–7.

61. Adler, K. B., Schwartz, J. E., Anderson, W., and Welton, A. F. (1987). Platelet activating factor stimulates secretion of mucin by explants of rodent airways in organ culture. *Exp. Lung Res.*, 13, 25–43.

62. Alpert, S. E., Kramer, C. M., Braseler, J. R., and Bach, M. K. (1990). Generation of lipoxygenase metabolites of arachidonic acid by monolayer cultures of tracheal epithelial cells and intact tracheal segments from rabbits. *Exp. Lung Res.*, 16, 207–230.

63. Ullman, A., Ciabottoni, G., Lofdahl, C.-G., Linden, A., Svedmyr, N., and Skoogh, B.-E. (1990). Epithelium-derived $PGE_2$ inhibits the contractile response to cholinergic nerve stimulation in isolated ferret trachea. *Pulm. Pharmacol.*, 3, 155–160.

64. Ullman, A., Lofdahl, C.-G., Svedmyr, N., and Skoogh, B.-E. (1990). Nerve stimulation releases mucosa-derived inhibitory factors, both prostanoids and nonprostanoids, in isolated ferret trachea. *Am. Rev. Respir. Dis.*, 141, 748–751.

65. Xie, Z., Hakoda, H., and Ito, Y. (1992). Airway epithelial cells regulate membrane potential, neurotransmission and muscle tone of the dog airway smooth muscle. *J. Physiol.*, 449, 619–639.

66. Shoji, S., Rickard, K. A., Ertl, R. F., Robbins, R. A., Linder, J., and Rennard, S. I. (1989). Bronchial epithelial cells produce lung fibroblast chemotactic factor: fibronectin. *Am. J. Respir. Cell Mol. Biol.*, 1, 13–20.

67. Robbins, R. A., Koyama, S., Nelson, K., Gossman, G., Rickard, K., and Rennard, S. I. (1990). Neutrophil adherence to bronchial epithelial cells. *Am. Rev. Respir. Dis.*, 141, A910.

68. Shoji, S., Ertl, R. F., Linder, J., and Romberger, D. J. (1990). Bronchial epithelial cells produce chemotactic activity for bronchial epithelial cells. *Am. Rev. Respir. Dis.*, 141, 218–225.

69. Brinkman, G. L. (1968). The mast cell in normal human bronchus and lung. *J. Ultrastruct. Res.*, 23, 115–123.

70. Cutz, E., Levison, H., and Cooper, D. M. (1978). Ultrastructure of airways in children with asthma. *Histopathology*, 2, 407–421.

71. Marin, M. G., Davis, B., and Nadel, J. A. (1977) Effect of histamine on electrical and ion transport properties of tracheal epithelium. *J. Appl. Physiol.*, 42, 735–738.

72. Majno, G., Shea, S. M., and Leventhal, M. (1969). Endothelial contraction induced by histamine-type mediators: an electron microscopic study. *J. Cell Biol.*, 42, 647–672.

73. McDonald, D. M. (1990). The ultrastructure and permeability of tracheobronchial blood vessels in health and disease. *Eur. Respir. J.*, 3 (Suppl. 12), 572s–585s.

74. Persson, C. G. A. (1986). Role of plasma exudation in asthmatic airways. *Lancet*, 2, 1126–1129.

75. White, M. V., Slater, J. E., and Kaliner, M. A. (1987). Histamine and asthma. *Am. Rev. Respir. Dis.*, 135, 1165–1176.

76. Chand, N. and Eyre, P. (1975). Classification and biological distribution of histamine receptor subtypes. *Agents Actions*, 5, 277–295.

77. Eiser, N. M. (1983). Hyperreactivity — its relationship to histamine receptors. *Eur. J. Respir. Dis.*, 64 (Suppl. 131), 99–114.

78. Knight, D. A., Stewart, G. A., and Thompson, P. J. (1992). Histamine tachyphylaxis in human airway smooth muscle. The role of $H_2$-receptors and bronchial epithelium. *Am. Rev. Respir. Dis.*, 146, 137–140.

79. Shelhamer, J. H., Marom, Z., and Kaliner, M. (1980) Immunologic and neuropharmacologic stimulation of mucous glycoprotein release from human airway *in vitro*. *J. Clin. Invest.*, 66, 1400–1408.

80. Ichinose, M. and Barnes, P.J. (1989). Inhibitory histamine $H_3$-receptors on cholinergic nerves in human airways. *Eur. J. Pharmacol.*, 163, 383–386.

81. Ichinose, M., Stretton, C. D., Schwartz, J.-C., and Barnes, P. J. (1989). Histamine $H_3$-receptors inhibit cholinergic neurotransmission in guinea-pig airways. *Br. J. Pharmacol.*, 97, 13–15.

82. Ichinose, M. and Barnes, P. J. (1989). Histamine $H_3$-receptors modulate nonadrenergic, noncholinergic neural bronchoconstriction in guinea-pig *in vivo*. *Eur. J. Pharmacol.*, 174, 49–55.

83. Ichinose, M., Belvisi, M. G., and Barnes, P. J. (1990). Histamine H₃-receptors inhibit neurogenic microvascular leakage in airways. *J. Appl. Physiol.*, 68, 21–25.
84. Ichinose, M. and Barnes, P. J. (1990). Histamine H₃-receptors modulate antigen-induced bronchoconstriction in guinea-pigs. *J. Allergy Clin. Immunol.*, 86, 491–495.
85. Marini, M., Vittori, E., Halemborg, J., and Mattoli, S. (1992). Expression of the potent inflammatory cytokines granulocyte-macrophage-colony-stimulating factor and interleukin-6 and interleukin-8 in bronchial epithelial cells of patients with asthma. *J. Allergy Clin. Immunol.*, 89, 1001–1009.
86. Mattoli, S., Colotta, F., Fincato, G., Mezzetti, M., Mantovani, A., Patalano, F., and Fasoli, A. (1991). Time course of IL1 and IL6 synthesis and release in human bronchial epithelial cell cultures exposed to toluene diisocynate. *J. Cell. Physiol.*, 149, 260–268.
87. Smith, S., Lee, D., Lacy, J., and Coleman, D. (1989). Rat tracheal epithelial cells in primary culture release granulocyte-macrophage colony-stimulating factor (GM-SCF). *Am. Rev. Respir. Dis.*, 139, A613.
88. Cox, G., Gauldie, J., and Jordana, M. (1992). Bronchial epithelial cell-derived cytokines (G-CSF and GM-CSF) promote the survival of peripheral blood neutrophils *in vitro*. *Am. J. Respir. Cell Mol. Biol.*, 7, 507–513.
89. Wills-Karp, M., Jinot, J., Lee, F., and Hirata, F. (1990). Interleukin-1 alters guinea-pig tracheal smooth muscle responsiveness to β-adrenergic stimulation. *Eur. J. Pharmacol.*, 183, 1185.
90. Van Oosterhout, A. J. M., Stam, W. B., Vanderschueren, R. G. J. R. J., and Nijkamp, F. P. (1992). Effects of cytokines on β-receptor function of human peripheral blood mononuclear cells and guinea-pig trachea. *J. Allergy Clin. Immunol.*, 90, 340–348.
91. Soloperto, M., Mattoso, V. L., Fasoli, A., and Mattoli, S. (1991). A bronchial epithelial cell-derived factor in asthma that promotes eosinophil activation and survival as GM-CSF. *Am. J. Physiol.*, 260, L530–L538.
92. Becker, S., Koren, H. S., and Henke, D. C. (1993). Interleukin-8 expression in normal nasal epithelium and its modulation by infection with respiratory syncytial virus and cytokines tumor necrosis factor, interleukin-1, and interleukin-6. *Am. J. Respir. Cell Mol. Biol.*, 8, 20–27.
93. Noah, T. L. and Becker, S. (1993). Respiratory syncytial virus-induced cytokine production by a human epithelial cell line. *Am. J. Physiol.*, 265, L472–L478.
94. McIntosh, K., Ellis, E. F., Hoffman, L. S., Lybass, T. G., Eller, J. J., and Fulginiti, V. A. (1973). The association of viral and bacterial infections with exacerbations of wheezing in young asthmatic children. *J. Pediatr.*, 82, 578–590.
95. Yanagisawa, M., Kurihara, H., Kimura, S., Tomobe, Y., Kobayashi, M., Mitsui, Y., Yazaki, Y., Goto, K., and Masaki, T. (1988). A novel potent vasoconstrictor peptide produced by vascular endothelial cells. *Nature*, 332, 411–415.
96. MacCumber, M. W., Ross, C. A., Glaser, B. M., and Snyder, S. H. (1989). Endothelin visualization of mRNAs by *in situ* hybridization provides evidence for local action. *Proc. Natl. Acad. Sci. U.S.A.*, 86, 7285–7289.
97. Springall, D. R., Howarth, P. H., Counihan, H., Djukanovic, R., Holgate, S. T., and Polak, J. M. (1991). Endothelin immunoreactivity of airway epithelium in asthmatic patients. *Lancet*, 337, 697–701.
98. Henry, P. J., Rigby, P. J., Self, G. J., Preuss, J. M. H., and Goldie, R. G. (1990). Relationship between endothelin-1 binding site densities and constrictor activities in human and animal airway smooth muscle. *Br. J. Pharmacol.*, 100, 786–792.
99. Hay, D. W. P., Luttmann, M. A., Hubbard, W. C., and Undem, B. J. (1993). Endothelin receptor subtypes in human and guinea-pig pulmonary tissues. *Br. J. Pharmacol.*, 110, 1175–1183.
100. Noveral, J. P., Rosenberg, S. M., Anbar, R. A., Pawlowski, N. A., and Grunstein, M. M. (1992). Role of endothelin-1 in regulating proliferation of cultured rabbit airway smooth muscle cells. *Am. J. Physiol.*, 263, L317–L324.

101. Tomlinson, P. R., Wilson, J. W., and Stewart, A. G. (1994). Inhibition by salbutamol of the proliferation of human airway smooth muscle cells grown in culture. *Br. J. Pharmacol.*, 111, 641–647.
102. Mullol, J., Chowdhury, B. A., and White, M. V. (1993). Endothelin in human nasal mucosa. *Am. J. Respir. Cell Mol. Biol.*, 8, 393–402.
103. Hay, D. W. P., Henry, P. J., and Goldie, R. G. (1993). Endothelin and the respiratory system. *Trends Pharmacol. Sci.*, 14, 29–32.
104. Mattoli, S., Mezzetti, M., Riva, G., Allegra, L., and Fasoli, A. (1990). Specific binding of endothelin on human bronchial smooth muscle cells in culture and secretion of endothelin-like material from bronchial epithelial cells. *Am. J. Respir. Cell Mol. Biol.*, 3, 145–151.
105. Black, P. N., Ghatei, M. A., Takahashi, K., Bretherton-Watt, D., Krausz, T., Dollery, C. T., and Bloom, S. R. (1989). Formation of endothelin by cultured airway epithelial cells. *FEBS Lett.*, 255, 129–132.
106. Ninomiya, H., Uchida, Y., Ishii, Y., Nomura, A., Kameyama, M., Saotome, M., Endo, T., and Hasegawa, S. (1991). Endotoxin stimulates endothelin release from cultured epithelial cells of guinea-pig trachea. *Eur. J. Pharmacol.*, 203, 299–302.
107. Rozengurt, N., Springall, D. R., and Polak, J. M. (1990). Localization of endothelin-like immunoreactivity in airway epithelium of rats and mice. *J. Pathol.*, 160, 5–8.
108. Sofia, M., Mormile, M., Faraone, S. M., Zofra, S., Romano, L., and Carratù, L. (1993). Increased endothelin-like immunoreactive material on bronchoalveolar lavage fluid from patients with bronchial asthma and patients with interstitial lung disease. *Respiration*, 60, 89–95.
109. Henry, P. J. and Goldie, R. G. (1994). Potentiation by endothelin-1 of cholinergic nerve-mediated contractions in mouse trachea via activation of $ET_B$ receptors. *Br. J. Pharmacol.*, 114, 563–569.
110. McKay, K. O., Armour, C. L., and Black, J. L. (1993). Endothelin-3 increases transmission in the rabbit pulmonary parasympathetic nervous system. *J. Cardiovasc. Pharmacol.*, 22 (Suppl. 8), S181–S184.
111. Tschirhart, E., Drijhout, J. W., Pelton, J. T., Miller, R. C., and Jones, C. R. (1991). Endothelins: functional and autoradiographic studies in guinea-pig trachea. *J. Pharmacol. Exp. Ther.*, 258, 381–387.
112. Goldie, R. G., Grayson, P. S., Knott, P. G., Self, G. J., and Henry, P. J. (1994). Predominance of endothelin$_A$ ($ET_A$) receptors in ovine airway smooth muscle and their mediation of ET-1-induced contraction. *Br. J. Pharmacol.*, 112, 749–756.
113. Wu, T., Rieves, D., Larivee, P., Logun, C., Lawrence, M. G., and Shelhamer, J. H. (1993). Production of eicosanoids in response to endothelin-1 and identification of specific endothelin-1 binding sites in airway epithelial cells. *Am. J. Respir. Cell Mol. Biol.*, 8, 282–290.
114. Advenier, C., Naline, E., Drapeau, G., and Regoli, D. (1987). Relative potencies of neurokinins in guinea pig trachea and human bronchus. *Eur. J. Pharmacol.*, 139, 133–137.
115. Martling, C. R., Theordorsson-Norheim, E., and Lundberg, J. M. (1987). Occurrence and effects of multiple tachykinins: substance P, neurokinin A, neuropeptide K in human lower airways. *Life Sci.*, 40, 1633–1643.
116. Naline, E., DeVillier, P., Drapeau, G., Toty, L. F., Bakdach, H., Regoli, D., and Advenier, C. (1989). Characterization of neurokinin effects and receptor selectivity in human isolated bronchi. *Am. Rev. Respir. Dis.*, 140, 679–686.
117. Barnes, P. J. (1986). Asthma as an axon reflex. *Lancet*, 1, 242–245.
118. Borson, D. B., Corrales, R., Varsano, S., Gold, W., Viro, N., Caughey, G., Ramachandran, J., and Nadel, J. A. (1986). Enkephalinase inhibitors potentiate SP-induced secretion of $^{35}SO_4$-macromolecules from ferret trachea. *Exp. Lung Res.*, 21, 21–36.
119. Shimura S., Sasaki, T., Okayama, H., Sasaki, H., and Takishima, T. (1987). Effect of SP on mucus secretion of isolated submucosal gland from feline trachea. *J. Appl. Physiol.*, 63, 646–653.

120. Andersson, R. G. G. and Grundström, N. (1983). The excitatory non-cholinergic, non-adrenergic nervous system of the guinea-pig airways. *Eur. J. Respir. Dis.*, 64 (Suppl. 131), 141–157.

121. Lundberg, J. M., Martling, C. R., and Saria, A. (1983). Substance P and capsaicin-induced contraction of human bronchi. *Acta Physiol. Scand.*, 119, 49–53.

122. Maggi, C. A. (1990). Tachykinin receptors in the airways and lung: what should we block? *Pharmacol. Res.*, 22, 527–540.

123. Brokaw, J. J., Hillenbrand, C. M., White, G. W., and McDonald, D. M. (1990). Mechanism of tachyphylaxis associated with neurogenic plasma extravasation in the rat trachea. *Am. Rev. Respir. Dis.*, 141, 1434–1440.

124. Payan, D. G. (1989). Neuropeptides and inflammation: the role of substance P. *Annu. Rev. Med.*, 40, 341–352.

125. Payan, D. G., Brewster, D. R., Missirian-Bastian, A., and Goetzl, E. J. (1984). Substance P recognition by a subset of human T-lymphocytes. *J. Clin. Invest.*, 74, 1532–1539.

126. Barnes, P. J. (1988). Neuropeptides and airway smooth muscle. *Pharmacol. Ther.*, 36, 119–129.

127. Rogers, D. F., Belvisi, M. G., Aursudkij, B., Evans, T. W., and Barnes, P. J. (1988). Effects and interactions of sensory neuropeptides on airway microvascular leakage in guinea-pigs. *Br. J. Pharmacol.*, 95, 1109–1116.

128. Shore, S. A., Stimler-Gerard, N. P., Coates, S. R., and Drazen, J. M. (1988). Substance P induced bronchoconstriction in guinea-pig. Enhancement by inhibitors of neutral metalloendopeptidase and angiotensin coverting enzyme. *Am. Rev. Respir. Dis.*, 137, 331–336.

129. Tucker, J. F., Brave, S. R., Charalambous, L., Hobbs, A. J., and Gibson, A. (1990). L-NG-nitro arginine inhibits non-adrenergic, non-cholinergic relaxations of guinea-pig isolated tracheal smooth muscle. *Br. J. Pharmacol.*, 100, 633–634.

130. Li, C. G. and Rand, M. J. (1991). Evidence that part of the NANC relaxant responses of guinea-pig trachea to electrical field stimulation is mediated by nitric oxide. *Br. J. Pharmacol.*, 102, 91–94.

131. Gao, Y. and Vanhoutte, P. M. (1993). Attenuation of contractions to acetylcholine in canine bronchi by an endogenous nitric oxide-like substance. *Br. J. Pharmacol.*, 109, 887–891.

132. Belvisi, M. G., Stretton, C. D., Yacoub, M., and Barnes, P. J. (1992). Nitric oxide is the endogenous neurotransmitter of bronchodilator nerves in humans. *Eur. J. Pharmacol.*, 210, 221–222.

133. Ellis, J. L. and Undem, B. J. (1992). Inhibition by L-NG-nitro-L-arginine of nonadrenergic, noncholinergic-mediated relaxations of human isolated central and peripheral airways. *Am. Rev. Respir. Dis.*, 146, 1543–1547.

134. Kobzik, L., Bredt, D. S., Lowenstein, C. J., Drazen, J., Gaston, B., Sugarbaker, D., and Stamler, J. S. (1993). Nitric oxide synthase in human and rat lung: immunocytochemical and histochemical localization. *Am. J. Respir. Cell Mol. Biol.*, 9, 371–377.

135. Filep, G., Battistini, B., and Sirois, P. (1993). Induction by endothelin-1 of epithelium-dependent relaxation of guinea-pig trachea: role of nitric oxide. *Br. J. Pharmacol.*, 109, 637–644.

136. Nijkamp, F. P., Van der Linde, H., and Folkerts, G. (1993). Nitric oxide sythesis inhibitors induce airway hyperresponsiveness in the guinea-pig *in vivo* and *in vitro*. *Am. Rev. Respir. Dis.*, 148, 727–734.

137. Knowles, R. G., Salter, M., Brooks, S. L., and Moncada, S. (1990). Anti-inflammatory glucocorticoids inhibit the induction by endotoxin of nitric oxide synthase in the lung, liver, and aorta of the rat. *Biochem. Biophys. Res. Commun.*, 172, 1042–1048.

138. Hamid, Q., Springall, D. R., Riveros-Moreno, V., Chanez, P., Howarth, P., Redington, A., Bousquet, J., Godard, P., Holgate, S. T., and Polak, J. M. (1993). Induction of nitric oxide synthase in asthma. *Lancet*, 342, 1510–1513.

139. Persson, M. G., Zetterström, O., Agrenius, V., Ihre, E., and Gustafsson, L. E. (1994). Single-breath nitric oxide measurements in asthmatic patients and smokers. *Lancet*, 343, 146–147.

140. Mulligan, M. S., Hevel, J. M., Marletta, M. A., and Ward, P. A. (1991). Tissue injury caused by deposition of immune complexes is L-arginine-dependent. *Proc. Natl. Acad. Sci. U.S.A.*, 88, 6338–6342.

141. Kharitonov, S. A., Yates, D., Robbins, R. A., Logan-Sinclair, R., Shinebourne, E. A., and Barnes, P. J. (1994). Increased nitric oxide in exhaled air of asthmatic patients. *Lancet*, 343, 133–135.

142. Gumbiner, B. (1987). Structure, biochemistry and assembly of epithelial tight junctions. *Am. J. Physiol.*, 253, C749–C758.

143. Farquhar M. G. and Palade, G. E. (1963). Junctional complexes in various epithelia. *J. Cell Biol.*, 17, 375–412.

144. Rennard, S. I., Beckmann, J. D., and Robbins, R. A. (1991), Biology of airway epithelial cells, in *The Lung: Scientific Foundations*, pp. 157–167, R. G. Crystal and J. B. West, Eds., Raven Press, New York.

145. Schneeberger, E. E. (1992). Alveolar type I cells, in *The Lung: Scientific Foundations*, pp. 229–234, R. G. Crystal and J. B. West, Eds., Raven Press, New York.

146. Pitts, J. D. and Finbow, M. E. (1986). The gap junction. J. Cell Sci., 4, (Suppl.), 239–266.

147. Revel, J. P., Nicholson, B. J., and Yancey, S. B. (1985). Chemistry of gap junctions. *Annu. Rev. Physiol.*, 47, 263–279.

148. Sheridan, J. D. and Atkinson, M. M. (1985). Physiological roles of permeable junctions: some possibilities. *Annu. Rev. Physiol.*, 47, 337–353.

149. Boat, T. F. and Matthews, L. W. (1973). Chemical composition of human tracheobronchial secretions, in *Sputum: Fundamentals and Clinical Pathology*, M. J. Dulfano, Ed., p. 243, C.C. Thomas, Springfield, IL.

150. Robinson, N. P., Kyle, H., Webber, S. E., and Widdicombe, J. G. (1989). Electrolyte and other chemical concentrations in the tracheal airway and mucus. *J. Appl. Physiol.*, 66, 2129–2135.

151. Mayrhofer, G. (1994). Epithelial disposition of antigen, in *Immunopharmacology of Epithelial Barriers*, pp. 19–70. R. G. Goldie, Ed., Academic Press, London.

152. Marin, M. G. and Culp, D. J. (1986). Isolation and culture of submucosal gland cells. *Clinics Chest Med.*, 7, 239–245.

153. Bhaskar, K. R., O'Sullivan, D. D., Seltzer, J., Rossing, T. H., Drazen, J. M., and Reid, L. M. (1985). Density gradient study of bronchial mucus aspirates from healthy volunteers (smokers and nonsmokers) and from patients with tracheostomy. *Exp. Lung Res.*, 9, 289–308.

154. Marin, M. G. (1986). Pharmacology of airway secretion. *Pharmacol. Rev.*, 38, 273–289.

155. Basbaum, C. B. and Finkbeiner, W. E. (1989). Mucus-producing cells of the airways, in *Lung Cell Biology*, pp. 37–79, D. Massaro, Ed., Marcel Dekker, New York.

156. Gundel, R. H. and Letts, L. G. (1994). Adhesion molecules and the modulation of mucosal inflammation, in *Immunopharmacology of Epithelial Barriers*, pp. 71–84, R. G. Goldie, Ed., Academic Press, London.

157. Glanville, A. R., Tazelaar, H. D., Theodore, J., Imoto, E., Rouse, R. V., Baldwin, J. C., and Robin, E. D. (1989). The distribution of MHC class I and II antigens on bronchial epithelium. *Am. Rev. Respir. Dis.*, 139, 330–334.

158. Kalb, T. H., Mayer, L. F., Teirstein, A. S., and Marom, Z. (1989). Human airway epithelial cells express functional MHC class II molecules. *Am. Rev. Respir. Dis.*, 139, A457.

159. Spurzem, J. R., Sacco, O., and Rennard, S. I. (1990). The expression of fibronectin and vitronectin receptors is regulated on bronchial epithelial cells. *Am. Rev. Respir. Dis.*, 141, A705.

160. McMenamin, C., Schön-Hegrad, M., Oliver, J., Girn, B., and Holt, P. G. (1991). Regulation of IgE responses to inhaled antigens: cellular mechanisms underlying allergic sensitization vs. tolerance induction. *Int. Arch. Allergy Appl. Immunol.*, 94, 78–82.

161. Sertl, K., Takemura, T., Tschachler, E. Ferrans, V. J., Kaliner, M. A., and Shevach, E. M. (1986). Dendritic cells with antigen-presenting capability reside in airway epithelium, lung parenchyma, and visceral pleura. *J. Exp. Med.*, 163, 436–451.

162. Holt, P. G., Schön-Hegrad, M. A., and Oliver, J. (1988). MHC class II antigen-bearing dendritic cells in pulmonary tissues of the rat: regulation of antigen presentation activity by endogenous macrophage populations. *J. Exp. Med.*, 167, 262–274.

163. Holt, P. G., Schon-Hegrad, M. A., Phillips, M. J., and McMenamin, P. G. (1989). Ia-positive dendritic cells form a tightly meshed network within the human airway epithelium. *Clin. Exp. Allergy*, 19, 597–601.

164. Johnson, A. R., Ashton, J., Schulz, W. W., and Erdos, E. G. (1985). Neutral metalloen-dopeptidases in human lung tissue and cultured cells. *Am. Rev. Respir. Dis.*, 132, 564–568.

165. Sekizawa, K., Tamaoki, J., Graf, P. D., Basbaum, C. B., Borson, D. B., and Nadel, J. A. (1987). Enkephalinase inhibitor potentiates mammalian tachykinin-induced contraction in ferret trachea. *J. Pharmacol. Exp. Ther.*, 243, 1211–1217.

166. Kerr, M. A. and Kenny, A. J. (1974). The purification and specificity of neutral endopep-tidase from rabbit kidney-brush border. *Biochem. J.*, 137, 477–88.

167. Bunnett, N. W., (1987). Release and breakdown: postsecretory metabolism of peptides. *Am. Rev. Respir. Dis.*, 136, S27–S34.

168. Dusser, D. J., Nadel, J. A., Sekizawa, K., Graf, P. D., and Borson, D. B. (1988). Neutral endopeptidase and angiotensin-converting enzyme inhibitors potentiate kinin-induced con-traction of ferret trachea. *J. Pharmacol. Exp. Ther.*, 244, 531–536.

169. Said, S. I. (1987). Effector actions: influence of neuropeptides on airway smooth muscle. *Am. Rev. Respir. Dis.*, 136, S52–S58.

170. Hay, D. W. P. (1989). Guinea-pig tracheal epithelium and endothelin. *Eur. J. Pharmacol.*, 171, 241–245.

171. Kondo, M., Tamaoki, J., and Takizawa, T. (1990). Neutral endopeptidase inhibitor poten-tiates the tachykinin-induced increase in ciliary beat frequency in rabbit trachea. *Am. Rev. Respir. Dis.*, 142, 403–406.

172. DeVillier, P., Advenier, C., Drapeau, G., Marsac, J., and Regoli, D. (1988). Comparison of the effects of epithelium removal and of an enkephalinase inhibitor on the neurokinin-induced contractions of guinea-pig trachea. *Br. J. Pharmacol.*, 94, 675–684.

173. Fine, J. M., Gordon, T., and Sheppard, D. (1989). Epithelium removal alters responsiveness of guinea pig trachea to substance P. *J. Appl. Physiol.*, 66, 232–237.

174. Frossard, N., Stretton, C. D., and Barnes, P. J. (1990). Modulation of bradykinin responses in airway smooth muscle epithelial forks. *Agents Actions*, 31, 204–209.

175. Fernandes, L. B., Preuss, J. M. H., and Goldie, R. G. (1992). Epithelial modulation of the relaxant activity of atriopeptides in rat and guinea-pig tracheal smooth muscle. *Eur. J. Pharmacol.*, 212, 187–194.

176. Farmer, S. G. and Togo, J. (1990). Effect of epithelium removal on relaxation of airway smooth muscle induced by vasoactive intestinal peptide and electrical field stimulation. *Br. J. Pharmacol.*, 100, 73–78.

177. Rhoden, K. J. and Barnes, P. J. (1990). Epithelial modulation of non-adrenergic, non-cholinergic and vasoactive intestinal peptide-induced responses: role of neutral endopep-tidase. *Eur. J. Pharmacol.*, 171, 247–250.

178. Lindström, E. G., Andersson, R. G. G., Granérus, G., and Grundström, N. (1991). Is the airway epithelium responsible for histamine metabolism in the trachea of guinea pigs? *Agents Actions*, 33, 1–2.

179. Yamauchi, K., Nakazawa, H., Sekizawa, K., Ohkawara, Y., Hiroki, H., Okayama, M., Tamura, G., Tanno, Y., Suzuki, H., Shibihara, S., Maeyama, K., Watanabe, T., Takamura, M., Sasaki, H., Takishima, T., and Shirato, K. (1993). The regulatory role of histamine-N-methyltrans-ferase in allergic reactions in the human airways. *Am. Rev. Respir. Dis.*, 147, A431.

180. Farmer, S. G., Fedan, J. S., Hay, D. W. P., and Raeburn, D. (1986). The effects of epithe-lium removal on the sensitivity of guinea-pig isolated trachealis to bronchodilator drugs. *Br. J. Pharmacol.*, 89, 407–414.

181. Advenier, C., DeVillier, P., Matran, R., and Naline, E. (1988). Influence of epithelium on the responsiveness of guinea-pig isolated trachea to adenosine. *Br. J. Pharmacol.*, 93, 295–302.

182. Goldenberg, H., Huttinger, M., Kollner, U., Kramar, R., and Pavelka, M. (1978). Catalase positive particles from pig lung. Biochemical preparations and morphological studies. *Histochemistry*, 56, 253–264.
183. Jones, K. G., Holland, J. R., Foureman, G. L., Bend, J. R., and Fouts, J. R. (1983). *J. Pharmacol. Exp. Ther.*, 225, 316–319.
184. Boyd, M. R. (1977). Evidence for the Clara cell as a site of cytochrome $P_{450}$-dependent mixed function oxidase activity in lung. *Nature*, 269, 713–715.
185. Gail, D. G. and Lenfant, C. J. M. (1983). Cells of the lung: biology and clinical implications. *Am. Rev. Respir. Dis.*, 127, 366–387.
186. Widdicombe, J. G. and Pack, R. J. (1982). The Clara cell. *Eur. J. Respir. Dis.*, 63, 202–220.
187. Beasley, R., Roche, W. R., Roberts, J. A., and Holgate, S. T. (1989). Cellular events in the bronchi in mild asthma and after bronchial provocation. *Am. Rev. Respir. Dis.*, 139, 806–817.
188. Laitinen, L. A., Heino, M., Laitinen, A., Kava, T., and Haahtela, T. (1985). Damage of the airway epithelium and bronchial reactivity in patients with asthma. *Am. Rev. Respir. Dis.*, 131, 599–606.
189. Lozewicz, S., Wells, C., Gomez, E., Ferguson, H., Richman, P., Devilia, J., and Davies, R. J. (1990). Morphological integrity of the bronchial epithelium in mild asthma. *Thorax*, 45, 12–15.
190. Heino, M., Monkare, S., Haahtela, T., and Laitinen, L. A. (1982). An electronmicroscopic study of the airways in patients with farmer's lung. *Eur. J. Respir. Dis.*, 36, 52–61.
191. Hers, J. F. P. H. (1966). Disturbances of the ciliated epithelium due to influenza virus. *Am. Rev. Respir. Dis.*, 93, 162–171.
192. Golden, J. A., Nadel, J. A., and Boushey, H. A. (1978). Bronchial hyperirritability in healthy subjects after exposure to ozone. *Am. Rev. Respir. Dis.*, 118, 287–294.
193. Holtzman, M. J., Fabbri, L. M., and O'Byrne, P. M. (1983). Importance of airway inflammation for hyperresponsiveness induced by ozone. *Am. Rev. Respir. Dis.*, 127, 686–690.
194. Mapp, C. E., Polato, R., Maestrelli, P., Hendrick, D. J., and Fabbri, L. M. (1985). Time course of the increase in airway responsiveness associated with late asthmatic reactions to toluene diisocyanate in sensitized subjects. *J. Allergy Clin. Immunol.*, 75, 568–572.
195. Boucher, R. C., Johnson, J., Inoue, S., Hulbert, W., and Hogg, J. C. (1980). The effect of cigarette smoke on the permeability of guinea pig airways. *Lab. Invest.*, 43, 94–100.
196. Hulbert, W. C., Walker, D. C., Jackson, A., and Hogg, J .C. (1981). Airway permeability to horseradish peroxidase in guinea pigs: the repair phase after injury by cigarette smoke. *Am. Rev. Respir. Dis.*, 123, 320–326.
197. Hulbert, W. C., McLean, H., and Hogg, J. C. (1985). The effect of acute airway inflammation on bronchial reactivity in guinea pigs. *Am. Rev. Respir. Dis.*, 132, 7–11.
198. Ilowite, J. S., Bennett, W. D., Sheetz, M. S., Groth, M. L., and Nierman, D. M. (1989). Permeability of the bronchial mucosa to $^{99m}$Tc-DPTA in asthma. *Am. Rev. Respir. Dis.*, 139, 1139–1143.
199. Elwood, R. K., Kennedy, S., Belzberg, A., Hogg, J. C., and Paré, P. D. (1983). Respiratory mucosal permeability in asthma. *Am. Rev. Respir. Dis.*, 128, 523–527.
200. O'Byrne, P. M., Dolovich, M., Dirks, R., Roberts, R. S., and Newhouse, M. T. (1984). Lung epithelial permeability: relation to nonspecific airway responsiveness. *J. Appl. Physiol.*, 57, 177–183.
201. Gleich, G. J., Frigas, E., Loegering, D. A., Wassom, D. L., and Steinmuller, D. (1979). Cytotoxic properties of eosinophil major basic protein. *J. Immunol.*, 123, 2925–2927
202. Horn, B. R., Robin, E. D., Theodore, J. A., and Van Kessel, A. (1975). Total eosinophil counts in the management of bronchial asthma. *N. Engl. J. Med.*, 292, 1152–1155.
203. Motojima, S., Frigas, E., Loegering, D. A., and Gleich, G. J. (1989). Toxicity of eosinophil cationic proteins for guinea-pig tracheal epithelium *in vitro*. *Am. Rev. Respir. Dis.*, 139, 801–805.
204. Flavahan, N. A., Slifman, N. R., Gleich, G. J., and Vanhoutte, P. M. (1988). Human eosinophil major basic protein causes hyperreactivity of respiratory smooth muscle. *Am. Rev. Respir. Dis.*, 138, 685–688.

205. Brofman, J. D., White, S. R., Blake, J. S., Munoz, N. M., Gleich, G. J., and Leff, A. R. (1989). Epithelial augmentation of trachealis contraction caused by major basic protein of eosinophils. *J. Appl. Physiol.*, 66, 1867–1873.

206. De Monchy, J. G. R., Kauffman, H. F., Venge, P., Koeter, G. H., Jansen, H. M., Sluiter, H. J., and De Vries, K. (1985). Bronchoalveolar eosinophilia during allergen-induced late asthmatic reactions. *Am. Rev. Respir. Dis.*, 131, 373–377.

207. Flavahan, N. A., Aarhus, L. L., Rimele, T. J., and Vanhoutte, P. M. (1985). Respiratory epithelium inhibits bronchial smooth muscle tone. *J. Appl. Physiol.*, 58, 834–838.

208. Goldie, R. G., Fernandes, L. B., Farmer, S. G., and Hay, D. W. P. (1990). Airway epithelium-derived inhibitory factor. *Trends Pharmacol. Sci.*, 11, 67–70.

209. Hay, D. W. P., Farmer, S. G., and Goldie, R. G. (1994). Inflammatory mediators and modulation of epithelial/smooth muscle interactions, in *Immunopharmacology of Epithelial Barriers*, pp. 119–146, R. G. Goldie, Ed., Academic Press, London.

210. Knight, D. A., Stewart, G. A., and Thompson, P. J. (1994). The epithelium and airway smooth muscle homeostasis: its relevance to asthma. *Clin. Exp. Allergy*, 24, 698–706.

211. Holroyde, M. C. (1986). The influence of epithelium on the responsiveness of guinea-pig isolated trachea. *Br. J. Pharmacol.*, 87, 501–507.

212. Small, R. C., Good, D. M., Dixon, J. S., and Kennedy, I. (1990). The effects of epithelium on the actions of cholinomimetic drugs in opened segments and perfused tubular preparations of guinea-pig trachea. *Br. J. Pharmacol.*, 100, 516–522.

213. Flavahan, N. A. and Vanhoutte, P. M. (1985). The respiratory epithelium releases a smooth muscle relaxing factor. *Chest*, 87, 189S–190S.

214. Barnes, P. J., Cuss, F. M., and Palmer, J. B. (1985). The effect of airway epithelium on smooth muscle contractility in bovine trachea. *Br. J. Pharmacol.*, 86, 685–691.

215. Knight, D. A., Adcock, J. A., Phillips, M. J., and Thompson, P. J. (1990). The effect of epithelium removal on human bronchial smooth muscle responsiveness to acetylcholine and histamine. *Pulm. Pharmacol.*, 3, 198–202.

216. Hay, D. W. P., Farmer, S. G., Raeburn, D., Robinson, V. A., Fleming, W. W., and Fedan, J. S. (1986). Airway epithelium modulates the reactivity of guinea-pig respiratory smooth muscle. *Eur. J. Pharmacol.*, 129, 11–18.

217. Hay, D. W. P., Raeburn, D., and Fedan, J. S. (1987). Regional differences in reactivity and the influence of the epithelium on canine bronchial smooth muscle. *Eur. J. Pharmacol.*, 141, 363–370.

218. Raeburn, D., Hay, D. W. P., Robinson, V. A., Farmer, S. G., Fleming, W. W., and Fedan, J. S. (1986). The effect of verapamil is reduced in isolated airways smooth muscle preparations lacking an epithelium. *Life Sci.*, 38, 809–816.

219. Butler, G. B., Adler, K. B., Evans, J. N., Morgan, D. W., and Szarek, J. L. (1987). Modulation of rabbit airway smooth muscle responsiveness by respiratory epithelium. *Am. Rev. Respir. Dis.*, 135, 1099–1104.

220. Goldie, R. G., Papadimitriou, J. M., Paterson, J. W., Rigby, P. J., Self, H. M., and Spina, D. (1986). Influence of the epithelium on responsiveness of guinea-pig isolated trachea to contractile and relaxant agonists. *Br. J. Pharmacol.*, 87, 5–14.

221. Tschirhart, E. and Landry, Y. (1986). Airway epithelium releases a relaxant factor: demonstration with substance P. *Eur. J. Pharmacol.*, 132, 103–104.

222. Grunstein, M. M., Chuang, S. T., Schramm, C. M., and Pawlowski, N. A. (1991). Role of endothelin-1 in regulating rabbit airway contractility. *Am. J. Physiol.*, 260, L75–L82.

223. Candenas, M.-L., Naline, E., Sarria, B., and Advenier, C. (1992). Effect of epithelium removal and of enkephalin inhibition of the bronchoconstrictor response to three endothelins of the human bronchus. *Eur. J. Pharmacol.*, 210, 291–297.

224. Hay, D. W. P., Farmer, S. G., Raeburn, D., Muccitelli, R. M., Wilson, K. A., and Fedan, J. S. (1987). Differential effects of epithelium removal on the responsiveness of guinea-pig tracheal smooth muscle to bronchoconstrictors. *Br. J. Pharmacol.*, 92, 381–388.

225. Hisayama, T., Takayanagi, I., Nakazato, F., and Hirano, K. (1988). Epithelium selectively controls hypersensitization of the response of smooth muscle to leukotriene $D_4$ by endogenous prostanoid(s) in guinea-pig trachea. *Naunyn-Schmiedebergs Arch. Pharmacol.*, 337, 296–300.

226. Brunelleschi, S., Haye-Legrand, I., Labat, C., Norel, X., and Benveniste, J. (1987). Platelet-activating factor-acether-induced relaxation of guinea-pig airway muscle: role of prostaglandin $E_2$ and the epithelium. *J. Pharmacol. Exp. Ther.*, 243, 356–363.

227. Conroy, D. M., Samhoun, M. N., and Piper, P. J. (1990). Relaxations of guinea-pig isolated trachea induced by platelet activating factor are epithelium-dependent and are antagonized by WEB 2086. *Eur. J. Pharmacol.*, 186, 315–318.

228. Preuss, J. M. H., Henry, P. J., and Goldie, R. G. (1992). Influence of age on epithelium-dependent responsiveness of guinea-pig and rat tracheal smooth muscle to spasmogens. *Eur. J. Pharmacol. (Environ. Pharmacol. Toxicol.)*, 228, 3–8.

229. Murlas, C. (1986). Effects of mucosal removal on guinea-pig airway smooth muscle responsiveness. *Clin. Sci.*, 70, 571–575.

230. Prié, S., Cadieux, A., and Sirois, P. (1990). Removal of guinea pig bronchial and tracheal epithelium potentiates the contractions to leukotrienes and histamine. *Eicosanoids*, 3, 29–37.

231. Manning, P. J., Jones, G. L., Otis, J., Daniel, E. E., and O'Byrne, P. M. (1990). The inhibitory influence of tracheal mucosa mounted in close proximity to canine trachealis. *Eur. J. Pharmacol.*, 178, 85–89.

232. Montano, L. M., Selman, M., Ponce-Monter, H., and Vargas, M. H. (1988). Role of airway epithelium on the reactivity of smooth muscle from guinea pigs sensitized to ovalbumin by inhalatory method. *Res. Exp. Med.*, 188, 167–173.

233. Aizawa, H., Miyazaki, N., Shigematsu, N., and Tomooka, M. (1988). A possible role of airway epithelium in modulating hyperresponsiveness. *Br. J. Pharmacol.*, 93, 139–145.

234. Fernandes, L. B., Preuss, J. M. H., Paterson, J. W., and Goldie, R. G. (1990). Epithelium-derived inhibitory factor in human bronchus. *Eur. J. Pharmacol.*, 187, 331–336.

235. Hay, D. W. P., Muccitelli, R. M., Horstmeyer, D. L., and Raeburn, D. (1988). Is the epithelium-derived inhibitory factor in guinea-pig trachea a prostanoid? *Prostaglandins*, 35, 625–638.

236. Güc, M. O., Ilhan, M., and Kayaalp, S. O. (1988). Epithelium-dependent relaxation of guinea-pig tracheal smooth muscle by histamine: evidence for non-$H_1$- and non-$H_2$-histamine receptors. *Arch. Int. Pharmacodyn.*, 296, 57–65.

237. Morrison, K. J. and Vanhoutte, P. M. (1992). Characterization of muscarinic receptors that mediate contraction of guinea-pig isolated trachea to choline esters: effect of removing epithelium. *Br. J. Pharmacol.*, 106, 672–676.

238. Lev, A., Christiansen, G. C., Zhang, R.-A., and Kelsen, S. G. (1990). Epithelial effects on tracheal smooth muscle tone: Influence of muscarinic agonists. *Am. J. Physiol.*, 258, L52–L56.

239. Stuart-Smith, K. and Vanhoutte, P. M. (1987). Heterogeneity in the effects of epithelium removal in the canine bronchial tree. *J. Appl. Physiol.*, 63, 2510–2515.

240. Stuart-Smith, K. and Vanhoutte, P.M. (1988). Arachidonic acid evokes epithelium-dependent relaxations in canine airways. *J. Appl. Physiol.*, 65, 2170–2180.

241. Gao, Y. and Vanhoutte, P. M. (1988). Removal of the epithelium potentiates acetylcholine in depolarizing canine bronchial smooth muscle. *J. Appl. Physiol.*, 65, 2400–2405.

242. Sekizawa, K., Caughey, S. C., Lazarus, S. C., Gold, W. M., and Nadel, J. A. (1989). Mast cell tryptase causes airways smooth muscle hyperresponsiveness in dogs. *J. Clin. Invest.*, 83, 175–179.

243. Franconi, G. M., Rubinstein, I., Levine, E. H., Ideda, S., and Nadel, J. A. (1990). Mechanical removal of airway epithelium disrupts mast cells and releases granules. *Am. J. Physiol.*, 259, L372–L377.

244. Buckner, D. K., Fedyna, J. S., Robertson, J. L., Will, J. A., England, D. M., Krell, R. D., and Saban, R. (1990). An examination of the influence of the epithelium on contractile responses to peptidoleukotrienes and blockade by ICI 204,219 in isolated guinea pig trachea and human intralobar airways. *J. Pharmacol. Exp. Ther.*, 252, 77–85.

245. Farmer, S. G. (1991). Role of kinins in airway diseases. *Immunopharmacology,* 22, 1–20.
246. Bewley, J., Bhoola, K. D., Crothers, D. M., and Cingi, M. I. (1988). Biphasic responses of the isolated guinea-pig tracheal muscle strip to kallidin and bradykinin. *Br. J. Pharmacol.,* 92, 597P.
247. Bramley, A. M., Samhoun, M. N., and Piper, P. J. (1990). The role of the epithelium in modulating the responses of guinea-pig trachea induced by bradykinin *in vitro. Br. J. Pharmacol.,* 99, 762–766.
248. Farmer, S. G., Burch, R. M., Meeker, S. N., and Wilkins, D. E. (1989). Evidence for a pulmonary bradykinin B, receptor. *Mol. Pharmacol.,* 36, 1–8.
249. Aizawa, T., Sekizawa, K., Aikawa, T., Maruyama, N., Itabashi, S., Tamura, G., Sasaki, H., and Takishima, T. (1990). Eosinophil supernatant causes hyperresponsiveness of airway smooth muscle in guinea pig trachea. *Am. Rev. Respir. Dis.,* 142, 133–137.
250. Liu, M. C., Bleecker, E. R., Lichtenstein, L. M., Kagey-Sobotka, A., Niv, Y., McLemore, T. L., Permutt, S., Proud, D., and Hubbard, W. C. (1990). Evidence for elevated levels of histamine, prostaglandin D$_2$, and other bronchoconstricting prostaglandins in the airways of subjects with mild asthma. *Am. Rev. Respir. Dis.,* 142, 126–132.
251. Walters, E. H., O'Byrne, P. M., Fabbri, L. M., Graf, P. D., Holtzman, M. J., and Nadel, J. A. (1988). Control of neurotransmission by prostaglandins in canine trachealis smooth muscle. *J. Appl. Physiol.,* 57, 129–134.
252. Frossard, N., Rhoden, K. J., and Barnes, P. J. (1989). Influence of epithelium on guinea pig airway responses to tachykinins: role of endopeptidase and cyclooxygenase. *J. Pharmacol. Exp. Ther.,* 248, 292–299.
253. Djokic, T. D., Nadel, J. A., Dusser, D. J., Sekizawa, K., Graf, P. D., and Borson, D. B. (1989). Inhibitors of neutral endopeptidase potentiate electrically and capsaicin-induced noncholinergic contraction in guinea pig bronchi. *J. Pharmacol. Exp. Ther.,* 247, 7–11.
254. Maggi, C. A., Patacchini, R., Perretti, F., Meini, S., Manzini, S., Santicioli, P., Del Bianco, E., and Meli, A. (1990). The effect of thiorphan and epithelium removal on contractions and tachykinin release produced by activation of capsaicin-sensitive afferents in the guinea-pig isolated bronchus. *Naunyn-Schmiedebergs Arch. Pharmacol.,* 341, 74–79.
255. Black, J. L., Johnson, P. R. A., and Armour, C. L. (1988). Potentiation of the contractile effects of neuropeptides in human bronchus by an enkephalinase inhibitor. *Pulm. Pharmacol.,* 1, 21–23.
256. Fagny, C., Michel, A., Léonard, I., Berkenboom, G., Fontaine, J., and Deschodt-Lanckman, M. (1991). *In vitro* degradation of endothelin-1 by endopeptidase 24.11 (Enkephalinase). *Peptides,* 12, 773–778.
257. Vijayaraghavan, J., Scicli, A. G., Carretero, O. A., Slaughter, C., Moomaw, C., and Hersh, L. B. (1990). The hydrolysis of endothelins by neutral endopeptidase 24.11 (enkephalinase). *J. Biol. Chem.,* 265, 14150–14155.
258. Adams, G. K. and Lichtenstein, L. (1979). *In vitro* studies of antigen-induced bronchospasm: effect of antihistamine and SRS-A antagonist on response of sensitized guinea pig and human airways to antigen. *J. Immunol.,* 122, 555–562.
259. Hay, D. W. P., Raeburn, D., Farmer, S. G., Fleming, W. W., and Fedan, J. S. (1986). Epithelium modulates the reactivity of ovalbumin-sensitized guinea-pig airway smooth muscle. *Life Sci.,* 38, 2461–2468.
260. Undem, B. J., Raible, D. G., Adkinson, N. F., and Adams, G. K. III. (1988). Effect of removal of epithelium on antigen-induced smooth muscle contraction and mediator release from guinea-pig isolated trachea. *J. Pharmacol. Exp. Ther.,* 244, 659–665.
261. Wessler, I., Hellwig, H., and Racké, K. (1990). Stimulation-induced over-flow of [$^3$H]-phosphorylcholine and [$^3$H]-acetylcholine from the isolated guinea-pig trachea: inhibitory role of the epithelium. *Br. J. Pharmacol.,* 99, 54P.
262. Ullman, A., Lofdahl, C.-G., Svedmyr, N., Bernsten, L., and Skoogh, B.-E. (1988). Mucosal inhibition of cholinergic contractions in ferret trachea can be transferred between organ baths. *Eur. Respir. J.,* 1, 908–912.

263. Lundblad, K. A. and Persson, C. G. A. (1988). The epithelium and the pharmacology of guinea-pig tracheal tone *in vitro. Br. J. Pharmacol.*, 93, 909–917.

264. Stuart-Smith, K. and Vanhoutte, P. M. (1990). Epithelium, contractile tone and responses to relaxing agonists in canine bronchi. *J. Appl. Physiol.*, 69, 678–685.

265. Hulsmann, A. R., Jongejan, R. C., Raatgeep, H. R., Stijnen, T., Bonta, I. L., Kerrebijn, K. F., and DeJongste, J. C. (1993). Epithelium removal and peptidase inhibition enhance relaxation of human airways to vasoactive intestinal peptide. *Am. Rev. Respir. Dis.*, 147, 1483–1486.

266. O'Donnell, M., Garippa, R., and Welton, A. F. (1985). Relaxant activity of atriopeptins in isolated guinea-pig airway and vascular smooth muscle. *Peptides*, 6, 597–601.

267. Ishii, K. and Murad, F. (1989). ANP relaxes bovine tracheal smooth muscle and increases cGMP. *J. Appl. Physiol.*, 256, C495–C500.

268. Sasaki, T., Shimura, S., Sasaki, H., and Takishima, T. (1989). Effect of epithelium on mucus secretion from feline tracheal submucosal glands. *J. Appl. Physiol.*, 66, 764–770.

269. Al-Bazzaz, F. J., Yadava, V. P., and Westenfelder, C. (1981). Modification of Na and Cl transport in canine tracheal mucosa by prostaglandins. *Am. J. Physiol.*, 240, F101–F105.

270. Finkbeiner, W. E. and Widdicombe, J. H. (1989). Control of nasal airway secretions, ion transport, and water movement, in *Defence Capillaries of the Respiratory Tract*, pp. 287–362, R. B. Schlesinger, Ed., Raven Press, New York.

271. Cox, G., Ohtoshi, T., Gauldie, J., Denburg, J., and Jordana, M. (1990). Human bronchial epithelial cells cause differentiation of HL-60 cells and prolong the *in vitro* survival of eosinophils. *Am. Rev. Respir. Dis.*, 141, A108.

272. Jordana, M., Vancheri, C., Ohtoshi, T., Tsuda, T., Cox, G., Harnish, D., Dolovich, J., Denburg, J., and Gauldie, J. (1989). Hemopoietic function of fibroblasts and epithelial cells derived from normal and inflamed upper respiratory airway tissues. *Am. Rev. Respir. Dis.*, 139, A251.

273. Tosi, M. F., Stark, M. J., Hamedani, A., Smith, C. W., Gruenert, D. C., and Huang, Y. T. (1991). Increased adhesion by neutrophils to human tracheal epithelial cells infected with parainfluenza virus type 2: role of epithelial ICAM-1 and neutrophil CD11/CD18 adhesions. *Pediatr. Res.*, 29, A186.

274. Varsano, S., Lazarus, S. C., Gold, W. M., and Nadel, J. A. (1988). Selective adhesion of mast cells to tracheal epithelial cells *in vitro. J. Immunol.*, 140, 2184–2192.

275. Wegner, C. D., Rothlein, R., and Gundel, R. H. (1991). Adhesion molecules in the pathogenesis of asthma. *Agents Actions*, 34 (Suppl.), 529–544.

276. Güc, M. O., Ilhan, M., and Kayaalp, S. O. (1988). Epithelium-dependent relaxation of guinea-pig tracheal smooth muscle by carbachol. *Arch. Int. Pharmacodyn.*, 294, 241–247.

277. Munakata, M., Mitzner, W., and Menkes, H. (1988). Osmotic stimuli induce epithelial-dependent relaxation in the guinea-pig trachea. *J. Appl. Physiol.*, 64, 466–471.

278. Vanhoutte, P. M. (1988). Epithelium-derived relaxing factor(s) and bronchial reactivity. *Am. Rev. Respir. Dis.*, 138, S24–S30.

279. Fernandes, L. B., Paterson, J. W., and Goldie, R. G. (1989). Co-axial bioassay of an epithelial relaxant factor from the guinea-pig trachea. *Br. J. Pharmacol.*, 97, 117–124.

280. Fernandes, L. B. and Goldie, R. G. (1990). Pharmacological evaluation of guinea-pig tracheal epithelium-derived inhibitory factor (EpDIF). *Br. J. Pharmacol.*, 100, 614–618.

281. Güc, M. O., Ilhan, M., and Kayaalp, S. O. (1988). The rat anococcygeus muscle is a convenient bioassay organ for the airway epithelium-derived relaxant factor. *Eur. J. Pharmacol.*, 148, 405–409.

282. Ilhan, M. and Sahin, I. (1986). Tracheal epithelium releases a vascular smooth muscle relaxant factor: demonstration by bioassay. *Eur. J. Pharmacol.*, 131, 293–296.

283. Fernandes, L. B. and Goldie, R. G. (1991). Antigen-induced release of airway epithelium-derived inhibitory factor. *Am. Rev. Respir. Dis.*, 143, 567–571.

284. Goldie, R. G. (1990). Receptors in asthmatic airways. *Am. Rev. Respir. Dis.*, 141, S151–S156.

285. Munakata, M., Masaki, Y., and Sakuma, I. (1990). Pharmacological differentiation of epithelium-derived relaxing factor from nitric oxide. *J. Appl. Physiol.*, 69, 665–670.

286. Hay, D. W. P., Muccitelli, R. M., Page, C. P., and Spina, D. (1992). Correlation between airway epithelium-induced relaxation of rat aorta in the co-axial bioassay and cyclic nucleotide levels. *Br. J. Pharmacol.*, 105, 954–958.

287. Gunn, L. K. and Piper, P. J. (1991). Potential sources of artifact in the co-axial bioassay. *Eur. J. Pharmacol.*, 203, 405–412.

288. Spina, D., Fernandes, L. B., Preuss, J. M. H., Hay, D. W. P., Muccitelli, R. M., Page, C. P., and Goldie, R. G. (1992). Evidence that epithelium-dependent relaxation of vascular smooth muscle detected by co-axial bioassays is not attributable to hypoxia. *Br. J. Pharmacol.*, 105, 799–804.

289. Iriarte, C. F., Pascual, R., Villanueva, M. M., Román, M., Cortijo, J., and Morcillo, E. J. (1990). Role of epithelium in agonist-induced contractile responses of guinea-pig trachealis: influence of the surface through which drug enters the tissue. *Br. J. Pharmacol.*, 101, 257–262.

290. Fedan, J. S., Nutt, M. E., and Frazer, D. G. (1990). Reactivity of guinea-pig isolated trachea to methacholine, histamine and isoproterenol applied serosally vs. mucosally. *Eur. J. Pharmacol.*, 190, 337–345.

291. Pavlovic, D., Fournier, M., Aubier, M., and Pariente, R. (1989). Epithelial vs. serosal stimulation of tracheal muscle: role of epithelium. *J. Appl. Physiol.*, 67, 2522–2526.

292. Sparrow, M. P. and Mitchell, H. W. (1991). Modulation by the epithelium of the extent of bronchial narrowing produced by substances perfused through the lumen. *Br. J. Pharmacol.*, 103, 1160–1164.

293. Fisher, J. T., Gray, P. R., Mitchell, H. W., and Sparrow, M. P. (1994). Epithelial modulation of neonatal and fetal porcine bronchial contractile responses. *Am. J. Respir. Crit. Care Med.*, 149, 1304–1310.

294. Mitchell, H. W., Fisher, J. T., and Sparrow, M. P. (1993). The integrity of the epithelium is a major determinant of the responsiveness of the dog bronchial segment to mucosal provocation. *Pulm. Pharmacol.*, 6, 263–268.

295. Omari, T. I., Sparrow, M. P., and Mitchell, H. W. (1993). Responsiveness of human isolated bronchial segments and its relationship to epithelial loss. *Br. J. Clin. Pharmacol.*, 35, 357–365.

296. Hogg, J. C. and Eggleston, P. A. (1984). Is asthma an epithelial disease? *Am. Rev. Respir. Dis.*, 129, 207–208.

297. Sant' Ambrogio, G. (1982). Information arising from the tracheobronchial trees of mammals. *Physiol. Rev.*, 62, 531–569.

298. Holtzman, M. J. (1985). Inflammation of the airway epithelium and the development of airway hyperresponsiveness, in *Progress in Respiratory Research, Asthma and Bronchial Hyperreactivity*, pp. 165–172, H. Herzog and A. P. Perruchoud, Eds., S. Karger, Basel.

Chapter 6

# HEPARIN AND RELATED MOLECULES: ANTIPROLIFERATIVE AND ANTI-INFLAMMATORY EFFECTS IN THE AIRWAYS

Stephen A. Kilfeather and Clive Page

## CONTENTS

0-8493-7813-3/97/$0.00+$.50
© 1997 by CRC Press, Inc.

# I. INTRODUCTION

Airway remodelling in asthma involves increased smooth muscle mass,[1-3] changes in bronchial vascular anatomy,[4] epithelial layer damage,[5] and subepithelial fibrosis with epithelial basement membrane reticular collagen deposition.[6] Enhanced inflammatory responses underlie the development of asthma, but the relationship between airway inflammation and the origin of structural changes is not understood. Glycosaminoglycans (GAGs) are saccharide polymers incorporated into proteins on cell surfaces and extracellular matrices. Free GAGs are secreted by many cells and released from extracellular sites by leukocyte-derived enzymes.

GAGs have high anionic charge and interact with extracellular matrix (ECM) proteins, cell surface receptors, and several groups of cytokines and growth factors. GAGs can be endocytosed, compartmentalised intracellularly, and secreted in altered, but biologically effective forms. GAGs influence many aspects of tissue remodelling and inflammation through effects on cell–ECM interaction, cell migration, and division. This review will provide an overview of the potential involvement of heparin and related heparan sulphate in regulation of inflammation and cell proliferation in the airways.

# II. ORIGIN OF GLYCOSAMINOGLYCANS

## A. GLYCOSAMINOGLYCAN STRUCTURE

GAGs are polymers of repeated alternating amine sugars (D-glucosamine or galactosamine) and a uronic acid (D-glucuronic acid or iduronic acid) with chain lengths varying from 2 to approximately 20 disaccharide units. The sugar residues are variably *O-* and *N*-sulphated or *N*-acetylated, providing dense anionic charge. The most common GAGs include heparin, heparan sulphate, chondroitin sulphate, dermatan sulphate, hyaluronic acid, and keratan sulphate. Heparin and heparan sulphate are members of the GAG family and have received most attention concerning GAG influence over cell behaviour, independent of their anticoagulant properties (for reviews see References 7 and 8). Heparin chains carry large regions composed of the disaccharide L-iduronic acid 2-*O*-sulphate ↦ D-glucosamine-*N*-6-*O*-sulphate (Figure 1). Heparan sulphate is composed of the disaccharide units D-glucuronic acid ↦ *N*-acetyl-D-glucosamine, but has far fewer substitutions enriched in *N-* and *O*-sulphation (Figure 2). The reduced substitution in heparan sulphate accounts for the lower density of anionic charge. Further variability in substitution provides a range of species within the heparin and heparan sulphate families.

## B. GLYCOSAMINOGLYCAN INCORPORATION
## INTO PROTEOGLYCANS

GAGs including heparin are linked to proteins at synthesis (for review see Reference 9). The resulting proteoglycan structures are ubiquitous in mammalian tissues and exist as cytoplasmic (granular), secreted, ECM, and cell-surface forms. proteoglycans can attain large mass, such as the ECM proteoglycan perlican (400–600 kDa) and an endothelial-derived heparan sulphate proteoglycan (HS proteoglycan) (600–800 kDa) (Figure 3). Large proteoglycans aggregate producing regions of high charge density generated from the attached anionic 300 amino acids and one to two GAG chains (approximately 40 kDa), including decorin (331 amino acids, two GAG chains) and biglycan (329 amino acids, one GAG chain). GAGs are classified according to acetylation, which together with variation in chain length and protein attachment confers specificity of action of proteoglycan species.[10-12] Proteoglycans usually contain more than one GAG species and are further classified according to the one predominating. The most common cell surface proteoglycans are HS proteoglycans with a high heparan sulphate content.

## C. DISTRIBUTION OF PROTEOGLYCANS
## IN THE LUNG

Heparin is present in connective tissue mast cells, while heparan sulphate is present in ECM and cell surface HS proteoglycans. Connective tissue mast cells are present in the lungs and provide a source of heparin proteoglycan, leading to heparin release during mast cell degranulation. Secretion of anticoagulant GAG, probably heparin, can be demonstrated in passively sensitised lung parenchyma following antigen challenge.[13] The concentration of GAG attained in parenchymal effluent under these conditions is within a range adequate for demonstration of several effects of heparin on cellular behaviour (1–100 µg/ml).[13] A systematic examination of chondroitin sulphate proteoglycan (CS proteoglycan) and HS proteoglycan distribution in the airways has

# Antithrombin III binding site

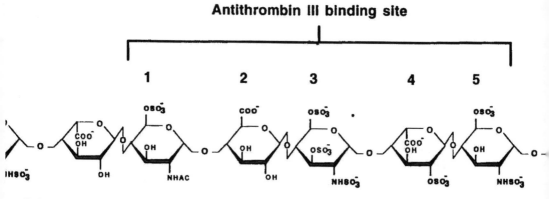

**FIGURE 1** Heparin octasaccharide. Saccharides 1–5 show the antithrombin III–binding site of heparin and heparan sulpha

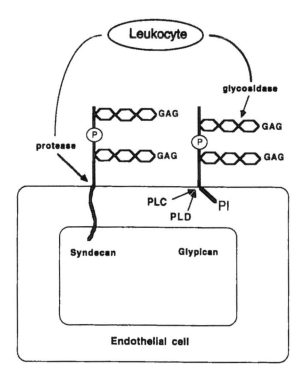

**FIGURE 2** Endothelial heparan sulphate proteoglycan. Proteoglycans are linked to endothelial cells by membrane-spanning regions for syndecans and by linkage to inositol phosphate (PI) as a glycosylphosphatidylinositol for glypicans. The transmembrane region of syndecans is vulnerable to cleavage by trypsin-like serine proteases, while glypicans are vulnerable to PLC and PLD. GAG chains such as heparan sulphate incorporated into proteoglycans (P) are released and excised by leukocyte-derived glycosidases.

been conducted in developing and adult rats.[14] Distribution of these proteoglycans was specific with respect to location and developmental stage. CS proteoglycan and HS proteoglycan demonstrated similar patterns of distribution, apart from a relatively lower HS proteoglycan content of smooth muscle external laminae. Basement membranes of airway epithelium and alveoli exhibited a large content of HS proteoglycan as previously observed,[15,16] suggesting an influence over basement membrane or reticular layer formation and behaviour of epithelial cells. Notably, HS proteoglycan content was dense in arterial, but not in venular vessels. The latter finding is of relevance to the passage of leukocytes through postcapillary venules at inflammatory sites, since HS proteoglycan and the GAG chains influence leukocyte adhesion to endothelial cells[8] (Section VII.A.5). The changing content of proteoglycans in the airway during development provides an indication of their potential influence over cell division, differentiation, and tissue repair.[14]

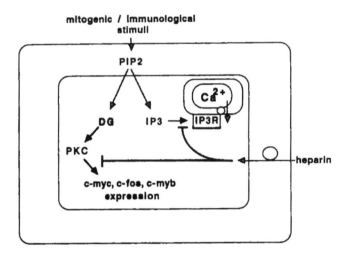

**FIGURE 3**   Intracellular sites of action of GAGs. GAGs such as heparin are internalised by high-affinity uptake sites. Phospholipase-initiated signal transduction results in phospholipid hydrolysis such as inositol bisphosphate (PIP$_2$) to diacylglycerol (DG) and inositol trisphosphate (IP$_3$), which activate PKC and Ca$^{2+}$ mobilisation, respectively. PKC-dependent pathways including oncogene (c-myb, c-fos, c-myb) expression, and IP$_3$ receptor (IP$_3$R) provide sites of GAG inhibition of mitogenic and inflammatory stimuli.

## D.  RELEASE OF FREE GAG AND PROTEOGLYCANS

Free GAG chains are derived by glycosidase excision from proteoglycans involving both heparanase and heparatinase[7,17] (see Figure 2). Two modes of HS proteoglycan anchorage to plasma membranes have been identified, and both are vulnerable during inflammatory responses. The syndecan group of HS proteoglycans possess a transmembrane section of the protein core that is sensitive to cleavage by trypsin-like serine proteases[7] (Figure 2). Leukocyte elastase alone can remove a large proportion of endothelial HS proteoglycan.[18] Members of the glypican family of HS proteoglycan are attached to a phosphatidylinositol as a glycosylphosphatidylinositol,[19-21] which is sensitive to hydrolysis by phospholipases (see Figure 2). Glypican HS proteoglycan linkages are hydrolysed by phospholipases C (PLC) and D (PLD) during signal transduction, and PLC has been used to remove cell surface glypican.[19]

The expression and release of glycosidases that liberate GAGs directly from proteoglycans and conduct further GAG excision to smaller chain lengths is increased from all activated circulating leukocytes and platelets.[22,23] Glycosidases thereby contribute to removal of endothelial heparan sulphate by activated leukocytes. GAG could be released efficiently from endothelial cells by the action of serine proteases and glycosidases from neutrophils alone,[18] acting in concert with elevated activity of PLC and PLD in endothelial membranes at inflammatory sites. The question remains, whether the release of free heparan sulphate and potential further reduction in chain length of heparan sulphate provides a predominantly pro- or antiproliferative and -inflammatory source of GAG. Furthermore, the removal of proteoglycans from smooth muscle by macrophage-derived enzyme activity appears to be primarily attributable to protease, as opposed to glycosidase, activity.[24] Subsequent degradation of heparan sulphate could be conducted by lysosomal glycosidase, in addition to extracellular glycosidase, following ingestion of GAG into macrophages (see Figure 3). The temporal relationship between leukocyte activation and glycosidase expression[22] may also reflect a capacity of leukocytes to degrade GAG intracellularly.

# III. MECHANISMS OF ACTION
# OF GLYCOSAMINOGLYCANS

## A. CELLULAR EFFECTS

Heparin has been investigated primarily for its anticoagulant property involving inhibition of thrombin through binding to antithrombin III at the specific GAG-binding site required for anticoagulant activity (see Figure 1). More recently, a growing range of activities of GAGs has been documented. Two major areas of activity of heparin and heparin analogues have been identified, including antiproliferative activity in several cell types[25,26] and potential anti-inflammatory or immunomodulatory activity.[27]

## B. CELLULAR UPTAKE

Heparin possesses several potential intracellular and extracellular sites of action. The dense anionic charge of heparin and related chains underlies the interaction between heparin and several groups of peptides and proteins, including heparin-binding growth factors and ECM proteins. GAG action on cell behaviour cannot, however, be considered as derived solely from extracellular charge effects. Heparin enters cells that express high-affinity cell surface uptake sites with estimated $t_{1/2}$ values ranging from 15 to 60 min. Smooth muscle cells can express $10\text{--}100 \times 10^3$ high-affinity uptake sites for heparin (dissociation constant of approximately 1 nM), depending upon their state of differentiation and stage of division.[25,28]

## C. INHIBITION OF Ca²⁺ MOBILISATION AND PROTEIN
## KINASE C–DEPENDENT PATHWAYS

Heparin is an established inhibitor of inositol trisphosphate ($IP_3$)-induced $Ca^{2+}$ mobilisation from intracellular stores,[29,30] suggesting that cellular responses involving PLC-induced generation of $IP_3$ are in general sensitive to heparin following acute exposure (minutes) (Figure 4). Inhibition of smooth muscle division by heparin has been demonstrated against mitogen-stimulated division dependent upon protein kinase C (PKC)-activated signal transduction pathways.[25] The range of PKC-dependent pathways that are sensitive to heparin has not been established, but could involve interference with expression of protooncogenes c-fos, c-myc, and c-myb[31-33] (see Figure 3). In addition,

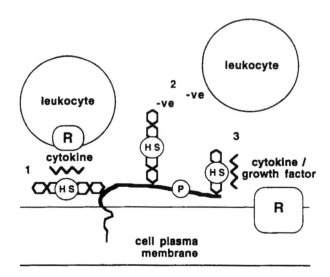

**FIGURE 4**   Leukocyte–proteoglycan (P) interaction. 1. Many heparin binding cytokines (including the chemokines MIP-1β, IL-8, and RANTES) provide stimuli for leukocyte migration through endothelial barriers. Cell surface heparan sulphate (HS) proteoglycans (P) provide sites of attachment and presentation of chemokines to leukocytes. 2. The dense negative charge of heparan sulphate facilitates endothelial barrier function. 3. HBGFs such as FGF are presented to endothelial cell surface receptors (R) by localised heparan sulphate proteoglycan.

heparin inhibition of AP-1 transactivation of the phorbol myristate acetate (TPA) response element (TRE) and inhibition of mitogen-activated $Na^+/H^+$ antiporter in rat VSMC have been observed.[34,35]

## D.   REQUIREMENTS OF CHARGE AND CHAIN LENGTH

Heparin is active when released from mast cells as a free GAG, whereas heparan sulphate is effective in regulation of cell function as a free GAG, bound to ECM proteins or incorporated into either cell surface or ECM HS proteoglycans. Heparan sulphate possesses less sulphation and correspondingly less anionic charge than heparin. Differences in overall charge density and fine structure contribute to differences in potency between these compounds under conditions in which their cellular effects are qualitatively similar, such as regulation of smooth muscle division. Thus, inhibition of smooth muscle is dependent upon a minimum GAG chain length and related to charge density.[35]

## E.   INHIBITION OF GLYCOSIDASES

Excision of GAG from proteoglycan provides a route for generation of free GAG, while reduction of chain length by glycosidases could provide a route for removal of GAG activity in which chain length is crucial (see Figure 2). The similarity between GAG species provides a source of competition between GAGs for glycosidases. Both heparin and chondroitin sulphate exhibit potent inhibition of tumour-derived heparanase activity against heparan sulphate[37-39] and, thereby, preserve heparan sulphate on HS proteoglycan in the presence of glycosidases (see Figure 2). Such an action could be exhibited by heparin released at high concentrations from mast cells at inflammatory sites.

## F. INTERACTION WITH MEDIATORS

A range of peptide mediators exhibits high affinity for heparin, resulting in modulation of activity through interaction with heparin or heparan sulphate (Table 1). A prominent example is the interaction with the serine protease inhibitor, antithrombin III, responsible for anticoagulant activity of heparin. Interaction with heparin for certain peptide cytokines can interrupt or facilitate their attachment to HS proteoglycan and storage or presentation by HS proteoglycan to adjacent cells or cell surface receptors (reviewed in References 7 and 40) (see Figure 4).

### TABLE 1
### Heparin Binding Chemokines
### and Growth Factors

#### Chemokines[a]

Macrophage inflammatory proteins (MIP-1α and MIP-1β)
Monocyte chemoattractant protein 1 (MCP-1)
NAP-1 (interleukin 8)
NAP-2
Platelet factor 4
RANTES

#### Growth factors[b]

Acidic and basic fibroblast growth factor
Hepatocyte growth factor
Kaposi sarcoma fibroblast growth factor
Platelet-derived growth factor
Transforming growth factor beta
Vascular endothelial growth factor

[a]   Reviewed in Reference 207.
[b]   Reviewed in Reference 208.

# IV. EFFECTS OF GLYCOSAMINOGLYCANS ON CELL ATTACHMENT AND MIGRATION

## A. CELL–MATRIX INTERACTION AND ATTACHMENT

Cell division and migration are fundamental characteristics of tissue remodelling and inflammation, and both aspects are dependent upon cell–ECM interaction. For an understanding of the influence of GAGs on cell division and migration, examination of GAG interaction with ECM is essential.

Predominant cells within the airways, including smooth muscle, fibroblast, epithelial, and endothelial cells, secrete several classes of proteoglycans.[7,40] Proteoglycans accumulate in ECMs and basement membranes, where they act in concert with cell surface proteoglycans to influence cell function. GAG binding is observed with most interstitial collagens (I, II, III, and IV)[41-44] and, as indicated in Table 2, GAG binding of collagen and other ECM proteins exhibits high affinity. HS proteoglycan binding to collagen is displaceable by heparin,[42] and inhibition of cell adhesion to ECM substrata by heparin could involve specific interference with HS proteoglycan–ECM interaction between ECM and cell surface HS proteoglycan and corresponding binding sites. This specificity is also reflected in the selective inhibition of fibroblast attachment to collagen substrata by certain GAGs.[45]

### TABLE 2
### High-Affinity Binding Sites for Heparin
### on Cell Attachment Proteins

| Cell attachment protein | kDa, nM |
|---|---|
| Collagen[202] | 5–25 |
| Fibronectin[203] | 4–100 |
| Vitronectin[204] | 10 |
| Laminin[205] | 34 |
| Thrombospondin[206] | 80 |

CS proteoglycan restricts cell attachment by inhibiting cellular HS proteoglycan interaction with fibronectin, vitronectin, laminin, and collagen.[46] Chondroitin sulphate chains also attached to the protein core of HS proteoglycan inhibit HS proteoglycan–fibronectin binding.[46] These findings illustrate the balance between GAG subtype content in cell surface proteoglycan in the control of cell proteoglycan–matrix interaction.

Cell attachment can, however, be achieved with low concentrations of collagen in the substratum.[48] This implies that saturation of collagen or, indeed, other ECM-binding sites may be required for inhibition of attachment through HS proteoglycan-binding sites by free GAG. This is endorsed by the higher (tenfold) concentrations of heparin required for inhibition of cell attachment to a type I collagen substrata than the affinity of heparin for type I collagen (5–25 nM).[45] Concentrations of free heparan sulphate in tissues in the presence or absence of inflammatory cell infiltration are unknown, and the influence of free heparan sulphate or other GAGs on cell attachment to collagen *in vivo* cannot be estimated at present. Anticoagulant GAGs, probably heparin, in the supernatants of sensitised lung undergoing an inflammatory response reach concentrations in the region of the heparin binding affinities for collagen.[13]

The possibility exists, therefore, that heparin concentrations in the vicinity of the mast cell could attain higher levels sufficient to influence HS proteoglycan–ECM interaction and cell attachment.

## B. CELL MIGRATION

In asthma, directional smooth muscle cell migration is not an obvious feature of the smooth muscle hypertrophy characteristic of the condition, but expansion of smooth muscle cell populations or mass requires adjustment of local contacts with ECM. There are, however, changes in the bronchial capillary network within the thickened airways of individuals with asthma,[4] requiring disruption of ECM by proliferating capillary endothelial cells. Similarly, maintenance of inflammation in the airways requires movement of leukocytes through the submucosa from postcapillary venules towards airway epithelia. GAGs could influence the movement of these cell types by interference with cell–matrix interaction, matrix effects on cytoskeletal organisation, and the activity of proteolytic enzymes in disruption of ECM and proteoglycans. Evidence for effects of GAGs on cell migration is provided by inhibition of vascular smooth muscle migration by heparin *in vitro*[50] and *in vivo*.[51,52]

HS proteoglycan accumulates at focal sties of attachment during migration. Close adhesive contacts formed during the initial stages of cell attachment during migration have been termed *reattachment substratum attached material* (R-SAM).[53,54] These are formed within 1 h, contain principally HS proteoglycan, and could signify dependency on HS proteoglycan and sensitivity to competition by free GAG, such as heparan sulphate or heparin. Examination of the effect of heparanase on fibroblast and endothelial cell reattachment suggests that HS proteoglycan is important at least in the initial attachment of cells, but loss of 85–90% of proteoglycans does not influence the maintenance of cell attachment.[55] The focal sites developed following initial cell attachment have been termed *long-term substratum attached material* (L-SAM) and contain increased chondroitin sulphate and hyaluronic acid and less heparan sulphate.[53] The reduction in HS proteoglycan content could reflect the independence of prolonged attachment on HS proteoglycan. Inhibition of migration by heparin appears more likely, therefore, to influence early attachment through R-SAM than through L-SAM.

## C. CYTOSKELETAL ORGANISATION

In addition to direct extracellular charge–based interference, GAG manipulation of intracellular pathways could contribute to GAG effects on cell attachment. The ECM communicates with the cell cytoplasm through interaction with cell surface integrins.[56] Interaction between integrins and the ECM relies upon the presence of an Arg-Gly-Asp (RGD) sequence in the ECM component and a proteoglycan-binding site (often HS proteoglycan or CS proteoglycan) within the ECM.[57] HS proteoglycan, while forming attachment sites, may also contribute to organisation of cell cytoskeleton during changes in cell shape following attachment.[58] This is evident from the influence of HS proteoglycan on cytoskeletal organisation.[58-61] GAG interference with HS proteoglycan–ECM interaction may therefore affect substratum–cell cytoskeletal communication through competition with HS proteoglycan in addition to or independent of effects on cell attachment. Not discussed here, but certainly of importance in this context, is the potential effect of GAGs on cell surface signalling involving PLC activation and $Ca^{2+}$ mobilisation that are involved in signal transduction mediating responses to several classes of chemotactic agents.

## D. INHIBITION OF PROTEASE AND GLYCOSIDASE ACTIVITY

Collagenase, elastase, and glycosidase are active in cell migration and tissue remodelling, and GAGs are involved in regulation of these enzymes. Inhibition of smooth muscle interstitial collagenase expression by heparin appears to involve interference with a PKC-dependent pathway.[62-64] This is not necessarily the case with inflammatory cells in which heparin has been found to increase collagenase expression.[65,66] Heparin is also a potent inhibitor of neutrophil elastase activity,[67-69] particularly important in regulation of leukocyte migration and the removal of cell surface proteoglycans by leukocytes. Within this context, removal of anionic charge (probably heparan sulphate) is observed at intestinal inflammatory sites, and GAG loss under these conditions possibly facilitates cell infiltration.[70] Migration and loss of anionic charge through disruption of GAG are also assisted by glycosidases.[22,71] Heparin is a direct competitive substrate for glycosidases[72] and inhibits heparanase expression in lymphocytes, albeit at a narrow and relatively low concentration range.[73] Removal of heparan sulphate from HS proteoglycan by glycosidases or the core protein of proteoglycans by proteases and phospholipases may affect not only cell migration and inflammatory cell infiltration, but also communication between intercalated HS proteoglycan and cell cytoskeletal activity (see Figure 2). Effects of GAG on cell attachment and migration therefore appear to be a complex of direct competition among HS proteoglycan, heparin, and free heparan sulphate for attachment sites and the integration of these interactions with events involving serine protease and glycosidases.

## V. GLYCOSAMINOGLYCAN EFFECTS ON MUSCLE AND ENDOTHELIAL CELL DIVISION

Changes in smooth muscle and endothelial cell function are involved in increased airway smooth muscle mass in asthma. These cell types are under facilitatory and inhibitor influences of endogenous GAGs. Antiproliferative activity of GAGs against smooth muscle appears to be exerted intracellulary,[25] while effects in endothelial cells are mediated by facilitation of heparin-binding factors such as fibroblast growth factor (FGF).[126] Both endothelial and smooth muscle cells secrete GAGs[74-69] and growth factors[80-82] that would be expected to influence division within endothelial and smooth muscle cell populations in the region of the submucosa. Both heparin and HS proteoglycan enhance FGF-induced endothelial cell mitogenesis (reviewed in Reference 7), while heparanase disrupts heparan sulphate–FGF complexes.[83] FGF stimulates endothelial production of tissue-plasminogen activator (t-PA), resulting in plasmin generation, which through destruction of ECM assists endothelial cell migration.[84] In addition, FGF in association with heparin reduces plasminogen activator inhibition (PAI-1).[85,86] Proteolysis-insensitive HS proteoglycan–FGF complexes are released by plasmin, thereby further facilitating plasmin generation and endothelial migration. These processes could contribute to the angiogenesis associated with airway wall thickening in asthma.[87,88] This proliferative action of GAGs in endothelial cells demonstrates the cell specificity of GAG action, since GAGs have been consistently found to inhibit smooth muscle proliferation.

The extent of smooth muscle proliferation in asthmatic airways appears to be slow, since the mass of smooth muscle tissue increases by a factor of twofold to threefold over decades,[89] and, therefore, on average cell division is achieved over years. Alternatively, more rapid airway smooth muscle cell proliferation could be localised to a small population of cells exhibiting a disproportionately high rate of turnover. Histochemical evidence does not support the latter case,[89] and the condition of airway smooth muscle cells in general in individuals with asthma could be considered relatively quiescent compared with the rapid rate of cell division in smooth muscle cells at subconfluence *in vitro* (division over 24–36 h) or following invasive procedures in arteries.

The rate of smooth muscle division is related to the degree of cell differentiation, which also affects the nature of protein synthesis and secretion from smooth muscle and the sensitivity to antiproliferative effects of GAGs.[25,90] Quiescent differentiated cells, termed *contractile,* express greater quantities of contractile proteins, including smooth muscle actin, and are more contractile *in vitro* (Figure 5). Dedifferentiated cells, termed *synthetic,* secrete larger quantities of growth factors and matrix proteins and are less responsive to contractile stimuli (reviewed in Reference 90). Cells in the synthetic state express increased α1 and α2 type I procollagen and increased α1 type III procollagen compared with the contractile state cells.[91,92] There is also an increase in chondroitin sulphate levels[93] that could contribute to the reduction in capacity of these cells to attach to fibronectin (see Section IV.A). Heparin redifferentiates synthetic state smooth muscle cells involving restoration of α-actin content and reduction in collagen synthesis[94-96] (see Figure 5). This is consistent with the inhibitory effect of heparin on collagen production *in vivo.* Thus, elevation of collagen and elastin levels in cells of repairing arteries following balloon catheterisation is lowered in heparin-treated animals.[97] Although heparin reduces the synthetic behaviour of smooth muscle through induction of differentiation, the effect on collagen expression has not always been consistent. In overconfluent smooth muscle cells, which attain high levels of differentiation, GAGs have altered the distribution of collagen between the different types, as opposed to total collagen content.[98] Heparin has also increased the expression of a 60,000-kDa collagen in vascular smooth muscle cells.[99]

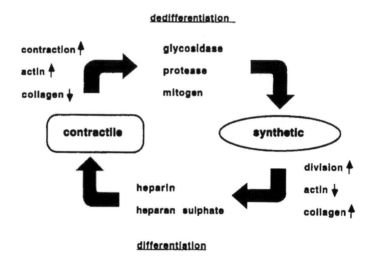

**FIGURE 5**   The balance between factors regulating smooth muscle differentiation and proliferation.

Differentiation can also be induced by heparin in cell populations with evolved insensitivity to the antiproliferative effects of heparin.[100] Inhibition of airway smooth muscle division by heparan sulphate has been observed without changes in phenotypic expression.[101] These findings suggest that differentiation and inhibition of cell division are not completely interdependent. The differential effects of heparan sulphate and chondroitin sulphates endorse the significance of changes in GAG content of matrix and cell proteoglycans during development.[14] An increase in HS proteoglycan content occurs with development to adult stage in rat airways,[14] and increased HS proteoglycan content could reflect a more differentiated state within tissues at advanced stages of development. This concept would be consistent with the reduced HS proteoglycan content of dedifferentiated smooth muscle cells and their increased mobility and propensity for division.[91-94]

The presence of other cell types, endothelial, fibroblastic, and inflammatory cells, further complicates the consequences of smooth muscle–GAG interaction. In an initial investigation of local regulation of airway smooth muscle cell proliferation, we have found that bovine airway smooth muscle explants maintained in culture release factors that both reduce and enhance high and low airway smooth muscle cell mitogenic responses, respectively.[102] Examination of antithrombin III–binding activity suggested that anticoagulant GAGs were absent from the smooth muscle explant-conditioned media. This excludes the possibility that anticoagulant heparin or related heparan sulphate was responsible for the inhibitory effect. The possibility remains that nonanticoagulant GAGs are released from the smooth muscle mass and that capillary endothelial cells within airway smooth muscle tissue are also a source of antiproliferative GAGs.

The antiproliferative activity of heparin against vascular smooth muscle is dependent upon both charge and chain length of the molecule without requiring the antithrombin III–binding site.[25,35] Hyaluronic acid, dermatan sulphate, protamine sulphate, and chondroitin sulphate do not inhibit VSMC division,[103,104] indicating that chain length, charge, and sulphation together are insufficient and specific distribution of charged groups is required for expression of antiproliferative activity. Tetrasaccharides generated from nitrous acid treatment of heparin are not antiproliferative,[35] but antiproliferative tetrasaccharides lacking the pentasaccharide antithrombin III–binding site can be released from endothelial cells.[105] This demonstrates the importance of uptake and subsequent secretion of modified GAGs and shows that observed antiproliferative effects of smooth muscle tissue-conditioned media[102] could be endothelial derived. The expansion of vascular and endothelial networks in asthmatic airways and potential reciprocal regulation between airway smooth muscle and endothelial cells warrant exploration.

# VI. MECHANISMS OF GLYCOSAMINOGLYCAN INHIBITION OF SMOOTH MUSCLE DIVISION

## A. INHIBITION AT PRE-S PHASE

Heparin inhibits vascular smooth muscle division if administered before S phase of the division cycle and before 18 h after carotid injury.[106-108] This reflects inhibition of smooth muscle division in G1 phase of the cell cycle.[30] In hepatocytes and smooth muscle cells there is a reduction in sulphate incorporation into GAG when the cells enter the mitotic phase and loss of heparan sulphate and HS proteoglycan from the cells.[109,110]

## B. INHIBITION OF PROTEIN KINASE C–DEPENDENT PATHWAYS

As described in Section III.C, heparin is an established inhibitor of $IP_3$-induced $Ca^{2+}$ mobilisation and indicates sensitivity of PLC-dependent pathways to inhibition by heparin. Activation of PKC is another consequence of PLC activation, and heparin inhibits mitogenesis stimulated by direct PKC activation.[111] Heparin reduces smooth muscle cell surface receptors for epidermal growth factor (EGF),[112] but vascular proliferative responses to EGF *in vitro* appear to be insensitive to heparin. This finding has been interpreted as demonstration of the selective inhibition of PKC-dependent division by heparin, since EGF-induced division does not require PKC activation.[113,114] Insensitivity of EGF-induced proliferation to heparin in bovine airway smooth muscle cells has also demonstrated, while mitogenic responses to serum and transforming growth factor beta (TGFβ) were significantly inhibited[102] (Figure 6).

## C. INHIBITION OF TRANSCRIPTION FACTORS

One potential mode of antiproliferative action of GAG is interruption of DNA binding by fos and jun families of transcription factors involved in

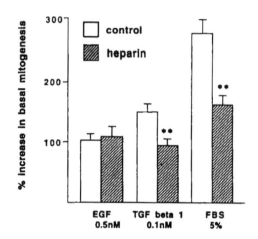

**FIGURE 6**   Effect of heparin on bovine airway smooth muscle division in response to fetal bovine serum (FBS), TGFβ1 (TGF beta 1), and EGF. **, P < 0.01 compared with control response.

proliferation. The DNA-binding domains of fos and jun both exhibit high affinity for heparin, and heparin inhibits fos and jun binding to DNA-promoter elements.[114,115] This would provide a route for inhibition of serum and phorbol ester-induced mitogenesis involving oncogene action in addition to inhibition of fos, myc, and myb oncoprotein expression[31-33] (see Figure 3). Interruption of signals mediated by PKC and its response element (AP-1) leading to expression of fos and jun could account for the relative selectivity for heparin for PKC-dependent mitogenic signalling in smooth muscle.

## D. INTERACTION WITH HEPARIN-BINDING GROWTH FACTORS

HS proteoglycan and heparin exhibit high affinity for certain growth factors (see Table 1) and thus influence their interaction with cell surface receptors and the ECM. These growth factors include: FGF, platelet-derived growth factor (PDGF), and heparin binding-epidermal growth factor (HB-EGF).[116-118] Heparan sulphate increases the affinity of basic FGF (bFGF) for its cell surface receptor, and this accounts for the necessity of HS proteoglycan for bFGF–receptor binding[119,120] (see Figure 4). A similar relationship exists among HS proteoglycan, HB-EGF, and its receptor.[121,122]

Reduction of heparin-binding growth factor (HBGF) storage at ECM HS proteoglycan can be achieved through direct competition with other GAGs or through the action of heparanase against HS proteoglycan.[123-126] This could provide a source of growth factor for cell surface receptors distant from an ECM storage site, but also reduce presentation of the growth factor to cell surface receptors adjacent to the ECM. The latter point is of particular relevance to endothelial cells, where heparin and HS proteoglycan facilitate mitogenic responses to FGF. Heparin inhibits formation of FGF–ECM complexes, but does not disrupt a preformed FGF–HS proteoglycan complex in ECM.[125,126] Therefore, GAGs are more likely to redirect HBGF as opposed to increase the free concentration through a releasing action.

Heparin inhibits exogenous FGF-induced vascular smooth muscle mitogenesis *in vivo*, suggesting that at least in the vasculature the balance of heparin activity towards FGF-induced mitogenesis is antiproliferative.[127] Therefore, the significance of displacement of HBGF from ECM HS proteoglycan by free GAG and potential elevation of free HBGF concentrations is unclear. Certainly, heparin can facilitate FGF–receptor mitogenic signals, but antimitogenic activity of heparin not involving binding of HBGF or manipulation of HBGF–receptor interaction is predominant in regulation of smooth muscle cell division. This is endorsed by the capacity of heparin to inhibit division following exposure of cells to PDGF and of serum to support division following removal of HBGFs.[128,129]

## E. INTERACTION BETWEEN GAG AND TGFβ

TGFβ provides a major contribution to tissue repair processes and could play a significant role in airway remodelling.[130] TGFβ is a potential regulator of smooth muscle division and ECM composition (reviewed in References 7 and 131). TGFβ stimulates both vascular[132,133] and airway smooth muscle division,[102] and upregulates HS proteoglycan. Upregulation of HS proteoglycan could contribute to the increase in binding of bFGF following exposure of smooth muscle cells to TGFβ.[137] TGFβ is carried by a α2-macroglobulin and displaced by heparin to increase free TGFβ levels.[134] The proteoglycan biglycan containing chondroitin and dermatan sulphate (Section II.B) is synthesised by interstitial fibroblasts and is present in ECM.[135,136] TGFβ increases biglycan expression in fibroblasts and epithelial cells,[137-139] and the ubiquitous distribution of TGFβ receptors suggests that induction of biglycan synthesis by TGFβ[137] could be widespread. Both biglycan and related decorin proteoglycans[140] bind and inactivate TGFβ activity.[141,142] The increased expression of the proteoglycans biglycan and decorin and the inhibitory effect of these proteoglycans on TGFβ binding suggest a major pathway for TGFβ regulation. Heparin inhibits TGFβ-induced airway smooth muscle division in a concentration-dependent fashion within the same concentration range required for inhibition of serum-induced division ($0.1–100$ μg/ml)[102] (see Figure 6). This could involve a direct effect of heparin on cellular responses to TGFβ, but equally possible is heparin inhibition of the mitogenic action of other growth factors, such as PDGF, that are induced by TGFβ.[81] TGFβ increases the chondroitin sulphate content of syndecan proteoglycan and, by reducing the heparan sulphate content, reduces the affinity for fibronectin.[49] This action would influence cell attachment mediated by syndecan interaction with ECM (see Section IV).

# VII. IMMUNE REGULATION BY GLYCOSAMINOGLYCANS

GAGs affect leukocyte function *in vitro* and demonstrate immunomodulation *in vivo*. Certain actions of heparin are mediated through direct effects of heparin at the cell surface or within cells, while others could be mediated through interaction with heparin-binding cytokines or inhibition of glycosidases and serine proteases.

## A. EFFECT OF GAG ON LEUKOCYTE ACTIVATION *IN VITRO*

### 1. GAG Inhibition of Mast Cells

The inhibitory effect of heparin on mast cell degranulation has been recognised for several decades and has been demonstrated against immunologic (anti-IgE) and nonimmunologic stimuli in circulating, peritoneal, and uterine mast cells.[143,144] This demonstrates the potential for negative feedback inhibition of mast cells and particularly connective tissue mast cells that release heparin. Heparin inhibition of serine proteases extends beyond facilitation of antithrombin III inhibition of thrombin. Thus, heparin inhibits human lung mast cell tryptase activity, in addition to inhibition of mast cell tryptase release.[145]

### 2. GAG Inhibition of Superoxide and Basic Proteins

Heparin and certain other related GAGs inhibit neutrophil superoxide release, and inhibition appears to be related to the nature of sulphation.[146,147] Effects of GAG on superoxide production from eosinophils, monocytes, and macrophages have not been investigated. Heparin binds superoxide dismutase (SOD),[148] which would facilitate location of SOD at proteoglycan-binding sites and provide a site for SOD removal. The dense GAG anionic charge provides a sink for eosinophil cationic proteins, including eosinophil cationic protein and major basic protein.[149] Neutralisation of these proteins by GAG released at inflammatory sites is relevant to the elevated eosinophil presence in the asthmatic airway.

### 3. GAG Effects on Lymphocyte Activation

Examination of GAG regulation of lymphocyte activation has concentrated on effects of heparan sulphate and heparin on lymphocyte mitogenesis and cytotoxicity. The effects on lymphocyte division differ between heparin and heparan sulphate and are dependent upon the conditions of assessment of lymphocyte division. In these aspects the effects of GAG on lymphocyte division differ considerably from the effects on smooth muscle and fibroblast division. Preincubation with heparin for 24 h inhibits lymphocyte mitogenesis in response to Con A and pokeweed mitogen conducted in a 5-day mixed lymphocyte reaction.[150,151] This inhibitory action is concentration dependent between 0.1 and 100 µg/ml and is not reproduced by either *N*-desulphated heparin or a sulphated disaccharide of heparin demonstrating minimum charge and chain length requirements (Kilfeather, unpublished observations). The inhibitory effect is reproduced by peritoneal mast cell–derived granules and, therefore, provides indication that mast cell–derived products, particularly heparin, can exhibit an antiproliferative effect against lymphocytes. In mixed lymphocyte reactions conducted over 2 days, however, heparin at 10–100 µg/ml markedly increases lymphocyte division, while heparin at 0.01 µg/ml is inhibitory. The latter effects observed during 2-day reactions do not require 24-h preincubation and, together with effects observed in 5-day reactions, are not reproduced by heparan sulphate.[152]

The facilitation of murine[153] and human lymphocyte[151] mitogenesis by heparan sulphate is dependent upon the duration of exposure and appears to be related to the balance of facilitatory effects of heparan sulphate on monocyte-derived IL-1 and prostaglandin.[153-154] The facilitatory effect of heparan sulphate on mitogenesis extends to T cell cytotoxicity with similar involvement of IL-1, while heparin under similar conditions is without effect on lymphocyte cytotoxicity.[155]

These findings raise the question of which GAG and conditions predominate *in vivo* in regulation of lymphocyte mitogenesis. In most tissues, ECM and basement membrane proteoglycan are the major sources of GAG. During inflammatory reactions free heparan sulphate is released from HS proteoglycan under the action of glycosidases secreted from activated circulating leukocytes including T-lymphocytes.[156-159] Where connective tissue mast cells are present, a balance of heparin and heparan sulphate–derived effects on lymphocyte proliferation would prevail. Additional factors in this balance include the inhibitory effect of heparin on glycosidase-mediated release of free heparan sulphate,[37-39,160-161] the potential for cells to endocytose and release modified forms of GAG, and the variation in time and concentration of exposure to differing GAGs.

## 4. GAG Effects on Macrophage Function

Macrophages comprise approximately 80% of cells resident in the airway lumen, but little examination of effects of GAG on macrophage function has been conducted. Heparan sulphate, at least, influences the production of IL-1 and prostaglandin $E_2$ from monocytic cells.[153-154] Macrophages provide an efficient route for removal of free GAG and those bound to eosinophil-derived basic proteins.[162]

## 5. GAG Effects on Endothelial Adhesion

The initial stages of cell adhesion involve deceleration of leukocytes rolling across adhesive molecules on the endothelial surface. This is followed by tighter adhesion preceding migration of leukocytes through the endothelial barrier.[163] Heparin-related GAGs inhibit leukocyte migration from the vasculature to inflammatory sites, and this appears to involve effects of GAG on leukocyte adhesion to the endothelium.[164-170] Heparin increases lymphocytes in the circulation consistent with inhibition of lymphocyte trafficking.[171] With relevance to airways and development of asthma, inhibition of allergen-induced eosinophil accumulation has been observed in the airways by exogenous administration of heparin.[172] Inhibition of allergen-induced eosinophil accumulation in the skin has also been observed, demonstrating a possibly generalised effect of heparin against eosinophil accumulation.[173]

Initial interaction between leukocytes and endothelium is mediated by cell surface lectin receptor (selectin)–carbohydrate interactions. Of the three selectins involved in cell adhesion (L, leukocyte, P and E, endothelial), L- and P-selectins are bound by heparin.[174-175] Anionic charge appears to be a requirement of P-selectin–binding sites, and this is consistent with the presence of a sulphated GAG-binding site present on neutrophils that binds P-selectin.[174] Pulmonary artery endothelial cells express a heparan sulphate proteoglycan that interacts with L-selectin.[175] Furthermore, heparin derivatives inhibit neutrophil migration dependent upon L- and P-selectin.[167]

Inhibition of leukocyte adhesion by GAG is dependent upon sulphation,[168-169,176] reflecting the requirement for anionic charge in selectin binding and providing further indication of competition between anionic charge of exogenous and endogenous GAG chains. Anionic charge is insufficient, however, since specific orientation of sulphation is required for inhibition of adhesive processes and linear-charged polymers, such as polyglutamic acid, are ineffective.

Effects of heparin on adhesive processes reliant upon β2-integrin molecules are less well understood. The integrins include Mac-1, LFA-1, p150.95, and VLA4 and are involved in generation of tighter binding of cells to the endothelial surface. Expression of integrins is stimulated by cytokines, many of which are heparin binding and can therefore be presented by attachment to endothelial surface HS proteoglycan to leukocytes already rolling under selectin-dependent adhesion. Several chemokine cytokines exhibit high affinity for heparin (see Table 1). Chemokines, including MIP-1β,[165] IL-8,[166] and RANTES,[176] activating lymphocytes, neutrophils, and eosinophils, respectively, bind to endothelial HS proteoglycan. The capacity for free GAG to interfere directly with integrin-mediated adhesion has not been demonstrated so far, but interference with accumulation of proadhesive cytokines at cell surface HS proteoglycan is a possibility.

## B. EFFECTS OF GLYCOSAMINOGLYCANS ON INFLAMMATORY RESPONSE *IN VIVO*

Examination of GAG effects on inflammation *in vivo* has been dominated by examination of effects of exogenously administered heparin. Specific examples *in vivo* include inhibition of delayed-type hypersensitivity (DTH) in the skin, bronchoconstriction in asthmatic individuals and allo- and xenograft rejection.

## 1. Effect of Heparin on Delayed-Type Hypersensitivity

The inhibitory effect of heparin against DTH observed in mice occurred at a dose of 5 mg/kg, but not 20 mg/kg.[177] Inhibition of DTH was also associated with inhibition of *ex vivo* T-lymphocyte heparanase release. A similar relationship between the narrow effective heparin-concentration range and inhibition of lymphocyte heparanase expression was observed *in vitro* in which heparin at 0.1 µg/ml, but not 0.001 or 10 µg/ml, was inhibitory.[178] Similarly, we have observed inhibition of lymphocyte division over a 2-day mixed lymphocytes reaction in the region of 0.001–0.01 µg/ml, but not at higher concentrations, when cells are exposed to a mitogenic stimulus and heparin simultaneously (see Section VII.A.3). The coincident fall in heparanase expression and reduction in DTH by heparin could be an indication of a role of heparanase in mediation of DTH. A clear example of the significant GAG loss that occurs during execution of inflammatory responses was provided by examination of GAG at intestinal inflammation sites.[70] From studies involving models of allograft and xenograft rejection, however, the pattern of GAG removal during reprofusion is indicative of the action of proteases prior to subsequent glycosidase reduction of free GAG.[17] The loss of inhibitory effect of heparin against DTH at higher concentrations indicates that direct antagonism of heparanase activity by substrate inhibition with heparin is not the only mechanism for inhibition of DTH, since inhibition through that route would be maintained at higher heparin concentrations.

## 2. Inhibition of Bronchoconstriction of Heparin

Investigation of the effects of heparin on bronchoconstriction will provide valuable information concerning the role of GAG in regulation of cells involved in airway inflammation and, therefore, the influence of GAG over the interaction between inflammatory response and airway remodelling. Inhalation of unfractionated heparin (1000 u/kg) has resulted in inhibition of airway responses to antigen challenge in certain studies in sensitised sheep[179] and asthmatic subjects[180] and in exercise-induced bronchoconstriction in asthmatic subjects.[181] Other studies in sensitised sheep and asthmatic subjects have shown no effect of inhalation of heparin (300–1000 u/kg) on either the early asthmatic response (EAR) or late asthmatic response (LAR) to allergen in sheep[182] and asthmatic subjects.[183-184] Pharmacodynamic studies have demonstrated that inhibition of airway responses to allergen by heparin are sensitive to dosage, timing, and route of administration.[179,180,185] Thus, inhibition of LAR in asthmatic subjects in one study was maintained during repeated administration of heparin 1000 u/kg, but LAR ensued within 1 h after cessation of heparin administration.[180]

The possible mechanisms of action involved in the observed inhibition of airway responses are difficult to estimate. Rapid inhibition of exercise-induced airway responses have been observed in individuals with asthma. Furthermore, inhibition by heparin of responses to antigen in sensitised sheep was reproduced with inhibitions of responses to the mast cell degranulating agent 48/80, but not to histamine or carbachol.[179] Heparin under these conditions is therefore not acting as a direct bronchodilator. Inhibition of mast cell degranulation[186] through inhibition of $IP_3$ activity is a possible contributory mechanism (Section III.C), although the current evidence does not support this mode of action as exclusive. EAR in response to allergen is considered dependent upon IgE-induced mast cell degranulation,[187] and significant inhibition of the LAR has been observed in the absence of a significant effect on EAR.[180] There is also the issue of access to mast cell cytoplasm following inhalation. The dense anionic charge and molecular size of heparin (approximately 12,000 kDa) would provide considerable restriction to passive movement across the epithelial barrier. The $t_{1/2}$ for uptake of heparin into epithelial cells has been estimated at approximately 60 min,[188] and significant inhibitory effects of heparin against mast cell release *in vitro* at 20–40 u/ml require approximately 20-min preincubation with optimum inhibition being attained at 60 min.[185] Therefore, estimation of the concentration of heparin attained in the subepithelial region at approximately 45 min following heparin inhalation is required to predict the relative contribution of inhibition of mast cell degranulation. In view of the rapid and marked inhibition of exercise-induced bronchoconstriction by inhaled heparin,[181] involvement of heparin inhibition of neuronal pathways should be considered in addition to other cell types.

There is considerable evidence supporting the role of infiltrating immunocompetent cells in mediation of LAR in response to allergen, which occurs several hours after antigen challenge. Inhibition of cell infiltration, migration, and subsequent inflammatory responses of both infiltrating and resident inflammatory cells could therefore provide additional routes for heparin activity following inhalation, particularly in reduction of the LAR. In this context, inhaled heparin has been found to inhibit eosinophil recruitment into nasal passages following antigen challenge in subjects with allergic rhinitis[189] and into guinea pig airways 24 h after heparin inhalation and allergen challenge.[190]

## VIII. INTEGRATION OF INFLAMMATORY CELL BEHAVIOUR AND AIRWAY REMODELLING

Persistent inflammatory cell activity within the submucosa and associated glycosidase and protease release could undermine heparan sulphate in that region. The HS proteoglycan-degrading actions of these enzymes release smooth muscle cells from their differentiated contractile state towards dedifferentiated synthetic and proliferative states.[24] On the other hand, heparin released from mast cells inhibits smooth muscle and fibroblast division and matrix protein secretion.[25] Heparin also provides negative feedback against mast cell degranulation[186] and direct inhibition of protease and glycosidase. Leukocytes involved with airway inflammation, including eosinophils, release an array of mediators that interact with GAGs and influence fibroblast and airway smooth muscle proliferation and protein secretion. These include PDGF,[191-193] EGF,[102,194-196] TGFβ and α,[102,197-200] and IL-1.[201] The relationship between leukocyte release of these growth factors and airway remodelling is not immediately apparent, since increased expression of TGFβ and PDGF have not been observed in asthmatic airways.[192,193,197]

The high content of HS proteoglycan in basement membranes of both airway and alveolar epithelia[14] suggests that HS proteoglycan could influence basement membrane composition, epithelial activity and communication, and cell migration between the submucosa and airway lumen. Release of heparin from mast cells and liberation of free heparan sulphate in the region of the epithelium during inflammation could influence remodelling of the basement membrane reticular layer in asthma. However, the increases in reticular layer thickness without increase in epithelial basement membrane do not suggest a universal disinhibition of collagen synthesis in this region.

## IX. CONCLUSION

The heparin and heparan sulphate GAGs influence the development of airway inflammatory responses and airway remodelling. GAGs exert effects on cell division, secretion, and migration and provide competitive inhibition of proteases and glycosidases for which they are substrates. They exhibit specificity and high affinity for a range of ECM proteins and cytokines, demonstrating that arrangement of charge substitutions in addition to high charge density is an important component of their activity. Through ubiquitous distribution and both extracellular and intracellular actions, GAGs have the potential to influence most cells involved in airway inflammation and remodelling. The observed effects of GAG on inflammatory and mitogenic processes and wide range of permutations in GAG structure suggest that development of compounds with specificity for certain cell functions could provide routes for therapeutic intervention. Further investigation of factors influencing GAG distribution in the airways is required to elucidate their role in regulation of inflammatory processes and remodelling.

## REFERENCES

1. Dunnill, M. S., Masarella, G. R., and Anderson, J. A., A comparison of the quantitative anatomy of the bronchi in normal subjects, in status asthmaticus, in chronic bronchitis, and in emphysema, *Thorax*, 24, 176, 1969.
2. Hossain, S., Quantitative measurement of bronchial muscle in men with asthma, *Am. Rev. Resp. Dis.*, 107, 99, 1973.
3. Ebina, M., Takahashi, T., Chiba, R., and Mitomya, M., Hyperactive site of the airway tract of asthmatic patients revealed by thickening of bronchial muscles: a morphological study. *Am. Rev. Resp. Dis.*, 141, 1327, 1990.
4. Laitinen, A., Laitinen, L. A., Vascular beds in the airways of normal subjects and asthmatics, *Eur. Respir. J. Suppl.*, 12, 658s, 1990.

5. Messer, J., Peters, G. A., and Bennet, W. A., Cause of death and pathological findings in 304 cases of bronchial asthma, *Dis. Chest*, 13, 27, 1960.
6. Roche, W. R., Williams, J. H., Beasley, R., and Holgate, S. T., Subepithelial fibrosis in the bronchi of asthmatics, *Lancet*, 1, 520, 1989.
7. Jackson, R. L., Busch, S. J., and Cardin, A. D., Glycosaminoglycans: molecular properties, protein interactions, and role in physiological processes, *Physiol. Rev.*, 71, 481, 1991.
8. Tyrrell, D. J., Kilfeather, S., and Page, C. P., Therapeutic uses of heparin beyond its traditional role as an anticoagulant, *Trends Pharmacol. Sci.*, 16, 198, 1995.
9. Lindahl, U., Lidholt, K., Spillmann, D., and Kjellen, L., More to "heparin" than anticoagulation, *Thromb. Res.*, 75, 1, 1994.
10. Fransson, L.-A., Structure and function of cell-associated proteoglycans, *Trends Biochem. Sci.*, 12, 406, 1987.
11. Gallagher, J. T., Lyon, M., and Steward, W. P., Structure and function of heparan sulphate proteoglycans, *Biochem. J.*, 236, 313, 1986.
12. Poole, A. R., Proteoglycans in health and disease: structures and functions, *Biochem. J.*, 236, 1, 1986.
13. Green, W. F., Konnaris, K., and Woolcock, A. J., Effect of salbutamol, fenoterol and sodium chromoglycate on the release of heparin from sensitized human lung fragments challenged with dermatophagoites pteronyssinus antigen, *Am. J. Resp. Cell Mol. Biol.*, 8, 518, 1993.
14. Sannes, P. L., Burch, K. K., Khosla, J., McCarthy, K. J., and Couchman, J. R., Immunohistochemical localization of chondroitin sulfate, chondroitin sulfate proteoglycan, heparan sulfate proteoglycan, entactin, and laminin in basement membranes of postnatal developing and adult rat lungs, *Am. J. Respir. Cell Mol. Biol.*, 8, 245, 1993.
15. Sannes, P. L., Cytochemistry and immunocytochemistry of basement membranes and other extracellular matrices, in *A Comprehensive Treatise on Pulmonary Toxicology: Vol. I. Comparative Pulmonary Biology of the Normal Lung*, Parent, R., Ed., Telford Press, Caldwell, NJ, 1992, 129.
16. Laurie, G., Leblond, C. P., and Martin, G. R., Light microscopic immunolocalization of type IV collagen, laminin, heparan sulphate proteoglycan, and fibronectin in basement membranes of a variety of rat organs, *Am. J. Anat.*, 167, 71, 1983.
17. Ihrcke, N. S., Wrenshall, L. E., Lindman, B. J., and Platt, J. L., Role of heparan sulphate in immune system-blood vessel interactions, *Immunol. Today*, 14, 500, 1993.
18. Key, N. S., Platt, J. H., and Vercellotti, G. M., Vascular endothelial cell proteoglycans are susceptible to cleavage by neutrophils, *Arterioscler. Thromb.*, 12, 836, 1992.
19. Carey, D. J. and Evans, D. M., Membrane anchoring of heparan sulphate proteoglycans by phosphatidylinositol and kinetics of synthesis of peripheral and detergent-solubilized proteoglycans in Schwann cells, *J. Cell Biol.*, 108, 1891, 1989.
20. Ishihara, M., Fedarko, N. S., and Conrad, H. E., Correlations between heparan sulphate metabolism and hepatoma growth, *J. Cell. Physiol.*, 138, 467, 1989.
21. Low, M. G., Glycosyl-phosphatidylinositol: a versatile anchor for cell surface proteins, *FASEB J.*, 3, 1600, 1989.
22. Vlodavsky, I., Eldor, A., Haimovitz-Fiedman, A., Matzner, Y., Ishai-Michaeli, R., Lider, O., Naperstek, Y., Cohen, I. R., and Fuks, Z., Expression of heparanase by platelets and circulating cells of the immune system: possible involvement in diapedesis and extravasation, *Invasion Metastasis*, 122, 112, 1992.
23. Oldberg, A., Heldin, C., Wasteson, A., Busch, C., and Hook, M., Characterization of a platelet endoglycosidase degrading heparin-like polysaccharides, *Biochemistry*, 19, 5755, 1980.
24. Campbell, J. H., Rennick, R. E., Kalevitch, S. G., and Campbell, G. R., Heparan sulphate-degrading enzymes induce modulation of smooth muscle phenotype, *Exp. Cell. Res.*, 200, 156, 1992.
25. Karnovsky, M. J. and Edelman, E. R., Heparin/heparan sulphate regulation of vascular smooth muscle behaviour, in *Airways and Vascular Remodelling in Asthma and Cardiovascular Disease — Implications for Therapeutic Intervention*, Black, J. and Page, C. P., Eds., Academic Press, New York, 1994, 45.

26. Kilfeather, S. A., Tagoe, S., Perez, A. C., Okona-Mensah, K., Matin, R., and Page, C. P., Inhibition of serum-induced proliferation of bovine tracheal smooth muscle cells in culture by heparin and related glycosaminoglycans, *Br. J. Pharmacol.*, 114, 1442, 1995.

27. Castellot, J. J., Jr., Wong, K., Herman, B., Hoover, R. L., Albertini, D. F., Wright, T. C., Caleb, B. L., and Karnovsky, M. J., Binding and internalisation of heparin by vascular smooth muscle cells, *J. Cell. Physiol.*, 124, 13, 1985.

28. Ghosh, T. K., Eis, P. S., Mullaney, J. M., Ebert, C. L., Gill, D. L., Competitive, reversible and potent antagonism of inositol 1,4,5-triphosphate-activated calcium release by heparin, *J. Biol. Chem.*, 263, 11075, 1988.

29. Koboyashi, S., Kitazawa, T., Somlyo, A. V., and Somlyo, A. P., Cytosolic heparin inhibits muscarinic and $\alpha$-adrenergic $Ca^{2+}$ release in smooth muscle, *J. Biol. Chem.*, 264, 17997, 1989.

30. Reilly, C. F., Kindy, M. S., Brown, K. E., Rosenberg, R. D., and Sonenshein, G. E., Heparin prevents vascular smooth muscle cell progression through the $G_1$ phase of the cell cycle, *J. Biol. Chem.*, 264, 6990, 1989.

31. Wright, T. C., Pukac, L. A., Castellot, J. J., Karnovsky, M. J., Levine, R. A., Kim-Park, G. H., and Campisi, J., Heparin suppresses the induction of c-fos and c-myc mRNA in murine fibroblasts by selective inhibition of a protein kinase C-dependent pathway, *Proc. Natl. Acad. Sci. U.S.A.*, 86, 3199, 1989.

32. Pukac, L. a., Castellot, J. J., Wright, T. C., Caleb, B. L., and Karnovsky, M., Heparin inhibits c-fos and c-myc mRNA expression in vascular smooth muscle cells, *Cell Regul.*, 1, 435, 1990.

33. Busch, S. L., Martin, G. A., Barnhart, R. L., Mano, M., and Cardin, A. D., Trans-repressor activity of nuclear glycosaminoglycans on fos and jun/AP-1 oncoprotein-mediated transcription, *J. Cell Biol.*, 116, 31, 1992.

34. Zaragosza, R., Stebel, F., and Owen, N. E., Heparin inhibits Na(+)-H+ exchange in vascular smooth muscle cells, *J. Cell Biol.*, 105, 104a, 1987.

35. Wright, T. C., Jr., Castellot, J. J., Jr., Petitou, M., Lormeau, J.-C., Chaoay, J., and Karnovsky, M. J., Structural determinants of heparin's growth inhibitory activity. Interdependence of oligosaccharide size and charge, *J. Biol. Chem.*, 264, 1534, 1989.

36. Bar-ner, M., Eldor, A., Wasserman, L., Matzner, Y., Cohen, I. R., Fuks, Z., and Vlodavsky, I., Inhibition of heparanase-mediated degredation of extracellular matrix heparan sulphate by non-anticoagulant heparin species, *Blood*, 70, 551, 1987.

37. Nakajima, M., Irimura, T., and Nicholson, G. L., Heparanses and tumor metastasis, *J. Cell Biochem.*, 36, 157, 1988.

38. Parish, C. R., Coombe, D. R., Jakobsen, K. B., Bennet, F. A., and Underwood, P. A., Evidence that sulphated polysaccharides inhibit tumour metastasis by blocking tumour cell-derived heparanases, *Int. J. Cancer*, 40, 511, 1987.

39. Skubitz, A. P., McCarthy, J. B., Charonis, A. S., and Furcht, L. T., Localization of three distinct heparin-binding domains of laminin by monoclonal antibodies, *J. Biol. Chem.*, 263, 4861, 1988.

40. Yabkowitz, R., Iowe, J. B., and Dixit, V. M., Expression and initial characterisation of a recombinant human thrombospondin heparin binding domain, *J. Biol. Chem.*, 264, 10888, 1989.

41. Stamatoglou, S. C. and Keller, J. M., Interactions of cellular glycosaminoglycans with plasma fibronectin and collagen, *Biochim. Biophys. Acta*, 719, 90, 1982.

42. Koda, J. E. and Bernfield, M., Heparan sulfate proteoglycans from mouse mammary epithelial cells. Basal extracellular proteoglycan binds specifically to native type I collagen fibrils, *J. Biol. Chem.*, 259, 11763, 1984.

43. Keller, K. M., Keller, J. M., and Kuhn, K., The C-terminus of type I collagen is a major binding site for heparin, *Biochem. Biophys. Acta*, 882, 1, 1986.

44. LeBaron, R. G., Hook, A., Esko, J. D., Gay, S., and Hook, M., Binding of heparan sulphate to type V collagen. A mechanism of cell substrate adhesion, *J. Biol. Chem.*, 264, 7950, 1989.

45. San Antonio, J. D., Lander, A. D., Wright, T. C., and Karnovsky, M. J., Heparin inhibits the attachment and growth of Balb/c-3T3 fibroblasts on collagen substrata, *J. Cell. Physiol.*, 150, 8, 1992.
46. Preissner, K. T. and Muller-Berghaus, G., Neutralisation and binding of heparin by S protein/vitronectin in the inhibition of factor Xa by antithrombin III, *J. Biol. Chem.*, 262, 12247, 1987.
47. Skorstengaard, K., Jensen, M. S., Petersen, T. E., and Magnusson, S., Purification and complete primary structures of the heparin, cell and DNA binding domains of bovine plasma fibronectin, *Eur. J. Biochem.*, 154, 15, 1986.
48. Yamagata, M., Susuki, S., Akiyama, S. K., Yamada, K. M., and Kimata, K., Regulation of cell-substrate adhesion by proteoglycans immobilised on extracellular substrates, *J. Biol. Chem.*, 264, 8012, 1989.
49. Rapraeger, A., Transforming growth factor (type β) promotes the addition of chondroitin sulphate chains to the cell surface proteoglycan (syndecan) of mouse mammary epithelia, *J. Cell Biol.*, 109, 2509, 1989.
50. Kleinman, H. K., Hewitt, A. T., Murray, J. C., Liotta, L. A., Rennard, S. I., Pennypacker, J. P., McGoodwin, E. B., Martin, G. R., and Fishman, P. H., Cellular and metabolic specificity in the interaction of adhesion proteins with collagen and with cells, *J. Supramol. Struct.*, 11, 69, 1979.
51. Majack, R. A. and Clowes, A. W., Inhibition of vascular smooth muscle migration by heparin-like glycosaminoglycans, *J. Cell. Physiol.*, 118, 253, 1984.
52. Clowes, A. W. and Clowes, M. M., Kinetics of cellular proliferation after arterial injury. II. Inhibition of smooth muscle growth by heparin, *Lab. Invest.*, 52, 611, 1985.
53. Clowes, A. W. and Clowes, M. M., Kinetics of cellular proliferation after arterial injury. IV. Heparin inhibits rat smooth muscle mitogenesis and migration, *Circ. Res.*, 58, 839, 1986.
54. Rollins, B. J. and Culp, L. A., Preliminary characterization of the proteoglycans in the substrate adhesion sites of normal and virus-transformed murine cells, *Biochemistry*, 18, 141, 1979.
55. Lark, M. W. and Culp, L. A., modification of proteoglycans during maturation of fibroblast substratum adhesion sites, *Biochemistry*, 22, 2289, 1983.
56. Gill, P. J., Silbert, C. K., and Silbert, J. E., Effects of heparan sulphate removal on attachment and reattachment of fibroblasts and endothelial cells, *Biochemistry*, 25, 405, 1986.
57. Hynes, R. O., Integrins: a family of cell surface receptors, *Cell*, 48, 549, 1987.
58. Ruoslahti, E. and Pierschbacher, M. D., New perspectives in cell adhesion: RGD and integrins, *Science*, 238, 491, 1987.
59. Laterra, J., Silbert, J. E., and Culp, L. A., Cell surface heparan sulfate mediates some adhesive responses to glycosaminoglycan-binding matrices, including fibronectin, *Cell Biol.*, 96, 112, 1983.
60. Lark, M. W. and Culp, L. A., Matrix interactions of cell surface proteoglycans, in *Diseases of Connective Tissue: Pathology of the Extracellular Matrix*, Uitto, J. and Perejda, A., Eds., Marcel Dekker, New York, 1985.
61. Rapraeger, A. and Bernfield, M., in *Extracellular Matrix*, Hawkes, S. and Wang, J. L., Eds., Academic Press, New York, 1982, 265.
62. Au, Y. P., Montgomery, K. F., and Clowes, A. W., Heparin inhibits collagenase gene expression mediated by phorbol ester-responsive element in primate arterial smooth muscle cells, *Circ. Res.*, 70(5), 1062, 1992.
63. Au, Y. P., Kenagy, R. D., Clowes, M. M., and Clowes, A. W., Mechanisms of inhibition by heparin of vascular smooth muscle cell proliferation and migration, *Haemostasis*, 23 (Suppl. 1), 177, 1993.
64. Kenagy, R. D., Nikkari, S. T., Welgus, H. G., and Clowes, A. W., Heparin inhibits the induction of three matrix metalloproteinases (stromelysin, 92-kD gelatinase, and collagenase) in primate arterial smooth muscle cells, *J. Clin. Invest.*, 93(5), 1987, 1994.

65. Yoffe, J. R., Taylor, D. J., and Woolley, D. E., Mast-cell products and heparin stimulate the production of mononuclear-cell factor by cultured human monocyte/macrophages, *Biochem. J.*, 230(1), 83, 1985.

66. Hoffe, J. R., Taylor, D. J., and Wooley, D. E., Mast cell products stimulate collagenase and prostaglandin E production by cultures of adherent rheumatoid synovial cells, *Biochem. Biophys. Res. Commun.*, 122(1), 270, 1984.

67. Redini, F., Lafuma, C., Hornebeck, W., Choay, J., and Robert, L., Influence of heparin fragments on the biological activities of elastase(s) and alpha 1 proteinase inhibitor, *Biochem. Pharmacol.*, 37(22), 4257, 1988.

68. Redini, F., Tixier, J. M., Petitou, M., Choay, J., and Robert, L., Inhibition of leukocyte elastase by heparin and its derivatives, *Biochem. J.*, 252(92), 515, 1988.

69. Walsh, R. L., Dillon, T. J., Scicchitano, R., and McLennan, G., Heparin and heparan sulphate are inhibitors of human leukocyte elastase, *Clin. Sci. Colch.*, 81(3), 341, 1991.

70. Murch, S. H., MacDonald, T. T., Walker-Smith, J. A., Levin, M., Lionetti, P., and Klein, N. J., Disruption of sulphated glycosaminoglycans in intestinal inflammation, *Lancet*, 341(8847), 711, 1993.

71. Lider, O., Baharav, E., Mekori, Y. A., Miller, T., Naparstek, Y., Vlodavsky, I., and Cohen, I. R., Suppression of experimental autoimmune disease and prolongation of allograft survival by treatment of animals with low doses of heparins, *J. Clin. Invest.*, 83(3), 752, 1989.

72. Bitan, M., Mohsen M., Levi, E., Wygoda, M. R., Miao, H. Q., Lider, O., Svahn, C. M., Ekre, H. P., Ishai-Michaeli, R., Bar-Shavit, R., et al., Structural requirements for inhibition of melanoma lung colonization by heparanase inhibiting species of heparin, *Isr. J. Med. Sci.*, 31(2–3), 106, 1995.

73. Lider, O., Mekori, Y. A., Miller, T., Bar-Tana, R., Vlodavsky, I., Baharav, E., Cohen, I. R., and Naparstek, Y., Inhibition of T lymphocyte heparanase by heparin prevents T cell migration and T cell-mediated immunity, *Eur. J. Immunol.*, 20(3), 493, 1990.

74. Castellot, J. J., Jr., Addonizio, M. L., Rosenberg, R., and Karnovsky, M. J., Cultured endothelial cells produce a heparin-like inhibitor of smooth muscle cell growth, *J. Cell Biol.*, 90, 372, 1981.

75. Hamati, H. F., Britton, E. L., and Carey, D. J., Inhibition of proteoglycan synthesis alters extracellular matrix deposition, proliferation, and cytoskeletal organisation of rat aortic smooth muscle cells in culture, *J. Cell Biol.*, 108, 2495, 1989.

76. Kinsella, M. G. and Wight, T. N., Modulation of sulfated proteoglycan synthesis by bovine aortic endothelial cells during migration, *J. Cell Biol.*, 1032, 679, 1986.

77. Saku, T. and Futhmayr, H., Characterisation of the major heparan sulfate proteoglycan secreted by bovine aortic endothelial cells in culture. Homology to the large molecular weight molecule of basement membranes, *J. Biol. Chem.*, 264, 3514, 1989.

78. Schmidt, A. and Buddecke, E., Bovine arterial smooth muscle cells synthesise two functionally different proteoheparan sulfate species, *Exp. Cell Res.*, 189, 269, 1990.

79. Tan, E. M. L., Levine, E., Sorger, T., and Unger, G. A., Heparin and endothelial cell growth factor modulate collagen and proteoglycan production in human smooth muscle cells, *Biochem. Biophys. Res. Commun.*, 163, 84, 1990.

80. Gibbons, G. H., Pratt, R. E., and Dzau, V. J., Vascular smooth muscle cell hypertrophy vs. hyperplasia: autocrine transforming growth factor β1 expression determines growth response to angiotensinII, *J. Clin. Invest.*, 90, 456, 1992.

81. Battegay, E. J., Raines, E. W., Seifert, R. A., Bowen-Pope, D. F., and Ross, R., TGFβ induces bimodal proliferation of connective tissue cells via control of an autocrine PDGF loop, *Cell*, 63, 515, 1990.

82. Rubanyi, G. M. and Parker-Botelho, L. H., Endothelins, *FASEB J.*, 5, 2713, 1991.

83. Vlodavsky, I., Michaeli, R. I., Bar-ner, M., Fridman, R., Horowitz, A. T., Fuks, Z., and Biran, S., Involvement of heparanase in tumor metastasis and angiogenesis, *Isr. J. Med. Sci.*, 24, 464–470, 1988.

84. Montesano, R., Vassalli, J. D., Baird, A., Guillemin, R., and Orci, L., Basic fibroblast growth factor induces angiogenesis in vitro, *Proc. Natl. Acad. Sci. U.S.A.,* 83(19), 7297, 1986.
85. Tsuboi, R., Sato, C., Kurita, Y., Ron, D., Rubin, J. S., Ogawa, H., Keratinocyte growth factor (FGF-7) stimulates migration and plasminogen activator activity of normal human keratinocytes, *J. Invest. Dermatol.,* 101(1), 49, 1993.
86. Konkle, B. A. and Ginsburg, D., The addition of endothelial cell growth factor and heparin to human umbilical vein endothelial cell cultures decreases plasminogen activator inhibitor-1 expression, *J. Clin. Invest.,* 82, 579, 1988.
87. Saksela, O., Moscateli, D., Sommer, A., and Rifkin, D. B., Endothelial cell-derived heparan sulfate binds basic fibroblast growth factor and protects it from proteolytic degradation, *J. Cell Biol.,* 17, 743, 1988.
88. Saksela, O. and Rifkin, D. B., Release of fibroblast growth factor-heparan sulfate complexes from endothelial cells by plasminogen activator-mediated proteolytic activity, *J. Cell Biol.,* 110, 767, 1990.
89. Ebina, M., Takahashi, T., Chiba, R., and Motomiya, M., Cellular hypertrophy and hyperplasia of airways smooth muscle underlying bronchial asthma, *Am. Rev. Respir. Dis.,* 148, 720, 1993.
90. Campbell, J. H. and Campbell, G. R., Vascular smooth muscle in culture and its relevance to the study of atherogenesis, in *Airways and Vascular Remodelling in Asthma and Cardiovascular Disease — Implications for Therapeutic Intervention,* Black, J. and Page, C. P., Eds., Academic Press, New York, 1994.
91. Campbell, G. R., Tachas, G., Cockerill, G., Campbell, J. H., Bateman, J. F., and Gabbiani, F., Messenger RNA expression by smooth muscle cells of different phenotype, in *Atherosclerosis VIII,* Grepaldi, G. et al., Eds., Elsevier, Amsterdam, 1989, 67.
92. Ang, A. H., Tachas, G., Campbell, J. H., Bateman, J. F., and Campbell, G. R., Collagen synthesis by cultured rabbit aortic smooth-muscle cells. Alteration with phenotype, *Biochem. J.,* 265(2), 461, 1990.
93. Merrilies, M. J., Campbell, J. H., Spandidis, E., and Campbell, G. R., Glycosaminoglycan synthesis by smooth muscle cells of differing phenotype and their response to endothelial cell conditioned medium, *Atherosclerosis,* 81, 245, 1990.
94. Chamley-Campbell, J. H. and Campbell, G. R., What controls smooth muscle phenotype? *Atherosclerosis,* 40, 347, 1981.
95. Clowes, A. W., Clowes, M. M., Kocher, O., Ropraz, P., Chaponnier, C., and Gabbiani, G., Arterial smooth muscle cells in vivo: relationship between actin isoform expression and mitogenesis and their modulation by heparin, *J. Cell Biol.,* 107, 1939, 1988.
96. Desmouliere, A., Rubbia-Brandt, L., and Gabbiani, G., Modulation of actin isoform expression in cultured arterial smooth muscle cells by heparin and culture conditions, *Atherosclerosis Thrombosis,* 11, 244, 1991.
97. Snow, A. D., Bolender, R. P., Wight, T. N., and Clowes, A. W., Heparin modulates the composition of the extracellular matrix domain surrounding arterial smooth muscle cells, *Am. J. Pathol.,* 137, 313, 1990.
98. Asselot-Chapel, C., Kern, P., and Labat, R. J., Biosynthesis of interstitial collagens and fibronectin by porcine aorta smooth muscle cells. Modulation by low-molecular-weight heparin fragments, *Biochim. Biophys. Acta,* 993(2–3), 240, 1989.
99. Majack, R. A. and Bornstein, P., Heparin regulates the collagen phenotype of vascular smooth muscle cells: induced synthesis of an Mr 60,000 collagen, *J. Cell Biol.,* 100(2), 613, 1985.
100. San-Antonio, J. D., Karnovsky, M. J., Ottlinger, M. E., Schillig, R., and Pukac, L. A., Isolation of heparin-insensitive aortic smooth muscle cells. Growth and differentiation, *Arterioscler. Thromb.,* 13, 748, 1993.
101. Halayko, A. J., Delacruz, R., and Stephens, N. L., Heparan sulphate inhibits proliferation of cultured airway smooth muscle cells but does not prevent phenotypic modulation, *Am. J. Respir. Crit. Care Med.,* 149(4), A300, 1994.

102. Kilfeather, S. A., Okona-Mensah, K. B., Tagoe, S., Costello, J., and Page, C., Stimulation of airway smooth muscle cell mitogenesis by transforming growth factor beta (TGFβ1) and inhibition by heparin and smooth muscle explant-conditioned media, *Eur. Respir. J.*, 8(S19), 547s, 1995.

103. Castellot, J. J., Jr., Beeler, D. L., Rosenberg, R. D., and Karnovsky, M. J., Structural determinants of the capacity of heparin to inhibit the proliferation of vascular smooth muscle cells, *J. Cell. Physiol.*, 120, 315, 1984.

104. Castellot, J. J., Jr., Choay, J., Lormeau, J.-C., Petitou, M., Sache, E., and Karnovsky, M. J., Structural determinants of the capacity of heparin to inhibit the proliferation of vascular smooth muscle cells. II. Evidence for a pentasaccharide sequence that contains a 3-0-sulfate group, *J. Cell Biol.*, 102, 1979, 1986.

105. Herbert, J.-M. and Maffrand, J.-P., Heparin interactions with cultured human vascular endothelial and smooth muscle cells: influence on vascular smooth muscle proliferation, *J. Biol. Chem.*, 138, 424, 1989.

106. Hoover, R. L., Rosenberg, R., Haering, W. A., and Karnovsky, M. J., Inhibition of rat arterial smooth muscle cell proliferation by heparin. II. In vitro studies, *Circ. Res.*, 47, 578, 1980.

107. Majewsky, M. W., Schwartz, S. M., Clowes, A. W., and Clowes, M. M., Heparin regulates smooth muscle S phase entry in the injured rat carotid artery, *Circ. Res.*, 61, 296, 1987.

108. Castellot, J. J., Jr., Hoover, R. L., Harper, P. A., and Karnovsky, M. J., Heparin and glomerular epithelial cell-secreted heparin-like species inhibit mesangial-cell proliferation, *Am. J. Pathol.*, 120, 427, 1985.

109. Fidarko, N. S., Ishihara, M., and Conrad, H. E., Control of cell division in hepatoma cells by exogenous heparan sulfate proteoglycan, *J. Cell. Physiol.*, 139, 287, 1989.

110. Breton, M., Berrou, E., Brahimi-Horn, M.-C., Devdon, E., and Picard, J., Synthesis of sulfated proteoglycans throughout the cell cycle in smooth muscle cells from pig aorta, *Exp. Cell Res.*, 166, 416, 1986.

111. Wright, T. C., Pukac, L. A., Castellot, J. J., Karnovsky, M. J., Levine, R. A., Kim-Park, G. H., and Capisi, J., Heparin suppresses the induction of c-fos and c-myc mRNA in murine fibroblasts by selective inhibition of a protein kinase C-dependent pathway, *Proc. Natl. Acad. Sci. U.S.A.*, 86, 3199, 1989.

112. Reilly, C. F., Fritze, L. M. S., and Rosenberg, R. D., Heparin-like molecules regulate the number of epidermal growth factor receptors on vascular smooth muscle cells, *J. Cell. Physiol.*, 136, 23, 1988.

113. Pukac, L. A., Hirsch, G. M., Lormeau, J.-C., Petitou, M., Chaoy, J., and Karnovsky, M. J., Antiproliferative effects of novel, nonanticoagulant heparin derivatives on vascular smooth muscle cells in vitro and in vivo, *Am. J. Pathol.*, 139, 1501, 1991.

114. Pukac, L. A., Ottlinger, M. E., and Karnovsky, M. J., Heparin suppresses specific second messenger pathways for protooncogene expression in rat vascular smooth muscle cells, *J. Biol. Chem.*, 267, 3707, 1992.

115. Busch, S. J., Jackson, R. L., and Sassone-Corsi, P., Heparin inhibits transcriptional activation by fos and jun oncoproteins, *Trans. Assoc. Am. Physicians*, 103, 21, 1990.

116. Burgess, W. H. and Macaig, T., The heparin binding (fibroblast) growth factor family of proteins, *Annu. Rev. Biochem.*, 58, 575, 1989.

117. Klagsbrun, M. and Baird, A., A dual receptor system is required for basic fibroblast growth factor activity, *Cell*, 67, 229, 1991.

118. Ruoslahti, E. and Yamaguchi, Y., Proteoglycans as modulators of growth factor activities, *Cell*, 64, 867, 1991.

119. Yayon, A., Klagbrun, M., Esko, J. D., Leder, P., and Ornitz, D. M., An obligatory role for low affinity, heparin binding sites in basic fibroblast growth factor-receptor interactions (Abstract), *J. Cell Biol.*, 111, 137, 1990.

120. Nugent, M. A. and Edelman, E. R., Kinetics of basic fibroblast growth factor binding to its receptor and heparan sulfate proteoglycan: a mechanism for cooperactivity, *Biochemistry*, 31, 8876, 1992.

121. Aviezer, D. and Yayon, A., Heparin-dependent binding and autophosphorylation of epidermal growth factor (EGF) receptor by heparin-binding EGF-like growth factor but not by EGF, *Proc. Natl. Acad. Sci. U.S.A.*, 91, 12173, 1994.

122. Higashiyama, S., Abraham, J. A., and Klagsbrun, M., Heparin-binding EGF-like growth factor stimulation of smooth muscle cell migration: dependence on interactions with cell surface heparan sulfate, *J. Cell Biol.*, 122(4), 933, 1993.

123. Ishai-Michaeli, R., Eldor, A., and Vlodavsky, I., Heparanase activity expressed by platelets, neutrophils and lymphoma cells releases active fibroblast growth factor from extracellular matrix, *Cell Regul.*, 1, 833, 1990.

124. Bashkin, P., Doctrow, S., Klagsbrun, M., Svahn, C. M., Folkman, J., and Vlodavsky, I., Basic fibroblast growth factor binds to subendothelial extracellular matrix and is released by heparatinase and heparin-like molecules, *Biochemistry*, 28, 1737, 1989.

125. Presta, M., Maier, A. M., Rusnati, M., and Ragnotti, G., Basic fibroblast growth factor is released from endothelial extracellular matrix in a biologically active form, *J. Cell. Physiol.*, 140, 68, 1989.

126. Baird, A. and Ling, N., Fibroblast growth factors are present in the extracellular matrix produced by endothelial cells in vitro: implications for a role of heparinase-like enzymes in the neovascular response, *Biochem. Biophys. Res. Commun.*, 142, 428, 1987.

127. Edelman, E. R., Nugent, M. A., Smith, L. T., and Karnovsky, M. J., Basic fibroblast growth factor enhances the coupling of intimal hyperplasia and proliferation of vasa vasorum in injured rat arteries, *J. Clin. Invest.*, 89(2), 465, 1992.

128. Hoover, R. L., Rosenberg, R., Haering, W. A., and Karnovsky, M. J., Inhibition of rat arterial smooth muscle cell proliferation by heparin. II. In vitro studies, *Circ. Res.*, 47, 578, 1980.

129. Reily, C. F., Fritze, L. M. S., and Rosenberg, R. D., Heparin inhibition of smooth muscle cell proliferation: a cellular site of action, *J. Cell. Physiol.*, 129, 11, 1986.

130. Border, W. A. and Ruoslahti, E., Transforming growth factor-beta in disease: the dark side of tissue repair, *J. Clin. Invest.*, 90, 1, 1992.

131. Massaque, J., The transforming growth factor-β family, *Annu. Rev. Cell Biol.*, 6, 597, 1990.

132. Majack, R. A., Beta-type transforming growth factor specifies organisational behaviour in vascular smooth muscle cell cultures, *J. Cell Biol.*, 105, 465, 1987.

133. Assoian, R. K. and Sporn, M. B., Type β transforming growth factor in human platelets: release during platelet degranulation and action on vascular smooth muscle cells, *J. Cell Biol.*, 102, 1217, 1986.

134. McAffrey, T. A., Falcone, D. J., Brayton, C. F., Agarwal, L. A., Welt, F. G. P., and Weskler, B. B., Transforming growth factor-β activity is potentiated by heparin via dissociation of the transforming growth factor-β/$\alpha_2$ macroglobulin inactive complex, *J. Cell Biol.*, 109, 441, 1989.

135. Gallaher, J. T., The extended family of proteoglycans: social residents of the pericellular zone, *Curr. Opin. Cell Biol.*, 1, 1201, 1989.

136. Hardingham, T. and Fosang, A. J., Proteoglycans: many forms and many functions, *FASEB J.*, 6, 861, 1992.

137. Romaris, M., Heredia, A., Molist, A., Bassols, A., Differential effect of transforming growth factor-β on proteoglycan synthesis in human embryonic lung fibroblasts, *Biochim. Biophys. Acta*, 1093, 229, 1991.

138. Kahari, V. M., Larjava, H., and Uitto, J., Differential regulation of extracellular matrix proteoglycan gene expression, *J. Biol. Chem.*, 266, 10608, 1991.

139. Maniscalco, W. M. and Campbell, M. H., TGF-β1 increases specific proteoglycan synthesis by alveolar type II cells in vitro, *Am. Rev. Respir. Dis.*, 147, A759, 1993.

140. Fisher, L. W., Termine, D., and Young, M. F., Deduced protein sequence of bone small proteoglycan I (biglycan) shows homology with proteoglycan II (decorin) and several nonconnective tissue proteins in a variety of species, *J. Biol. Chem.*, 264, 4571, 1989.

141. Yamaguchi, Y., Mann, D. M., and Ruoslahti, E., Negative regulation of transforming growth factor-β by the proteoglycan decorin, *Nature*, 346, 281, 1990.

142. Ruoslahti, E., Yamaguchi, Y., Hildebrand, A., and Border, W. A., Extracellular matrix/growth factor interactions, *Cold Spring Harb. Symp. Quant. Biol.*, 57, 309, 1992.

143. Dragstedt, C. A., Wells, J. A., Silva, M., and Rocha, E., Inhibitory effect of heparin upon histamine release by trypsin, antigen and protease, *Proc. Soc. Exp. Biol. Med.*, 51, 191, 1942.

144. Higginbotham, R. D. and Dougherty, T. F., Mechanism of heparin protection against a histamine release (48/80), *Proc. Soc. Exp. Biol. Med.*, 92, 493, 1956.

145. Schwartz, L. B. and Bradford, T. R. B., Regulation of tryptase from human lung mast cells by heparin, *J. Biol. Chem.*, 261, 7372, 1986.

146. Bazzoni, G., Beltran-Nunez, A., Mascellani, G., Bianchini, P., Dejana, E., Del-Maschio-A., et al., Effect of heparin, dermatan sulfate, and related oligo-derivatives on human polymorphonuclear leukocyte functions, *J. Lab. Clin. Med.*, 121, 268, 1993.

147. Cerletti, C., Rajtar, G., Marchi, E., and de Gaetano, G., Effects of glycosaminoglycans on platelet and leucocyte function: role of N-sulfation, *Semin. Thromb. Haemostasis*, 20, 245, 1994.

148. Oyanagui, Y. and Sato, S., Heparin, a potent releasing agent of extracellular superoxide dismutase (EC-SOD C), suppresses ischaemic paw oedema in mice, *Free Radical Res. Commun.*, 9, 87, 1990.

149. Motojima, S., Frigas, E., Loegering, D. A., and Gleich, G. J., Toxicity of eosinophil cationic proteins for guinea pig tracheal epithelium in vitro, *Am. Rev. Respir. Dis.*, 139, 801, 1989.

150. Frieri, M. and Metcalfe, D. D., Analysis of the effect of mast cell granules on lymphocyte blastogenesis in the absence and presence of mitogens: identification of heparin as a granule-associated suppressor factor, *J. Immunol.*, 131, 1942, 1983.

151. Kilfeather, S. A., Wahid, S., Costello, J., and Page, C., Inhibition by heparin and stimulation by heparan sulphate of human lymphocyte mitogenesis, *Eur. Respir. J.*, 8(S19), 535s, 1995.

152. Kilfeather, S. A., Hailu, H., Wahid, S., Shteyner, F., Carew, B., Shittu, E., Costello, J., and Page, C., Effect of heparin on lymphocyte mitogenesis in a 2-day mixed lymphocyte reaction, *Am. J. Crit. Care Med.*, abstract, 1996.

153. Wrenshall, L. E., Cerra, A. F. B., Carlson, F. B., Bach, F., and Platt, J. L., Regulation of murine lymphocyte responses by heparan sulphate, *J. Immunol.*, 147, 455, 1991.

154. Wrenshall, L. E., Cerra, F. B., Singh, R. V., and Platt, J. L., Heparan sulfate initiates signals in murine macrophages leading to divergent biological outcomes, *J. Immunol.*, 154, 871, 1995.

155. Wrenshall, L. E., Cerra, A. F. B., Carlson, F. B., and Platt, J. L., Modulation of cytolitic T cell responses by heparan sulfate, *Transplantation*, 57, 1087, 1994.

156. Geller, R. L., Ihrcke, N. S., and Platt, J. L., The release of endothelial cell associated heparan sulphate proteoglycan by activated T cells, *Transplantation*, 57(5), 770, 1994.

157. Naperstek, Y., Cohen, I. R., Fuks, Z., and Vlodavsky, I., Activated T lymphocytes produce a matrix-degrading heparan sulphate endoglycosidase, *Nature*, 310, 241, 1984.

158. Savion, N., Fuks, Z., and Vlodavsky, L., Interaction of T lymphocytes and macrophages with cultured vascular endothelial cells: attachment, invasion, and subsequent degradation of the subendothelial extracellular matrix, *J. Cell. Physiol.*, 118, 169, 1984.

159. Fridman, R., Lider, O., Naperstek, Y., Fuks, Z., Vlodavsky, L., and Cohen, I. R., Soluble antigen induces T lymphocytes to secrete an endoglycosidase that degrades the heparan sulfate moiety of subendothelial extracellular matrix, *J. Cell. Physiol.*, 130, 85, 1987.

160. Nakajima, M., Irimura, T., De Ferrante, D., Di Ferrante, N., and Nicholson, G. L., Heparan sulfate degradation: relation to tumor invasive and metastatic properties of mouse B16 melanoma sublines, *Science*, 220, 611, 1983.

161. Nakajima, M., Irimura, T., Di Ferrante, N., and Nicholson, G. L., Metastatic melanoma heparanase. Characterisation of heparan sulphate degradation fragments produced by B16 melanoma endoglucuronidase, *J. Biol. Chem.*, 259, 2283, 1984.

162. Mahadoo, J. A., Pulmonary administration of heparin. Ph.D. thesis, University of Saskatchewan, Canada, 1992.

163. Pilewski, J. M. and Albelda, S. M., Adhesion molecules in the lung. An overview, *Am. Rev. Respir. Dis.*, 148, S31, 1993.
164. Arfors, K. E. and Ley, K., Sulfated polysaccharides in inflammation, *J. Lab. Clin. Med.*, 121, 201, 1993.
165. Tanaka, Y., Adams, D. H., and Shaw, S., Proteoglycans on endothelial cells present adhesion-inducing cytokines to leukocytes, *Immunol. Today*, 14, 111, 1993.
166. Rot, A., Endothelial cell binding of NAP-1/IL-8: role in neutrophil emigration, *Immunol. Today*, 13, 291, 1992.
167. Nelson, R. M., Cecconi, O., Roberts, W. G., Aruffo, A., Linhardt, R. J., and Bevilacqua, M. P., Heparin oligosaccharides bind L- and P-selectin and inhibit acute inflammation, *Blood*, 82, 3253, 1993.
168. Tangelder, G. J. and Arfors, K.-E., Inhibition of leukocyte rolling in venules by protamine and sulfated polysaccharides, *Blood*, 77, 1565, 1991.
169. Ley, K., Cerrito, M., and Arfors, K.-E., Sulfated polysaccharides inhibit leukocyte rolling in rabbit mesentery venules, *Am. J. Physiol.*, 260, 1667, 1991.
170. Silvestro, L., Viano, I., Macario, M., Colangelo, D., Montrucchio, G., Panico, S., and Fantozzi, R., Effects of heparin and its desulfated derivatives on leukocyte-endothelial adhesion, *Semin. Thromb. Haemostasis*, 20(3), 254, 1994.
171. Sasaki, S., Production of lymphocytosis by polysaccharide polysulphates (heparinoids), *Nature*, 214, 1041, 1967.
172. Seeds, E. A. M., Hanss, J., and Page, C. P., The effect of heparin and related proteoglycans on allergen and PAF-induced eosinophil infiltration, *J. Lipid Mediators*, 7, 269, 1993.
173. Texeira, M. M. and Hellewell, P. G., Suppression by intradermal administration of heparin of eosinophil accumulation but not oedema formation in inflammatory reactions in guinea-pig skin, *Br. J. Pharmacol.*, 110, 1496, 1993.
174. Skinner, M. P., Lucus, C. M., Burns, G. F., Chesterman, C. N., and Berndt, M. C., GMP-140 binding to neutrophils is inhibited by sulfated glycans, *J. Biol. Chem.*, 266, 5371, 1991.
175. Norgard-Sumnicht, K. E., Varki, N. M., and Varki, A., Calcium-dependent heparin-like ligands for L-selectin in nonlymphoid endothelial cells, *Science*, 261, 480, 1993.
176. Shute, J., Basophil migration and chemotaxis, *Clin. Exp. Allergy*, 22(3), 321, 1992.
177. Lider, O., Mekori, Y. A., Miller, T., Bar-Tana, R., Vlodavsky, I., Baharav, E., Cohen, I. R., and Naparstek, Y., Inhibition of T-lymphocyte heparanase by heparin prevents T cell migration and T-cell-mediated immunity, *Eur. J. Immunol.*, 20, 493, 1990.
178. Lider, O., Baharav, E., Mekori, Y. A., Miller, T., Naperstek, Y., and Cohen, I. R., Suppression of experimental autoimmune diseases and prolongation of allograft survival by treatment of animals with low doses of heparins, *J. Clin. Invest.*, 83, 752, 1989.
179. Ahmed, T., Abraham, W. M., D'Brot, J., Effects of inhaled heparin on immunologic and non-immunologic bronchoconstrictor responses in sheep, *Am. Rev. Respir. Dis.*, 145, 566, 1992.
180. Diamant, Z., Timmers, M. C., van der Veen, H., Page, C., van der Meer, F. J., and Sterk, P., Effect of inhaled heparin on allergen-induced early and late asthmatic responses in patients with atopic asthma, *Am. J. Crit. Care Med.*, in press.
181. Ahmed, T., Garrigo, J., and Danita, I., Preventing bronchoconstriction in exercise-induced asthma and inhaled heparin, *N. Engl. J. Med.*, 329, 90, 1993.
182. Ahmed, T., D'Brot, J., Abraham, W. M., Lucio, J., Robinson, M. J., Shakir, S., and San-Pedro, B., Heterogeneity of allergic airway responses: differences in signal transduction? *Am. J. Respir. Crit. Care Med.*, 151, A130, 1995.
183. Bowler, S. D., Smith, S. M., and Lavercombe, P. S., Heparin inhibits the immediate response to antigen in the skin and lungs of allergic subjects, *Am. Rev. Respir. Dis.*, 147, 160, 1993.
184. O'Donnell, W. J., Rosenberg, M. A., Kelleher, K., Drazen, J. M., and Israel, E., Inhaled heparin does not protect asthmatic against induced bronchoconstriction, *Am. Rev. Respir. Dis.*, 145, A422, 1992.

185. Ahmed, T., Syriste, T., Lucio, J., Abraham, W., Robinson, M., and D'Brot, J., Inhibition of antigen-induced airway cutaneous responses by heparin: a pharmacodynamic study, *J. Appl. Physiol.*, 74, 192, 1993.

186. Lucio, J., D'Brot, J., Guo, C.-B., Abraham, W. M., Lichtenstein, L. M., Kagey-Sabokta, A., and Ahmed, T., Immunological mast cell responses and histamine release are attenuated by heparin, *J. Appl. Physiol.*, 73, 1093, 1992.

187. Wenzel, S. E., Fowler, A. A., and Schwartz, L. B., Activation of pulmonary mast cells by bronchoalveolar allergen challenge in vivo release of histamine and tryptase in atopic subjects with and without asthma, *Am. Rev. Respir. Dis.*, 137, 1002, 1988.

188. Wilson, O., Jacobs, A. L., Stewart, S., and Carson, D. D., Expression of externally disposed heparin/heparan sulphate binding sites by uterine epithelial cells, *J. Cell. Physiol.*, 143, 60, 1990.

189. Crimi, N., Armato, F., Lamicela, M., Magri, S., Pistorio, M. P., Mastruzzo, C., and Vancheri, C., Inhibitory effect of heparin on eosinophils recruitment after nasal antigen challenge, *Eur. Respir. J.*, 8(19), 10s, 1995.

190. Seeds, E. A. M., Horne, A. P., Tyrrell, D. J., and Page, C. P., The effect of inhaled heparin and related glycosaminoglycans on allergen-induced eosinophil infiltration in guinea pigs, *Pulm. Pharmacol.*, in press.

191. Hirst, S. J., Barnes, P. J., and Twort, C. H., Quantifying proliferation of cultured human and rabbit airway smooth muscle cells in response to serum and platelet-derived growth factor, *Am. J. Respir. Cell Mol. Biol.*, 7(6), 574, 1992.

192. Aubert, J. D., Hayashi, S., Hards, J., Bai, T. R., Pare, P. D., and Hogg, J. C., Platelet-derived growth factor and its receptor in lungs from patients with asthma and chronic airflow obstruction, *Am. J. Physiol.*, 266(6 Pt. 1), L655, 1994.

193. Taylor, I. K., Sorooshian, M., Wangoo, A., Haynes, A. R., Kotecha, S., Mitchell, D. M., and Shaw, R. J., Platelet-derived growth factor-beta mRNA in human alveolar macrophages in vivo in asthma, *Eur. Respir. J.*, 7(11), 1966, 1994.

194. Sannes, P. L., Burch, K. K., and Khosla, J., Immunohistochemical localization of epidermal growth factor and acidic and basic fibroblast growth factors in postnatal developing and adult rat lungs, *Am. J. Respir. Cell Mol. Biol.*, 7(2), 230, 1992.

195. Powell, P. P., Klagsbrun, M., Abraham, J. A., and Jones, R. C., Eosinophils expressing heparin-binding EGF-like growth factor mRNA localize around lung microvessels in pulmonary hypertension, *Am. J. Pathol.*, 143(3), 784, 1993.

196. Tomlinson, P. R. T., Wilson, J. W., and Stewart, A. G., Inhibition by salbutamol of the proliferation of human airway smooth muscle cells grown in culture, *Br. J. Pharmacol.*, 111, 641–647,

197. Aubert, J. D., Dalal, B. I., Bai, T. R., Roberts, C. R., Hayashi, S., and Hogg, J. C., Transforming growth factor beta 1 gene expression in human airways, *Thorax*, 49(3), 225, 1994.

198. Pennington, D. W., Lopez, A. R., Thomas, P. S., Peck, C., and Gold, W. M., Dog mastocytoma cells produce transforming growth factor beta 1, *J. Clin. Invest.*, 90(1), 35, 1992.

199. Elovic, A., Wong, D. T., Weller, P. F., Matossian, K., and Galli, S. J., Expression of transforming growth factors-alpha and beta 1 messenger RNA and product by eosinophils in nasal polyps, *J. Allergy Clin. Immunol.*, 93(5), 864, 1994.

200. Ohno, I., Lea, R. G., Flanders, K. C., Clark, D. A., Banwatt, D., Dolovich, J., Denburg, J., Harley, C. B., Gauldie, J., and Jordana M., Eosinophils in chronically inflamed human upper airway tissues express transforming growth factor beta 1 gene (TGF beta 1), *J. Clin. Invest.*, 89(5), 1662, 1992.

201. De, S., Zelazney, E. T., Souhrada, J. F., and Souhrada, M., Interleukin-1b stimulates the proliferation of cultured airway smooth muscle cells via platelet-derived growth factor, *Am. J. Respir. Cell Mol. Biol.*, 9, 645, 1993.

202. San-Antonio, J. D., Karnovsky, M. J., Gay, S., Sanderson, R. D., and Lander, A. D., Interactions of syndecan-1 and heparin with human collagens, *Glycobiology*, 4(3), 327, 1994.

203. Yamada, K. M., Kennedy, D. W., Kimata, K., and Pratt, R. M., Characterization of fibronectin interactions with glycosaminoglycans and identification of active proteolytic fragments, *J. Biol. Chem.*, 255(13), 6055, 1980.
204. Preissner, K. T. and Muller-Bergaus, G., Neutralization and binding of heparin by S protein/vitronectin in the inhibition of factor Xa by antithrombin III, *J. Biol. Chem.*, 262, 12247, 1987.
205. Tarsio, J. F., Reger, L. A., and Furcht, L. T., Molecular mechanisms in basement membrane complications of diabetes. Alterations in heparin, laminin, and type IV collagen association, *Diabetes*, 37(5), 532, 1988.
206. Lawler, J. W. and Slayter, H. S., The release of heparin binding peptides from platelet thrombospondin by proteolytic action of thrombin, plasmin and trypsin, *Thromb. Res.*, 22(3), 267, 1981.
207. Miller, M. D. and Krangel, M. S., Biology and biochemistry of the chemokines: a family of chemotactic and inflammatory cytokines, *Crit. Rev. Immunol.*, 12, 17, 1992.
208. Bobik, A. and Campbell, J. H., Vascular-derived growth factors cell biology, pathophysiology and pharmacology, *Pharmacol. Rev.*, 45, 1, 1993.

Chapter 7

# *IN VIVO* MODELS OF SMOOTH MUSCLE GROWTH

James G. Martin and Tony R. Bai

## CONTENTS

## I. INTRODUCTION

A cardinal feature of asthma is airway hyperresponsiveness which manifests itself by exaggerated responses to a variety of stimuli, both pharmacological and physical. Hyperresponsiveness is usually, but not always, associated with symptomatic asthma, suggesting that the propensity for exaggerated airway narrowing may represent a risk for the development of clinical disease. In many asthmatic subjects there are structural changes in the airways which result in measurable increases in the thickness of the airway.[1-4] This remodelling process, which is presumably a consequence of chronic inflammation, may amplify the degree of airway narrowing[5] and, in the extreme case, may account for fixed obstruction. While it is possible that even subclinical disease is associated with structural changes of the airways, it also seems plausible that disease-related remodelling may compound a problem which has its origins elsewhere. For instance, asymptomatic airway hyperresponsiveness may reflect some alteration in airway smooth muscle function, whereas the expression of disease through airway narrowing may require airway inflammation. While acknowledging that the question of whether or not airway remodelling is at the root of airway hyperresponsiveness has not been answered, we have ample reason to suspect that airway changes of the kind described in chronic asthma are important.

## II. DETERMINANTS OF AIRWAY RESPONSIVENESS *IN VIVO*

Airway smooth muscle is presumed to be the major effector of the airway narrowing that occurs during bronchial provocation testing. The evidence frequently evoked in support of this notion includes the observation that inhaled airway smooth muscle relaxants, such as $\beta_2$-adrenergic receptor agonists, rapidly induce airway dilatation following bronchial provocation. The precise role that smooth muscle plays in the exaggerated airway narrowing of asthma has long been debated, and it is still not clear whether an abnormality of the airway smooth muscle or of its regulation by external modulating factors is responsible. Studies of potential determinants of airway responsiveness, such as altered neural control (exaggerated cholinergic activity, deficient inhibitory neural pathways) and epithelial influences (eicosanoids, nitric oxide), have revealed definite but small effects of insufficient magnitude to account for much of the variability in airway responsiveness in normal human subjects or animals and are, therefore, even less likely to explain the degree of hyperresponsiveness that is observed in asthma.

Recent observations have suggested that mechanical factors may be of primary importance in airway hyperresponsiveness. The sensitivity of induced bronchoconstriction to lung volume in humans[6] and animals[7] has been interpreted as indicating that the limitation of airway narrowing *in vivo* is caused by an inability of airway smooth muscle to overcome the impedance imposed by the parenchymal tethering. Combined physiological and morphometric measurements of the load applied by lung elastic recoil in canine lung during bronchoconstriction at varying lung volumes suggest that, *in situ*, airway smooth muscle contraction is opposed by substantial elastic loads.[8] Disrupting parenchymal attachments to the airways by administering elastase to animals causes significant augmentation of maximal bronchoconstriction.[9] The cartilage and other components of the airway wall are likely to provide an additional impedance to smooth muscle shortening in larger airways. Papain, which causes softening of cartilage, results in an augmentation of airway responses in rabbits,[10] presumably through effects on airway cartilage, which in the normal airway opposes excessive narrowing.[11] Curiously, it is the maximal degree of induced bronchoconstriction that is affected by changes in lung volume in human subjects and by intratracheal elastase in rats. Submaximal airway narrowing is little changed. This suggests that the factors determining submaximal and maximal levels of bronchoconstriction may be different.

Interspecies differences in airway responsiveness among normal animals are potentially accounted for by differences in airway smooth muscle.[12] The guinea pig, which has long been known for excessive responses to bronchoconstrictors, has much more muscle than a number of other species with lesser responses. Both sensitivity to inhaled methacholine and maximal narrowing seem to be related to the quantity of airway smooth muscle.[12] While the association of increased maximal narrowing to airway smooth muscle mass is intuitively obvious, the relationship of airway smooth muscle mass and sensitivity is not.

## III. MECHANISMS OF HYPERRESPONSIVENESS IN ASTHMA

### A. MECHANICAL DETERMINANTS

It has been postulated that changes in impedance to airway smooth muscle shortening through loss of the coupling between parenchyma and airway or through changes in the properties of the airway wall could account for hyperresponsiveness in asthma.[13] To date, there is little evidence in favour of such changes. The properties of the airway wall in asthmatic subjects do not appear to have been investigated. Loss of lung elastic recoil has been demonstrated in certain cases of asthma[14] and is associated with a poor prognosis. Even in normal subjects there is a relationship between the maximal degree of bronchoconstriction that can be induced and lung recoil.[15] However, loss of lung elastic recoil is not a generally observed phenomenon in asthma. Furthermore, hyperresponsiveness in asymptomatic subjects or normal animals seems unlikely to be entirely accounted for in this way. Alternative explanations for increased responsiveness include the possibility that airway smooth muscle may have increased force-generating capacity which overcomes the loads normally impeding smooth muscle shortening or that the ability of airway smooth muscle to shorten may be related to the elastance of extracellular matrix elements surrounding muscle fibres. A decrease in the load because of a change in the amount or nature of the extracellular matrix could potentially allow for increased shortening of otherwise normal muscle.[16]

There is considerable, albeit circumstantial, evidence suggesting that airway smooth muscle may provide the key to understanding airway hyperresponsiveness. There are several ways in which airway smooth muscle could lead to increases in airway narrowing for a given bronchoconstrictive stimulus. An alteration in the contractile properties of smooth muscle could result in more airway narrowing. To date, there is little agreement concerning contractile properties of asthmatic muscle, largely because of the lack of availability of tissues for study. Several reports have suggested an increased capacity for force generation.[17,18] Airway smooth muscle from allergic dogs has been reported to show an increased shortening capacity, as well as maximal velocity of shortening.[19] The significance of these changes for *in vivo* responsiveness has not been established, but it does indicate the potential for modification of smooth muscle properties by allergen. Some or all of the capacity for increased force generation by asthmatic airways may reflect the greater mass of muscle which is present. Increased mass should lead to greater force and, therefore, shortening and airway narrowing, assuming that the contractile properties of the muscle are not significantly different from normal muscle. This may not necessarily be the case. For example, although in resistive blood vessels absolute maximal force is increased by pathological increases in smooth muscle mass, the stress (force/cross-sectional area) generated by the muscle is actually less.[20]

As already mentioned, it is unknown whether the increased mass of muscle is acquired in the course of the disease or whether it represents the characteristic that permits the disease to express itself. It is plausible that an increased mass of muscle, conceivably an inherited characteristic, may precede the development of disease, which manifests itself only when the appropriate inflammation, another feature of asthma, is present. Asymptomatic hyperresponsiveness is a well-recognized entity, and it appears that when present it may predispose to the development of clinical disease. Whether or not an increase in airway smooth muscle is a feature of such subjects is not known.

An increased quantity of airway smooth muscle in asthmatic airways is but one feature of the remodelling that occurs. All compartments of the airway wall, the adventitia, and submucosa, as well as the smooth muscle, are affected.[4,21] Subepithelial basement membrane collagen deposition seems to occur uniquely in asthma[22] and suggests a repair process, perhaps related to epithelial damage. It therefore seems likely that airway smooth muscle increases in response to the chronic stimulation provided by inflammation. Much of the increase in muscle may be caused by hyperplasia.[2,5] However, few studies have addressed whether hyperplasia or hypertrophy is primarily responsible for the changes. Recent reports using careful morphometric approaches have focussed on muscle mass only. The issue is not without importance, given the fact that the contractility of hypertrophied muscle may not be normal.[20]

## IV. MECHANISMS OF SMOOTH MUSCLE GROWTH IN ASTHMA

The regulation of airway smooth muscle growth has received much attention in recent times. Most investigators have confined their studies to cultured smooth muscle. While providing considerable insight into the control of smooth muscle and providing information about the potential growth-promoting substances that may be involved, it will be necessary to confirm the relevance of such model systems *in vivo*. There are no studies that we are aware of directly testing the phenotypic changes that may have accompanied the increase in muscle mass in asthma. *In vitro* studies have clearly shown major phenotypic changes in smooth muscle in culture undergoing proliferation.[23] If such changes were also a feature of asthmatic airways, they could have profound effects on the responsiveness of the muscle. However, given the chronicity of the disease process, it seems likely that restoration of the contractile phenotype may occur.

A number of potentially interesting candidate growth-promoting substances have been identified by *in vitro* testing. Of particular interest are those associated with allergic inflammation since allergy is one of the best-characterised mechanisms by which asthma is induced. Thromboxane, endothelin, cysteinyl-leukotrienes, and histamine have been shown to have mitogenic activity.[24-26] The evidence for the synthesis and release of these substances in asthma is solid. The precise mechanisms by which such bronchoconstrictive mediators stimulate smooth muscle proliferation *in vitro* appear to be complex and to involve interactions among them. For example, endothelin causes phospholipase $A_2$ activation and thromboxane synthesis in cultured rabbit airway smooth muscle cells. Thromboxane, in turn, triggers cysteinyl-leukotriene synthesis.[24] The mitogenic activity of endothelin seems to mediated by leukotriene and so is indirect.

Information concerning more-classic growth factors, such as platelet-derived growth factor (PDGF), transforming growth factor $\beta$, insulin-like growth factors, and others is lacking at present. PDGF and B-PDGF receptor expression have been associated with interstitial macrophages surrounding airway smooth muscle cells in asthmatic airways.[27] However, there is no evidence that expression of mRNA levels is in excess in airways from individuals without airway remodelling. Perhaps the chronicity of the asthmatic process is associated with small differences in mRNA so that immunolocalisation techniques are too qualitative to allow detection of signals. Alternatively, other molecules singly or in combination with PDGF may be required for remodelling. *In vitro* experiments strongly suggest the plausibility of interactions between growth factors and contractile agonists in airway remodelling. For example, the cysteinyl-leukotriene $LTC_4$ stimulates fibroblast growth factor (FGF) release from macrophages, suggesting at least one possible pathway by which growth of airway smooth muscle might be triggered *in vivo*.[28] Macrophage-derived products with growth-promoting potential merit particular attention since the macrophage itself can be activated by allergen exposure by IgE-dependent mechanisms,[29] much as can mast cells.

## V. ANIMAL MODELS OF SMOOTH MUSCLE GROWTH: ALLERGEN-INDUCED CHANGE

The Brown Norway (BN) rat has been extensively characterised as a model of allergic bronchoconstriction. This animal is a high IgE producer in response to active sensitisation.[30] Following allergen (ovalbumin, OA) challenge, about 70% of the animals have early and late responses.[31] By 24 h after challenge, airway hyperresponsiveness to inhaled cholinergic substances occurs.[32,33] Airway inflammation occurs also and is strikingly eosinophilic.[34] All of these characteristics suggest that the BN rat has an atopic constitution and are manifest in the particular profile of lymphokines typically synthesised by T-lymphocytes of the Th2 type.[35] After as few as three allergen challenges this animal has a measurable increase in the area of airway smooth muscle in its airways (Plate 1*).

Several morphometric studies have documented consistent increases in muscle following allergen challenge.[36,37] The magnitude of the increase has been found by different observers to vary from less than a doubling to as much as a several-fold increase. Since the ability to distinguish muscle from adjacent connective tissue can potentially influence the results, there is variability in the outcome related to staining techniques, as well as to observer assessment of the tissues. Inter- and intraobserver correlations are highly significant, but the estimates of the absolute values of smooth muscle can show systematic differences from observer to observer.

Allergen-induced increase in muscle is observed throughout the airway tree, although the biggest changes occur in the larger airways. The preferential increase in smooth muscle in the larger airways is also consistent with the distribution of airway narrowing, which is greatest in central airways and least in the periphery.[38] The explanation is likely related to distribution of the aerosolised OA (allergen); most of the particles of aerosol are likely to have been deposited in large airways. However, mast cells are in greatest density in central airways and diminish in density towards the periphery.[38] It is probable that both the pattern of deposition of aerosol and the relatively greater mast cell density centrally contribute to the observed gradient in the intensity of the allergic reaction and the consequent changes in airway smooth muscle.

Recently, the effects of allergen challenge on airway tissues have been addressed by studying the incorporation of bromodeoxyuridine (BrdU) into cells in the airway wall. This measure of the number of cells passing through the S phase of the cell cycle is a useful way of identifying hyperplasia. Substantial incorporation of BrdU into airway myocytes and epithelial cells has been observed following allergen challenge. An illustrative photomicrograph is shown in Figure 1. Incorporation of BrdU into epithelial cells is quite apparent, but incorporation into cells lying under the epithelium with spindle-shaped nuclei is also evident. Similar studies have been performed on the sensitised guinea pig.[39] The protocol used differed, in that animals were challenged more frequently and with a larger total exposure to allergen. There was also a substantial incorporation of BrdU into airway cells in these animals. Curiously, these animals did not have any increase in the area of smooth muscle in the airways studied to date, namely, in noncartilaginous airways and trachea.

---

* Plate 1 follows page 80.

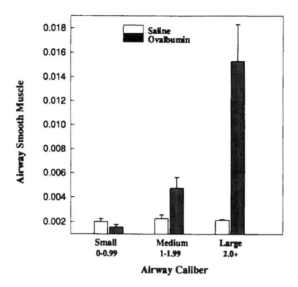

**FIGURE 1** OA challenges increases airway smooth muscle mass in the bronchi of sensitised animals. Airway smooth muscle is standardised for size by dividing measurements of Pbm². Airway smooth muscle shows no significant difference as a function of size in control animals but shows a marked gradient from large to small airways in OA-challenged animals. Airway smooth muscle is significantly greater in large and medium-sized airways but not small airways in OA-challenged animals. The means + 1 SE are shown. (From Panettieri, R. A. et al., *Am. J. Physiol.*, 259, L365, 1990. With permission.)

The explanation for this finding is not known, but it is possible that the BrdU may have arrested the cells in the S phase. It is also possible that the size of the cells after division may have been less than before, such that there was little increase in volume despite mitosis having taken place. Increased loss of cells, perhaps through apoptosis, is a further possibility which could account for these findings. If a preferential increase in muscle occurs in larger airways, as in the rat, it is possible that a similar phenomenon may be operative in the guinea pig and that morphometric analyses of cartilaginous airways may be necessary to reveal changes in mass.

Detection of cellular proliferation *in vivo* using BrdU requires consideration of the optimal administration of this nucleotide, particularly when the goal is to detect replication of stromal cells, such as smooth muscle cells that divide less frequently than epithelial cells. A variety of dosing schedules and routes of administration have been employed. In the rat model two injections of BrdU (25 mg/kg each; i.p.) were administered before and two after the final of three OA challenges. In the guinea pig antigen model, administration of BrdU via a subcutaneous osmotic pump throughout the period of the 6-week protocol yielded smooth muscle–labelling indices similar to an intermittent dosing schedule; a ninefold increase in proliferation index was detected with twice weekly intraperitoneal administration 1 h before antigen challenge for 5 weeks and then daily for 7 days prior to termination (Bai et al., unpublished observations). In a subsequent study, the latter protocol, without daily administration in the final week, detected only a fourfold increase in labelling.[40] The difference in labelling index between control and OA-challenged rats was greater, 35-fold in large airways and ninefold in small airways, suggesting that the duration of administration may have been excessive in the guinea pig or that true differences for propensity for muscle growth are present. An unresolved issue in relation to *in vivo* models of airway smooth muscle growth in response to antigen is the relationship between airway remodelling and length of challenge. Do prolonged periods of antigen challenge lead to greater remodelling than shorter periods?

The incorporation of BrdU into epithelial cells indicates a clear reaction of these cells to allergen challenge. Despite the absence of light microscopical alterations, it seems very likely that changes in cell function occur. It has been shown that the activity of acetylcholinesterase in the airway epithelium of chronically allergen-challenged dogs is reduced.[41] This change is a potential contributor to changes in cholinergic responsiveness, particularly when challenge is administered by inhalation. It does, however, raise questions about the possibility of other phenotypic changes in airway epithelium that may be of significance to remodelling.

## VI. MECHANISMS OF ALLERGEN-INDUCED AIRWAY SMOOTH MUSCLE GROWTH

Few studies are available that address the mechanisms of airway smooth muscle growth following allergen challenge *in vivo*. Wang et al.[37] have shown that MK-571, a selective $LTD_4$ antagonist, prevents the increase in airway smooth muscle in the BN rat following multiple allergen exposures. Although it seems somewhat surprising that a single antagonist could prevent airway smooth muscle growth, given the complex nature of the allergic responses, cysteinyl-leukotrienes and, in particular, $LTD_4$ are the most important mediators of the airway responses to allergen challenge in the rat.[42,43] $LTD_4$ antagonists markedly reduce the early response and abolish the late response in its entirety. It appears that cysteinyl-leukotrienes are therefore not only responsible for airway narrowing, but also for the more chronic changes associated with allergen challenge.

It has been shown that prolonged exposure to contractile agonists increases the probability that these substances will initiate cell proliferation.[44] In this regard, cysteinyl-leukotrienes are also more likely than other substances to cause smooth muscle proliferation. The prolonged synthesis of leukotrienes is suggested by studies to date.[43,45] The time course of excretion through the biliary tract, which is the major route of excretion of cysteinyl-leukotrienes, suggests that, at least in the rat, allergen challenge of sufficient magnitude to cause late responses is associated with prolonged synthesis of cysteinyl-leukotrienes. It is probable that the *in vivo* exposure of smooth muscle cells to bioactive amines, such as histamine and serotonin, both potential mitogens,[26,46] is relatively brief since these substances are involved in early but not late responses.

The increase in airway smooth muscle induced by allergen challenge is also attenuated by nedocromil, an antiallergic drug which effectively reduces allergic airway responses in the rat.[47] Interestingly, when the drug is administered before exposure to allergen, protection against smooth muscle growth is more complete than when it is administered after the early response has been allowed to occur. The drug still blocks late responses even when administered in this way. This finding suggests that mediators, presumably $LTD_4$, released during both early and late responses contribute to the growth of smooth muscle. While it is possible that $LTD_4$ itself may act as a mitogenic agent, it is also possible that it acts through release of other more-classic growth factors such as PDGF; as previously mentioned, release of FGF from macrophages has been reported to occur after exposure to $LTC_4$.[28] It will be of interest to establish if other leukotriene-related airway narrowing, such as exercise- or hyperpnea-induced bronchoconstriction,[48,49] are also associated with an increase in smooth muscle proliferation. This question is of some importance in view of the possibility that otherwise apparently benign triggers for bronchoconstriction may in some susceptible individuals cause growth of airway smooth muscle.

In addition to consideration of the possible effects of leukotriene released in association with hyperpnea- or exercise-induced airway narrowing, sensory neuropeptides themselves merit attention. Peptides released from sensory neurons could directly or indirectly induce smooth muscle growth. Direct proliferative effects have been demonstrated *in vitro* with related cell types, such as lung fibroblasts[50] and vascular smooth muscle cells.[51] Indirect effects could occur following tachykinin-induced increases in vascular permeability, with release of other mitogens such as thrombin, or following tachykinin-induced release of other mediators such as IL-8 or leukotrienes, as already mentioned. In the guinea pig model, the role of tachykinins in the induction of smooth muscle proliferation has been addressed by pretreating the animals with capsaicin, and it appears that they are not essential to the process. Prior neuropeptide depletion did not prevent the development of smooth muscle replication.[40]

The epithelium may also have a role to play in determining whether or not changes in smooth muscle mass take place. This structure is metabolically active and produces eicosanoids and other substances such as endothelin. Prostaglandin $E_2$ is a potent negative regulator of airway smooth muscle growth,[52] whereas endothelin is mitogenic,[25] at least *in vitro*.

## VII. NONALLERGIC MODELS OF AIRWAY SMOOTH MUSCLE GROWTH

### A. HYPEROXIA

Hyperoxic exposure of neonatal rats causes a variety of changes in airway structure and function.[53] Chronic exposure for a period of 8 days causes striking changes in both the epithelium and airway smooth muscle. There is measurable epithelial thickening, as well as an increase in smooth muscle by as early as 6 days after initiating exposure. The analysis of BrdU incorporation indicates an increased proportion of cells entering the S phase of the cell cycle in each of the layers of the airway.[54] The relative contributions of hyperplasia and hypertrophy to the increase in airway smooth muscle have not been established, but it seems reasonable to assume a substantial portion of the change is related to hyperplasia.

The mechanism of hyperoxia-induced changes in rat airways is not known. Although the effects of hyperoxia on the lung have been extensively investigated, the focus has been on alveolar wall remodelling. Hypertrophy and hyperplasia of a number of cell types lead to thickening of the alveolar-capillary membrane. PDGF is a known mitogen for mesenchymal cells, and both the ligand PDGF and its receptor are rapidly expressed in lung within hours of breathing oxygen.[55] PDGF is also a mitogen for smooth muscle, and even though no attempt to localise its expression to airway tissues was made in this study it seems quite possible that it will also be found to be expressed in this location.

The administration of acetylcholine by inhalation to guinea pigs has been used to test the hypothesis that "work hypertrophy" may be stimulated by repeated contraction of airway smooth muscle. Animals were challenged to the point of asphyxia repeatedly by administering acetylcholine as an aerosol into a chamber for a 15-min period about 10 times a day for 2 to 3 weeks. Subsequently, histologic examination of the airways was performed, and the quantity of airway smooth muscle in the membranous, but not the cartilaginous, airways increased after this rather extreme insult. These changes may have resulted from hyperplasia and not so-called work hypertrophy. Contractile agonists, which cause phospholipase C activation and phosphoinositide hydrolysis, have the potential to be mitogenic.[56] Diacylglycerol, which is also produced following hydrolysis of membrane phosphotidylinositol bisphosphate, activates protein kinase C similar to phorbol esters, which are known tumour-promoting substances. The prolonged exposure to acetylcholine is more likely to evoke cell proliferation than a more transient exposure.[44] It is also possible that cholinergic receptors on other cell types may have triggered intermediate cells to release more-specific growth-promoting substances.

The exposure of adult dogs to sulphur dioxide has been shown to cause a number of histological changes in the airways, of which an increase of smooth muscle is one.

## VIII. RELATIONSHIP OF AIRWAY SMOOTH MUSCLE GROWTH TO HYPERRESPONSIVENESS

It is logical to presume that an increase in airway smooth muscle may lead to hyperresponsiveness to bronchoconstrictive stimuli. It must be remembered that the link between the quantity of airway smooth muscle and responsiveness hinges on the notion that impedances to smooth muscle shortening *in vivo* determine the extent of airway narrowing for any given constrictive stimulus. Certain evidence supports a critical role for mechanical forces in determining airway narrowing. For example, it is true that differences in airway responsiveness between different strains of rat appear to be accounted for by differences in the quantity of smooth muscle in the airways.[57] Likewise, interspecies differences in responsiveness may be linked to airway smooth muscle mass.[12] The causal link between mass of smooth muscle and hyperresponsiveness is bolstered by the finding of changes in responsiveness, as well as muscle mass, in most of the experimental models developed thus far. There is one exception, namely, the sulphur dioxide–exposed dog. In these animals, responsiveness to inhaled histamine is reduced by exposure to the pollutant gas. These associations are not proof of causality. The experiments necessary to test directly the hypothesis that smooth muscle quantity and responsiveness are causally linked are not immediately obvious, so that it may be some time before definitive proof is obtained.

## IX. SUMMARY

Various insults to the airways have the potential to induce airway smooth muscle growth. It is not certain to what extent the mechanisms underlying smooth muscle growth are common among the various exogenous stimuli that have been documented to effect growth. A feature in common to most of these stimuli is airway inflammation. The pattern of inflammation has not been adequately compared among the various models to allow any speculation concerning possible responsible cells. Changes in the airway epithelium also are common to most of the models, but the changes are more striking in animals exposed to hyperoxia and sulphur dioxide, whereas allergen-challenged animals have light microscopically normal epithelium. Sulphur dioxide does not affect hyperresponsiveness, however. Even in allergen-challenged animals the epithelium shows signs of response to the exposure, raising the importance of phenotypic changes in the epithelium in evoking changes in the underlying muscle. There is much work to be done to elucidate the precise cellular and molecular mechanisms that cause the airway changes. There is the exciting prospect that careful evaluation of the processes that lead to airway remodelling *in vivo* may lead to new therapies designed at preventing, rather than palliating, airway disease.

## REFERENCES

1. Dunnill, M. S., Masarrella, G. R., and Anderson, J. A., A comparison of the quantitative anatomy of the bronchi in normal subjects, in status asthmaticus, in chronic bronchitis and in emphysema, *Thorax,* 24, 176, 1969.
2. Ebina, M., Yaegashi, H., Chiba, R., Takahashi, T., Motomiya, M., and Tanemura, M., Hyperreactive site in the airway tree of asthmatic patients revealed by thickening of bronchial muscles. A morphometric study, *Am. Rev. Respir. Dis.,* 141, 1327, 1990.

3. Ludwig, M. S., Dreshaj, I., Solway, J., Munoz, A., and Ingram, R. H., Jr., Partitioning of pulmonary resistance during constriction in the dog: effects of volume history, *J. Appl. Physiol.*, 62, 807, 1987.

4. Kuwano, K., Bosken, C. H., Pare, P. D., Bai, T. R., Wiggs, B. R., and Hogg, J. C., Small airways dimensions in asthma and in chronic obstructive pulmonary disease, *Am. Rev. Respir. Dis.*, 148, 1220, 1993.

5. Moreno, R. H., Hogg, J. C., and Pare, P. D., Mechanics of airway narrowing, *Am. Rev. Respir. Dis.*, 133, 1171, 1986.

6. Ding, D. J., Martin, J. G., and Macklem, P. T., Effects of lung volume on maximal methacholine induced bronchoconstriction in normal human subjects, *J. Appl. Physiol.*, 62, 1324, 1987.

7. Sly, P. D., Brown, K. A., Bates, J. H. T., Macklem, P. T., Milic-Emili, J., and Martin, J. G., The effect of lung volume on interrupter resistances in cats challenged with methacholine, *J. Appl. Physiol.*, 64, 360, 1988.

8. Okazawa, M., Bai, T. R., Wiggs, B. R., and Pare, P. D., Airway smooth muscle shortening in excised canine lung lobes, *J. Appl. Physiol.*, 74, 1613, 1993.

9. Bellofiore, S., Eidelman, D. H., Macklem, P. T., and Martin, J. G., Effects of elastase-induced emphysema on airway responsiveness to methacholine in rats, *J. Appl. Physiol.*, 66, 506, 1989.

10. Moreno, R. H., Lisboa, C., Hogg, J. C., and Pare, P. D., Limitation of airway smooth muscle shortening by cartilage stiffness and lung elastic recoil in rabbits, *J. Appl. Physiol.*, 75, 738, 1993.

11. Moreno, R. H. and Pare, P. D., Intravenous papain-induced cartilage softening decreases preload of tracheal smooth muscle, *J. Appl. Physiol.*, 66, 1694, 1989.

12. Martin, J. G., Opazo-Saez, A., Du, T., Tepper, R., and Eidelman, D. H., *In vivo* airway reactivity: predictive value of morphological estimates of airway smooth muscle. Review, *Can. J. Physiol. Pharmacol.*, 70, 597, 1992.

13. Macklem, P. T., Bronchial hyperresponsiveness, *Chest*, 87, 158S, 1985.

14. Woolcock, A. J. and Read, J., Lung volumes in exacerbation of asthma, *Am. J. Med.*, 41, 259, 1966.

15. Shardonofsky, F. R., Martin, J. G., and Eidelman, D. H., Effect of body posture on concentration-response curves to inhaled methacholine, *Am. Rev. Respir. Dis.*, 145, 750, 1992.

16. Bramley, A. M., Thomson, R. J., Roberts, C. R., and Schellenberg, R. R., Hypothesis: excessive bronchoconstriction in asthma is due to decreased airway elastance, *Eur. Respir. J.*, 7, 337, 1994.

17. Bai, T. R., Abnormalities in airway smooth muscle in fatal asthma, *Am. Rev. Respir. Dis.*, 141, 552, 1990.

18. Schellenberg, R. R. and Foster, A., In vitro responses of human asthmatic airway and pulmonary vascular smooth muscle, *Int. Arch. Allergy Appl. Immunol.*, 75, 237, 1984.

19. Antonissen, L. A., Mitchell, R. W., Kroeger, E. A., Kepron, W., Tse, K. S., and Stephens, N. L., Mechanical alterations of airway smooth muscle in a canine asthmatic model, *J. Appl. Physiol. Respir. Environ. Exercise Physiol.*, 46, 681, 1979.

20. Berner, P. F., Somlyo, A. V., and Somlyo, A. P., Hypertrophy-induced increase of intermediate filaments in vascular smooth muscle, *J. Cell Biol.*, 88, 96, 1981.

21. Saetta, M., Di Stefano, A., Rosina, C., Thiene, G., and Fabbri, L. M., Quantitative structural analysis of peripheral airways and arteries in sudden fatal asthma, *Am. Rev. Respir. Dis.*, 143, 138, 1991.

22. Roche, W. R., Beasley, R., Williams, J. H., and Holgate, S. T., Subepithelial fibrosis in the bronchi of asthmatics, *Lancet*, 1, 520, 1989.

23. Chamley-Campbell, J. H., Campbell, G. R., and Ross, R., Phenotype-dependent response of cultured aortic smooth muscle to serum mitogens, *J. Cell Biol.*, 89, 379, 1981.

24. Noveral, J. P. and Grunstein, M. M., Role and mechanism of thromboxane-induced proliferation of cultured airway smooth muscle cells, *Am. J. Physiol.*, 263, L555, 1992.

25. Noveral, J. P., Rosenberg, S. M., Anbar, R. A., Pawlowski, N. A., and Grunstein, M. M., Role of endothelin-1 in regulating proliferation of cultured rabbit airway smooth muscle cells, *Am. J. Physiol.*, 263, L317, 1992.
26. Panettieri, R. A., Yadvish, P. A., Kelly, A. M., Rubinstein, N. A., and Kotlikoff, M. I., Histamine stimulates proliferation of airway smooth muscle and induces c-fos expression, *Am. J. Physiol.*, 259, L365, 1990.
27. Aubert, J. D., Hayashi, S., Hards, J., Bai, T. R., Pare, P. D., and Hogg, J. C., Platelet-derived growth factor and its receptor in lungs from patients with asthma and chronic airflow obstruction, *Am. J. Physiol.*, 266, L655, 1994.
28. Phan, S. H., McGarry, B. M., Loeffler, K. M., and Kunkel, S. L., Regulation of macrophage-derived fibroblast growth factor release by arachidonate metabolites, *J. Leukocyte Biol.*, 42, 106, 1987.
29. Thorel, T., Joseph, M., Tsicopoulos, A., Tonnel, A. B., and Capron, A., Inhibition by nedocromil sodium of IgE-mediated activation of human mononuclear phagocytes and platelets in allergy, *Int. Arch. Allergy Appl. Immunol.*, 85, 232, 1988.
30. Pauwels, R., Bazin, H., Platteau, B., and van der Straeten, M., The influence of antigen dose on IgE production in different rat strains, *Immunology*, 36, 151, 1979.
31. Eidelman, D. H., Bellofiore, S., and Martin, J. G., Late airway responses to antigen challenge in sensitized inbred rats, *Am. Rev. Respir. Dis.*, 137, 1033, 1988.
32. Bellefiore, S. and Martin, J. G., Antigen challenge of sensitized rats increases airway responsiveness to methacholine, *J. Appl. Physiol.*, 65, 1642, 1988.
33. Elwood, W., Barnes, P. J., and Fan Chung, K., Airway hyperresponsiveness is associated with inflammatory cell infiltration in Brown-Norway rats, *Int. Arch. Allergy Immunol.*, 99, 91, 1992.
34. Renzi, P. M., Olivenstein, R., and Martin, J. G., Inflammatory cell populations in the airways and parenchyma after antigen challenge of the rat, *Am. Rev. Respir. Dis.*, 147, 967, 1993.
35. Watanabe, A., Mishima, H., Schotman, E., Renzi, P. M., Martin, J. G., and Hamid, Q., Adoptively transferred late allergic airway responses are associated with Th2 type cytokines in the rat, *ARCCM*, 152, 64, 1995.
36. Sapienza, S., Du, T., Eidelman, D. H., Wang, N. S., and Martin, J. G., Structural changes in the airways of sensitized brown Norway rats after antigen challenge, *Am. Rev. Respir. Dis.*, 144, 423, 1991.
37. Wang, C. G., Du, T., Xu, L. J., and Martin, J. G., Role of leukotriene D4 in allergen-induced increases in airway smooth muscle in the rat, *Am. Rev. Respir. Dis.*, 148, 413, 1993.
38. Du, T., Sapienza, S., Eidelman, D. H., Wang, N. S., and Martin, J. G., Morphometry of the airways during late responses to antigen challenge in the rat, *Am. Rev. Respir. Dis.*, 143, 132, 1991.
39. Wang, Z. L., Okazawa, M., Yarema, M., Weir, T., Roberts, C. R., Walker, B. W., Paré, P. D., and Bai, T. R., Effect of chronic antigen and B2 agonist exposure on airway remodelling in guinea pigs, *ARCCM*, 152, 2097, 1995.
40. Lau, E., Mckay, K. O., Paré, P. D., and Bai, T. R., Prior neuropeptide depletion does not prevent airway smooth muscle proliferation induced by antigen exposure *in vivo*, *ARCCM*, (in press).
41. Mitchell, R. W., Kelly, E., and Leff, A. R., Reduced activity of acetylcholinesterase in canine tracheal smooth muscle homogenates after active immune-sensitization, *Am. J. Respir. Cell Mol. Biol.*, 5, 56, 1991.
42. Sapienza, S., Eidelman, D. H., Renzi, P. M., and Martin, J. G., Role of leukotriene D4 in the early and late pulmonary responses of rats to allergen challenge, *Am. Rev. Respir. Dis.*, 142, 353, 1990.
43. Martin, J. G., Xu, L. J., Toh, M. Y., Olivenstein, R., and Powell, W. S., Leukotrienes in bile during the early and the late airway responses after allergen challenge of sensitized rats, *Am. Rev. Respir. Dis.*, 147, 104, 1993.

44. Berridge, M. T., Inositol phosphates and cell proliferation, *Biochim. Biophys. Acta*, 907, 33, 1987.
45. Powell, W. S., Xu, L. J., and Martin, J. G., Effects of dexamethasone on leukotriene synthesis and airway responses to antigen and leukotriene D4 in rats, *ARCCM*, (in press).
46. Panettieri, R. A., Eszterhas, A., and Murray, R. K., Agonist-induced proliferation of airway smooth muscle cells is mediated by alterations in cytosolic calcium, *Am. Rev. Respir. Dis.*, 145 (Abstr.), A15, 1992.
47. Du, T., Sapienza, S., Wang, C. G., Renzi, P. M., Pantano, R., Rossi, P., and Martin, J. G., Effect of nedocromil sodium on allergen-induced airway responses and changes in the quantity of airway smooth muscle in rats, *J. Allergy Clin. Immunol.*, 1996. (in press)
48. Manning, P. J., Watson, R. M., Margolskee, D. J., Williams, V. C., Schwartz, J. I., and O'Byrne, P. M., Inhibition of exercise-induced bronchoconstriction by MK-571, a potent leukotriene D4-receptor antagonist, *N. Engl. J. Med.*, 323, 1736, 1990.
49. Garland, A., Jordan, J. E., Ray, D. W., Spaethe, S. M., Alger, L., and Solway, J., Role of eicosanoids in hyperpnea-induced airway responses in guinea pigs, *J. Appl. Physiol.*, 75, 2797, 1993.
50. Bai, T. R. and Zhou, D., Substance P induces proliferation of human lung fibroblasts, *ARCCM*, 1996. (in press)
51. Nilsson, J., von Euler, A. M., and Dalsgaard, C. J., Stimulation of connective tissue cell growth by substance P and substance K, *Nature*, 315, 61, 1985.
52. Florio, C., Martin, J. G., Styhler, A., and Heisler, S., Antiproliferative effect of prostaglandin E2 in cultured guinea pig tracheal smooth muscle cells, *Am. J. Physiol.*, 266, L131, 1994.
53. Hershenson, M. B., Aghili, S., Punjabi, N., Hernandez, C., Ray, D. W., Garland, A., Glagov, S., and Solway, J., Hyperoxia-induced airway hyperresponsiveness and remodeling in immature rats, *Am. J. Physiol. Lung Cell Mol. Physiol.*, 262(6), L263, 1992.
54. Hershenson, M. B., Kelleher, M. D., Naureckas, E. T., Abe, M. K., Rubinstein, V. J., Zimmermann, A., Bendele, A. M., McNulty, J. A., Panettieri, R. A., and Solway, J., Hyperoxia increases airway cell S-phase traversal in immature rats in vivo, *Am. J. Respir. Cell Mol. Biol.*, 11(3), 298, 1994.
55. Powell, P. P., Wang, C. C., and Jones, R., Differential regulation of the genes encoding platelet-derived growth factor receptor and its ligand in rat lung during microvascular and alveolar wall remodeling in hyperoxia, *Am. J. Respir. Cell Mol. Biol.*, 7(3), 278, 1992.
56. Rozengurt, E. and Ober, S. S., The role of early signaling events in the mitogenic pathway, *News Physiol. Sci.*, 5, 21, 1990.
57. Eidelman, D. H., DiMaria, G. U., Bellofiore, S., Wang, N. S., Guttmann, R. D., and Martin, J. G., Strain-related differences in airway smooth muscle and airway responsiveness in the rat, *Am. Rev. Respir. Dis.*, 144, 792, 1991.

Chapter 8

# RELATIONSHIP BETWEEN SMOOTH MUSCLE SHORTENING AND RESISTANCE IN ISOLATED AIRWAYS

Howard W. Mitchell, Peter K. McFawn, John C. Marriott, and Malcolm P. Sparrow

## CONTENTS

## I. INTRODUCTION

The attention in recent years on restructuring of the inflamed bronchial wall and the potential importance of this to bronchial responsiveness underscore an important relationship among airway structure, airways resistance, and airflow. Studies show that the sensitivity and reactivity (responsiveness) of the airway to provocative stimulation of the smooth muscle is dominated by the structural components of the airway wall, or the arrangement of the

0-8493-7813-3/97/$0.00+$.50
© 1997 by CRC Press, Inc.

components in the intact airway, as much as by the pharmacological or physiological properties of the airway smooth muscle cells alone.[1-3]

There is a scarcity of experimental findings defining the actions of the smooth muscle in producing airway lumen narrowing. A number of studies have imaged narrowing of the airway lumen *in vivo* — in early studies using tantalum and most recently using high-resolution computed tomography[4-8] — but concurrent information on changes in smooth muscle length or on bronchial flow is not available. Computerised models have been used widely in order to fill this significant gap in knowledge about narrowing of the intact airway.[9-11] Models have been extended to examine the influence of airway wall dimensions on bronchial responsiveness, and model outputs support a hypothesis for a role of wall restructuring in the bronchial hyperresponsiveness of asthma.[12-14] In this chapter we will examine recent experimental findings carried out in live airways *in vitro*, which begin to define the responsiveness of airways from the activation of the smooth muscle through the sequence of events in the airway wall leading to a change in flow. The principal steps are outlined in Figure 1. The major topics to be addressed in this chapter are:

- How much smooth muscle contraction (force and shortening) is produced by physiological and maximum levels of muscle provocation in the intact airway *in vitro*,
- The extent of narrowing of the bronchial lumen and the reduction in flow brought about by the above muscle contraction,
- Use of findings from airways *in vitro* to examine some of the important assumptions made when simulating airway narrowing in mathematical models, and
- Assessment of the evidence linking the structure of the airway wall to the relationship between smooth muscle shortening and bronchial responsiveness.

## II. BRONCHIAL RESPONSIVENESS *IN VIVO* AND *IN VITRO*

The responsiveness of the bronchial tree is a useful marker of pulmonary disease and may provide clues to underlying abnormalities.[15] To understand mechanisms involved in individual bronchi, however, it would seem to be greatly advantageous to define responsiveness and bronchial narrowing *in vitro*. A number of recent studies have begun to do this by using segments of bronchus that are perfused through the lumen with Krebs solution, usually under a constant driving pressure, so that responsiveness can be defined from the lumen flow.[16,17] Flow can, however, be readily transformed to airway resistance as long as a pressure component in the system is known.[16,18] Airway resistance has been the variable most widely chosen to investigate responsiveness in the mathematical models of airway narrowing.[9-13] In isolated airways, responsiveness is defined from the position of the dose–flow response curve

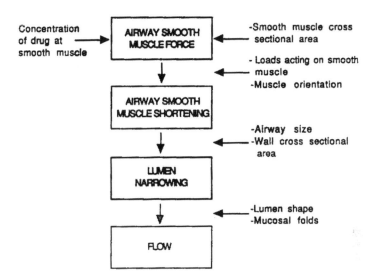

**FIGURE 1**   Main steps involved in airway narrowing and in the reduction of flow through the airway lumen. Several of the properties of the airway wall which have been either shown to be, or proposed to be, important in airway responsiveness are listed.

(e.g., $EC_{50}$), that is, "sensitivity," and from the "reactivity," which is the maximum flow reduction obtained, or the slope of the dose–response curve. These parameters can be used to provide information on the mechanisms that produce airway narrowing *in vitro*. *In vivo* the $PD_{20}$ from the provocation test is commonly used to investigate airway narrowing and its alteration by bronchoactive agents. An important difference in the information gained from *in vivo* and *in vitro* measurements, however, is that in the former responsiveness is measured at the mouth and it represents the response characteristics of airways throughout the bronchial tree — these cannot be individually controlled or monitored. In contrast, *in vitro* measurements provide information about the responsiveness of individual airways, and experimental conditions, such as the airway size and location, dose and site of drug delivery, airway transmural and driving pressures, can be largely controlled.

## A. CHARACTERISITCS OF LUMEN FLOW AND RESISTANCE IN ISOLATED AIRWAY SEGMENTS

The responsiveness of isolated perfused bronchial segments (2–3 mm i.d.) from pigs to bronchoconstrictor drugs is shown in Figure 2a as a percentage change in flow of fluid through the lumen, which is the equivalent of change in airway conductance (flow/pressure). Fluid flow was monitored at the distal end of the segment using a flow head similar to those used for detecting airflow. Carbachol or histamine was perfused through the lumen of the bronchus in increasing doses, and this caused the flow to reduce as the provocative dose was increased until, at high doses, it ceased. If the variable of flow is transformed to resistance (pressure/flow; Figure 2b), the dose–response curve takes on an entirely different appearance as the resistance rises at an increasing rate as high doses are approached. The shape of the resistance dose–response curve is due to the hyperbolic relationship between resistance and flow plotted in Figure 3a. Initially, as the bronchus starts to narrow, large changes in flow are produced by very small changes in airway resistance. As narrowing continues, progressively larger changes in resistance produce progressively smaller changes in flow until infinite changes in resistance produce only trivial changes in flow. For example, in Figure 3a an increase in resistance of only 0.2 cmH$_2$O/ml/min reduced flow by 20 ml/min — to reduce flow by another 20 ml/min, resistance had to increase an infinite amount.

Flow is controlled by the size and shape of the airway lumen, both of which change considerably as the airway constricts with deep folds appearing at the mucosal border. The area of the interstices between the mucosal folds in the constricted bronchus can be significant and in the pig amounts to some 25% of the total lumen area (unpublished data). Current models of airway narrowing take no account of the mucosal folds; instead, they consider the airway to be a cylindrical structure. In the real airway, fluid may be trapped in the interstices[19] between mucosal folds, significantly reducing the effective lumen area. The effect of large mucosal folds could then be to increase airway narrowing above that predicted by current models. The functional effects of the mucosal folds on flow have not been shown experimentally nor have they been simulated — but as airway restructuring could significantly change the pattern of folding in diseased airways such information is urgently needed.

*In vivo* lumen flow may be laminar or turbulent depending on airway division.[11] In isolated segments of airway discussed above, both the velocity of flow through the airway lumen and the Reynold's numbers are low, indicating that flow should be laminar. Figure 3b shows the pressure–flow plot for bronchial segments when they were either relaxed or partly contracted by carbachol indicating that flow was largely laminar and remained so during constriction. Bronchial flow *in vitro* might be assumed to be related to the fourth power of the radius ($r^4$); however, in liquid perfused segments of airway, which are relatively short (2–3 cm) and cannulated at both ends, flow tends to fit an $r^3$ relationship.[2] Under these conditions, measurements of flow may be less sensitive to changes in airway calibre than might be expected for Poiseuillian flow.

## 1.  Responsiveness of Airways from Different Locations in the Bronchial Tree

*In vivo* studies suggest that airway narrowing and flow may be inhomogeneous throughout the bronchial tree. Bronchial images in dogs show more narrowing at peripheral sites, than at central, in response to stimulation of the cervical vagi[4] and to intravenously administered drugs.[5,6] However, the apparent topographical differences in narrowing that are visualised from airway profiles *in vivo* could be related to the distribution of the stimulus within the bronchial tree, to the sensitivity of smooth muscle cells, or to morphological factors in airways from different locations or of different sizes. For example,

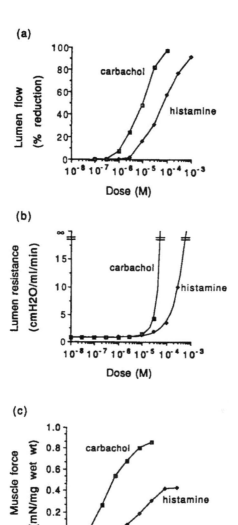

**FIGURE 2** Responsiveness of pig isolated airway preparations to carbachol and histamine. (a) Reduction in the flow of Krebs solution through the lumen of perfused 2–3-mm-i.d. bronchial segments in response to drugs added luminally. (b) Data transformed to resistance by dividing total pressure drop (system + airway) by flow. (c) Active force produced by strips of smooth muscle cells prepared from the same bronchi as in (a) and (b). (In part from Mitchell, H. W. et al., *J. Appl. Physiol.*, 66, 2704, 1989. With permission.)

the cross-sectional area of the inner airway wall (comprising the smooth muscle and the mucosa) and of the airway wall including the lumen may be of particular importance to narrowing.[20,21] The ratio of these two areas is termed the relative wall area (rWA), and it will be discussed further below.

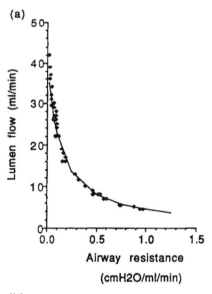

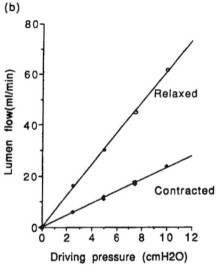

**FIGURE 3** Mechanics of fluid flow in isolated perfused bronchial segments (3 mm i.d) from the pig. (a) Data pooled from 13 bronchial segments indicating the effect of increasing airway resistance, by applying varying doses of acetylcholine, on bronchial lumen flow. Airway resistance was calculated from the pressure drop measured between the proximal and distal ends of the bronchus and from the flow measured by collecting perfusate. (b) Effect of changing the driving pressure on lumen flow. Results shown from a single experiment — first, in a relaxed bronchial segment, then after producing airway narrowing by adding a submaximal dose of acetylcholine. (From McFawn, P. K. et al., *Eur. Respir. J.*, 8, 161, 1995. With permission.)

We tested the hypothesis that airways from different locations exhibit differing responsiveness by comparing dose–flow curves of bronchial segments obtained from the peripheral (2–2.5 mm i.d.) and the central (5–6 mm i.d.) parts of the bronchial tree of the pig (Figure 4a).[2] Peripheral airways were nearly two orders of magnitude more sensitive to carbachol than were the central, and they always closed off with high doses of drug, whereas large airways did not, instead exhibiting a plateau. The difference in response between the two airways was not restricted to carbachol, but it was also seen with other bronchoconstrictor stimuli. The sensitivity shift was not caused by differences in the pharmacological responsiveness of the smooth muscle cells because the dose–response (force) curves of the proximal and the distal bronchus were the same (Figure 4b). Neither could the differences be attributed to the gross histology of the central and peripheral airway walls because the structural components — the epithelium, smooth muscle, and cartilage — are similar throughout the airways in this species.

However, in peripheral airways the inner airway wall forms a greater proportion of the total airway cross section (inner wall area/relaxed lumen area + inner wall area, i.e., rWA) than it does in central airways.[2,13] Mathematical simulations of airway narrowing suggest that the presence or absence of a plateau in the dose–resistance curve is due partly to the relative thickness of the inner wall, which upon constriction occupies the airway lumen and causes a progressive amplification of lumen narrowing, and also to the amount of smooth muscle shortening present when the airway is stimulated maximally.[9,11,12] The greater maximum flow reduction observed in perfused peripheral airways, compared with central, is consistent with the greater rWA in the smaller airways. Because the occupation of the lumen by the inner wall is progressive, the effect on responsiveness is most likely to be apparent in the upper parts of a dose–response curve, where the contraction of the smooth muscle is near maximal.

The great difference in sensitivity between large and small airways had not, however, been foreseen. There is evidence that it is due partly to differences in the permeability of the epithelium in central and peripheral airways, because the sensitivity difference was greatly reduced in airways from which the epithelium had been gently removed.[2] The importance of the epithelium in restricting drug access to the underlying smooth muscle and, therefore, on responsiveness is becoming increasingly clear.[22-25]

## B. RELATIONSHIP BETWEEN SMOOTH MUSCLE CONTRACTION AND AIRWAY NARROWING

### 1. Airway Smooth Muscle Force

How much force needs to be developed by the smooth muscle to produce airway narrowing and the reduced flow that has been described? The effect of bronchoconstrictor drugs (carbachol and histamine) on lumen flow and smooth muscle force are compared in Figure 2a and c, from which two general observations can be made.

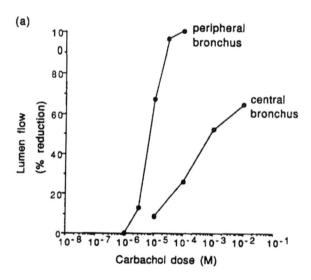

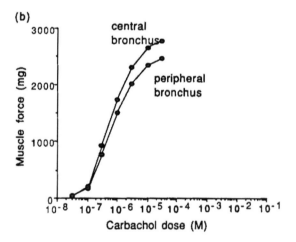

**FIGURE 4** Responsiveness of bronchi from central (5-6 mm i.d.) and peripheral (2-2.5 mm i.d.) parts of the bronchial tree of the pig. (a) Lumen flow in perfused segments of bronchus with carbachol applied to the lumen. (b) Active force produced by strips of smooth muscle from similar bronchi. (In part from Mitchell, H. W. and Sparrow, M. P., *Eur. Respir. J.*, 7, 298, 1994. With permission.)

First, the two drugs caused the same maximum effect on flow (functional airway closure), but they produced different forces in the smooth muscle, with histamine producing only half the maximum force as carbachol. This suggests that only half maximum muscle force (about 0.4 mN/mg or 0.5 kg/cm$^2$ stress[26]) is needed to effectively close off the bronchus. This finding applies to the

2–3 mm-i.d. bronchus only. There are no measurements of the stress producing the plateau observed at the top of the dose–response curve in large airways. The estimate of active muscle stress required to produce airway closure in pig perfused airways *in vitro* agrees quite closely with calculations of the stress required to produce major narrowing of airways in excised dog lungs.[27] Interestingly, the smooth muscle stress producing airway narrowing in the dog was also about one-half of the maximum stress that can be produced by canine airway smooth muscle.

A second observation from the experiments shown in Figure 2a and c was an apparent discrepancy between the sensitivity of the smooth muscle in producing force and the sensitivity of airway narrowing. For example, lower doses of carbachol were required to generate force compared with narrowing. This was expected, however, because in the intact bronchial tube the carbachol was administered only to the mucosal surface. With the establishment of a concentration gradient across the intact airway wall, the concentration at the smooth muscle would be less than that originally applied to the lumen,[25,28] leading to an apparent decrease in sensitivity.

Because the pharmacological responsiveness of smooth muscle from asthmatic airways does not appear to be different from controls, there has been a focus on possible alterations in the amount of smooth muscle or in its geometric arrangement in the airway wall. The airways of asthmatic subjects, studied post-mortem, exhibit a thickening of several components of the airway wall, including the mucosa, basement membrane, and smooth muscle.[14] It is probable that the increased muscle thickness allows more tension to be produced so that airway and parenchyma loads can be more readily overcome with more smooth muscle shortening resulting. This should increase the airway responsiveness,[29] but confirmation of this in animal models is not available.

## 2. Airway Smooth Muscle Shortening

There are no techniques described in the literature for establishing directly the effect of drug provocation on smooth muscle length in the bronchus, but morphometric techniques have permitted it to be estimated in fixed airway sections.[30] In the trachea, on the other hand, both morphometric techniques and the more direct sonomicrometry have been used to record smooth muscle length.[31] Findings in tracheal tubes and in the trachea *in situ* indicate that the smooth muscle shortens by about 30–40%[30-32] when it is stimulated. This level of smooth muscle shortening will, however, have only a minor effect on tracheal lumen diameter — i.e., 10–13% reduction assuming that the muscle band occupies about one-third of the tracheal circumference. This estimate has not been confirmed by direct measurement, but it agrees closely with calculations of lumen diameter made from the measurement of airway pressure drop in guinea pig perfused trachea.[18]

In the dog excised lung,[27] muscle shortening in response to high doses of carbachol aerosol varies widely in different airways, perhaps as a result in part

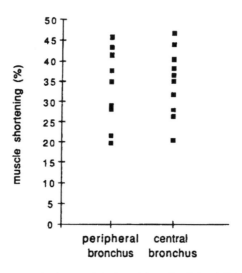

**FIGURE 5**   Muscle shortening in central (5–6 mm i.d.) and peripheral (3–4 mm i.d.) bronchial segments from pigs. Muscle shortening was induced by applying a range of submaximal to supramaximal doses of acetylcholine ($10^{-5}$ to $>5 \times 10^{-2}$ M), each to a different bronchial segment. Each airway was fixed in 4% buffered formaldehyde in the presence of acetylcholine; then it was embedded and cryosectioned for the measurement of muscle shortening using the method of morphometric reconstruction described by James et al.[30] Experiments were carried out at 5 cmH₂O transmural pressure. Muscle shortening in the contracted airway was corrected for muscle length in the relaxed airway by deducting 8% from measured values (see text for details).

of variable aerosol deposition, with maximum shortenings in some airways of as much as 60%. Smooth muscle shortening tended to be greater in large-bore airways than in small, but the mean muscle shortening for all airways was 41%. The dose of carbachol used produced an increase in total resistance of some twofold to 40-fold depending on the transpulmonary pressure. In contrast, transpulmonary pressure had very little effect on the muscle shortening, which is inconsistent with the pressure dependence of airway reactivity. In the pig airway, smooth muscle shortening was recorded in the isolated bronchus at approximately 5 cmH₂0 transmural pressure, using doses of acetylcholine from near threshold to "supramaximal" (approximately $10^{-5}$ M to $>5 \times 10^{-2}$ M; unpublished data). The muscle shortenings produced ranged from about 20 to 45% (Figure 5) and were similar in either peripheral or central bronchi. However, in neither of the above studies was there concurrent information on airway calibre or information enabling muscle shortening to be related to a physiological end point in an individual airway, such as to the top of a dose–response (flow) curve.

The morphometric technique for assessing smooth muscle length in a constricted airway relies heavily on an assumption that the smooth muscle is at its relaxed length when the lumen boundary is circular in shape — i.e., when the mucosal folds normally seen are absent. In general, however, this only occurs at high-inflation pressures. Airways studied at transmural pressures of 0–10 cmH$_2$O show that the mucosa has a folded or wrinkled appearance, even when the muscle is fully relaxed (e.g., in the presence of theophylline). By necessity, therefore, estimations of active muscle shortening produced in response to a stimulus are adjusted for the muscle length that is associated with the folded mucosa present in the relaxed state. This averaged 8% in the experiments carried out in the authors' laboratory on the pig bronchus, and it was deducted from all values of active muscle shortening. Whether or not disparities in morphometrically estimated muscle shortening described (e.g., in the dog lung[27]) are related to systematic errors is uncertain, but there is clearly a strong need for alternative, direct techniques. Sonomicrometry has been used to measure muscle length in the trachealis in large animal species,[32] but whether or not this technique might be adapted to physically smaller preparations of bronchus is uncertain.

### 3. Concurrent Measurement of Airway Lumen Narrowing by Direct Imaging and Smooth Muscle Shortening

The relationship between the shortening of the smooth muscle and the resulting narrowing of the airway is complex and nonlinear. Airway narrowing appears to be constrained by forces operating in the lung parenchyma and chest wall, and it varies at different locations and with the type of provocation used. Airway profiles obtained from lungs *in vivo* suggest that maximum narrowing to methacholine in the dog is around 50% in 2-mm airways at 20 cmH$_2$O transpulmonary pressure[5,33] and about 60% to stimulation of the vagal nerves.[4] In the pig lung at FRC, bronchograms suggest that maximum narrowing is less, about 30%.[6]

There is little experimental information on the extent of airway narrowing present in particular airways, and none that defines the relationship between smooth muscle shortening and airway narrowing. Several detailed models of this have been presented,[9-11] and their predictive value has been directed to understanding the basis of bronchial hyperresponsiveness.[12] In contrast to this theoretical approach, we sought experimental solutions by adapting fibreoptic endoscopy techniques to directly visualise the lumen of bronchial segments *in vitro* in order to study steps involved in airway narrowing.[34] Narrowing was produced either by electrical field stimulation (EFS) or by adding acetylcholine to the bath. The image of the lumen narrowing was recorded on videotape for subsequent measurement using image analysis software. At the conclusion of a run, the muscle was fixed for histological processing and estimation of muscle shortening.

At atmospheric pressure (i.e., zero transmural pressure) the lumen of 3.5-mm-i.d. bronchi narrowed promptly in response to EFS (Figure 6). With maximum stimulus parameters, the lumen diameter narrowed by about 28% diameter within 10–20 s, with relaxation as rapid. Acetylcholine produced dose-dependent narrowing, which was more gradual than EFS, taking 2–4 min for completion. Narrowing was present at transmural pressures operating in either direction across the airway wall. In absolute terms, narrowing was

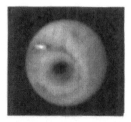 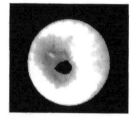 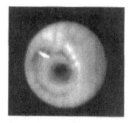

**FIGURE 6**  Lumen of a 3.5-mm-i.d. bronchial segment from a pig. The image was obtained with a fibreoptic endoscope inserted into the airway lumen. Visualisation of the margin of the lumen was aided by first applying a ring of blue dye to the mucosa. Left hand panel shows control, middle panel EFS (which produced approximately 30% lumen narrowing), and right hand panel 12 s after the end of EFS. Note the presence of mucosal folds and of a side branch.

greatest between 0 and 10 cmH₂O lumen pressure. But the resting inner diameter also increased with increasing transmural pressure, so that in percentage terms there was very little difference in response to provocation with transmural pressure.

Concurrent measurements of pig bronchial lumen narrowing and smooth muscle shortening to a range of submaximal to maximal doses of acetylcholine ($10^{-5}$–$10^{-2}$ M) is shown in Figures 7 and 8a. This dose range of acetylcholine caused the muscle to shorten by as much as 40% in individual bronchi and the lumen diameter to be more than halved. It is clear that the reduction of lumen diameter is always greater than muscle shortening. The line of best fit for the experimentally obtained points is very close to the predicted curve for airways of this inner wall area, suggesting that the airway wall encroaches on the airway lumen to restrict flow and that the airway wall behaves uniformly during narrowing.

The amount of narrowing produced by smooth muscle shortening might be influenced by the orientation of the smooth muscle layer in the bronchial wall. There is little quantitative information on this, but a recent study using imaging techniques suggests that the smooth muscle is pitched at some 30° in human airways.[35] Mathematical analysis indicates that more narrowing could be produced in an airway containing helically arranged smooth muscle,[10] and Wiggs et al.[36] commented that airway narrowing is "exaggerated" by an increased angle of spiral. But calculations also indicate that much more muscle tension is required to cause spiralled smooth muscle to shorten;[10] therefore, under conditions where smooth muscle tension is "normal," the most probable *physiological* effect of pitch is to reduce airway narrowing.

The data points obtained experimentally in the pig bronchus did not confirm the hypothesis that the muscle is pitched at 30°. Instead, the data are consistent with smooth muscle arranged very close to perpendicular to the long axis of the airway (see Figure 7). It is possible that there are important species differences, and more studies are needed to assess muscle orientation before a conclusion on its significance to bronchial responsiveness can be formed.

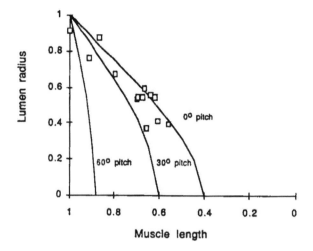

**FIGURE 7** Effect of muscle shortening on narrowing of the pig bronchial lumen. Data points were obtained from experiments in which the lumen radius was imaged with an endoscope connected to a video camera and the muscle shortening was estimated morphometrically. Each point is from one bronchial segment stimulated with a dose of acetylcholine in the submaximal to maximal range ($10^{-5}$ to $10^{-2}$ M). Lines show a predicted relationship between muscle shortening and lumen radius for the bronchi used; these were 3.5 mm resting lumen i.d., able to narrow, but having a fixed length of 20 mm and an rWA of 0.17. The pitch of the smooth muscle used in the calculation was 0°, 30°, or 60° from perpendicular. The experimental data best fitted a predicted relationship for airways in which the smooth muscle was perpendicular to the long axis. (Data adapted from Mitchell, H. W. and Sparrow, M. P., *Eur. Respir. J.*, 7, 1317, 1994.)

## 4. Airway Closure — Smooth Muscle Shortening and Lumen Narrowing

High doses of acetylcholine ($10^{-3}$–$10^{-2}$ M) caused a cessation of lumen flow in the perfused bronchial segments discussed above — that is, "functional" airway closure[2,34] (e.g., similar to that obtained to carbachol shown in Figure 2a). Direct imaging of the lumen of airways subjected to these high doses of drug showed that the lumen was reduced in diameter by 48%, or by 68% cross-sectional area. The muscle shortening which produced these effects was between 30 and 40%[34] (see Figures 7 and 8a). Yet, a calculation of airway narrowing in this size airway (3.5 mm i.d.) indicates that much more smooth muscle shortening is needed to eliminate the lumen. For example, extrapolation of the plot shown in Figure 8a indicates that the lumen will be closed off only when the muscle shortens by 59%, much more than the shortening actually associated with the cessation of flow in the experimental system. Since the halving of the lumen of the perfused airway caused the flow to be stopped (an observation reasonably consistent with a predicted effect where flow is proportional to the fourth power of the radius), further contraction of the smooth muscle and airway narrowing are probably unimportant.

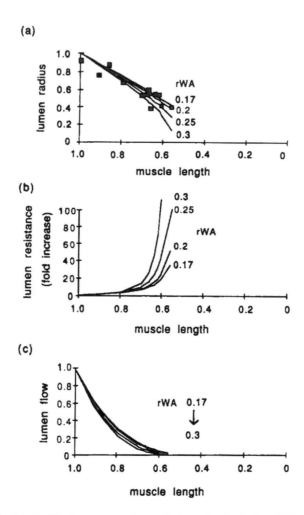

**FIGURE 8** Relationship between smooth muscle shortening in pig bronchial segments and lumen narrowing. Experimental data points shown in panel (a) are those shown in Figure 7. The predicted effect of muscle shortening measured experimentally on (a) lumen radius, (b) lumen resistance, and (c) lumen flow were calculated for bronchi with an rWA of 0.17, 0.20, 0.25, and 0.30. The actual rWA of the bronchus was 0.17.

## III. IMPLICATIONS OF EXPERIMENTAL FINDINGS ON ISOLATED BRONCHI FOR AIRWAY WALL RESTRUCTURING AND BRONCHIAL HYPERRESPONSIVENESS

In the foregoing, several structural properties of the airway wall that could contribute to bronchial hyperresponsiveness have been discussed. These include the thickness of the mucosal layers and the smooth muscle, the arrangement of the smooth muscle band in the airway wall, and the geometry of the airway lumen. The proposal[9,11-13,21] that airway wall thickening might cause hyperresponsiveness was based primarily on mathematical simulations of airway narrowing which showed that airway resistance was increased markedly when the rWA was increased. In hypertension, a thickening of the vessel wall had been proposed to be involved in raising total peripheral resistance and blood pressure.[37]

The influence of airway wall thickening on bronchial responsiveness is considered in detail elsewhere in this book. However, it will also be considered briefly here because our *in vitro* measurements in isolated bronchi may allow the influence of the inner wall to be further assessed.

We have used the actual inner wall and lumen dimensions of perfused bronchial segments and the measured values of muscle shortening to project an effect of rWA on airway narrowing, resistance, and flow using the equations of Moreno et al.[9] and Wiggs et al.[11] The data points in Figure 8a show the effect of muscle shortening on lumen diameter, as measured in our experiments. Superimposed are plots indicating the predicted relationship and the effect of different rWA. The effect of increasing rWA on lumen narrowing is most apparent in the upper regions of the plot, where muscle shortening approaches near maximum levels of 30 to 40%. These data were then transformed to resistance ($R = 1/r^4$) and to flow ($F = r^4$) in Figure 8b and c. The effect of increased rWA on resistance seems impressive but, again, only when the plot is extended to towards maximum contraction of the smooth muscle. The physiologically important parameter of flow shows very little dependence on these changes in rWA. When the resistance vs. muscle shortening curves for different rWAs begin to diverge, flow has already fallen by 90% and the physiological significance of additional narrowing brought about by increasing the rWA is somewhat questionable.

The effect of hypertrophy of the smooth muscle on flow has not been established, but its effect on resistance might be similar to the effect of wall area described above because it may produce an increase in the maximum resistance at the top of a dose–response curve.[29] However, there is also a predicted increase in the sensitivity of airway narrowing, which is of importance because the flows at submaximum levels of airway activation are probably more relevant to lung function than maximum changes. It may be possible to test this experimentally by combining isolated airway techniques with animal models of lung inflammation and hyperresponsiveness.

Findings in individual airways *in vitro* show that there is no single responsiveness in the lung, but rather responsiveness varies from one part of the bronchial tree to the next (see Figure 4a). This can be attributed to airway morphology and size. These findings indicate the importance of the site(s) of drug deposition in provocation tests on the responsiveness measured at the mouth. They also indicate the potential magnitude of hyperresponsiveness that could be produced by a process involving airway wall restructuring and the importance of the location(s) at which such changes take place.

Investigations into airway narrowing *in vitro* are still in their infancy. Most notable is a lack of information that defines relationships between smooth muscle shortening and lumen flow. These are necessary before current hypotheses about the relative importance of wall factors and smooth muscle shortening on responsiveness and hyperresponsiveness can be tested.

## ACKNOWLEGMENTS

Work in the authors' laboratory was supported by the National Health and Medical Research Council of Australia, the Australian Research Council, and the National SIDS Council of Australia.

## REFERENCES

1. Omari, T. I., Mitchell, H. W., and Sparrow, M. P., Epithelial damage and responsiveness of bronchial segments, *Clin. Exp. Pharmacol. Physiol.*, 18 (Suppl.), 47, 1991.
2. Mitchell, H. W. and Sparrow, M. P., Increased responsiveness to cholinergic stimulation of small compared to large diameter cartilaginous bronchi, *Eur. Respir. J.*, 7, 298, 1994.
3. Vincenc, K. S., Black, J. L., Yan, K., Armour, C. L., Donnelly, P. D., and Woolcock, A. J., Comparison of *in vivo* and *in vitro* responses to histamine in human airways, *Am. Rev. Respir. Dis.*, 128, 875, 1983.
4. Cabezas, G. A., Graf, P. D., and Nadel, J. A., Sympathetic vs. parasympathetic nervous regulation of airways in dogs, *J. Appl. Physiol.*, 3, 651, 1971.
5. Shioya, T., Solway, J., Munoz, N. M., Mack, M., and Leff, A. R., Distribution of airway contractile responses within the major diameter bronchi during exogenous bronchoconstriction, *Am. Rev. Respir. Dis.*, 135, 1105, 1987.
6. Murphy, T. M., Roy, L., Phillips, I. J., Mitchell, R. W., Kelly, E. A., Munoz, N. M., and Leff, A. R., Effect of maturation on topographic distribution of bronchoconstrictor responses in large diameter airway of young swine, *Am. Rev. Respir. Dis.*, 143, 126, 1991.
7. McNamara, A. E., Muller, N. L., Okazawa, M., Arntorp, J., Wiggs, B. R., and Pare, P. D., Airway narrowing in excised canine lungs measured by high-resolution computed tomography, *J. Appl. Physiol.*, 73, 307, 1992.
8. Brown, R. H., Herold, C. J., Hirshman, C. A., Zerhouni, E. A., and Mitzner, W., *In vivo* measurements of airway reactivity using high-resolution computed tomography, *Am. Rev. Respir. Dis.*, 144, 208, 1991.
9. Moreno, R. H., Hogg, J. C., and Pare, P. D., Mechanics of airway narrowing, *Am. Rev. Respir. Dis.*, 133, 1171, 1986.
10. Bates, J. H. T. and Martin, J. G., A theoretical study of the effect of airway smooth muscle orientation on bronchoconstriction, *J. Appl. Physiol.*, 69, 995, 1990.
11. Wiggs, B. R., Moreno, R., Hogg, J. C., Hilliam, C., and Pare, P. D., A model of the mechanics of airway narrowing, *J. Appl. Physiol.*, 69, 849, 1990.
12. Wiggs, B. R., Bosken, C., Pare, P. D., James, A. L., and Hogg, J. C., A model of airway narrowing in asthmatic and in chronic obstructive pulmonary disease, *Am. Rev. Respir. Dis.*, 145, 1251, 1992.
13. James, A. L., Pare, P. D., and Hogg, J. C., The mechanics of airway narrowing in asthma, *Am. Rev. Respir. Dis.*, 139, 242, 1989.

14. Carroll, N., Elliot, J., Morton, A., and James, A., The structure of large and small airways in nonfatal and fatal asthma, *Am. Rev. Respir. Dis.*, 147, 405, 1993.

15. Woolcock, A. J., Salome, C. M., and Yan, K., The shape of the dose–response curve to histamine in asthmatic and normal subjects, *Am. Rev. Respir. Dis.*, 130, 71, 1984.

16. Mitchell, H. W., Willet, K. E., and Sparrow, M. P., Perfused bronchial segment and bronchial strip: narrowing vs. isometric force by mediators, *J. Appl. Physiol.*, 66, 2704, 1989.

17. Hulsmann, A. R., Raatgeep, H. R., Bonta, I. L., Stijnen, T., Kerrebijin, K. F., and Dejongste, J. C., The perfused human bronchiolar tube characteristics of new model, *J. Pharmacol. Toxicol. Methods*, 28, 29, 1992.

18. Munakata, M., Huang, I., Mitzner, W., and Menkes, H., Protective role of epithelium in the guinea pig airway, *J. Appl. Physiol.*, 66, 1547, 1989.

19. Yager, D., Butler, J. P., Bastacky, J., and Israel, E., Amplification of airway constriction due to liquid filling of airway interstices, *J. Appl. Physiol.*, 66, 2873, 1989.

20. Freedman, B. J., The functional geometry of the bronchi, *Bull. Pathophysiol. Resp.*, 8, 545, 1972.

21. Ariens, E. J., Pharmacology of airway smooth muscle, in *Bronchial Hyperresponsiveness: Normal and Abnormal Control, Assessment and Therapy*, Nadel, J. A., Pauwels, R., and Snashall, P. D., Eds., Blackwell Publications, London, 1987, 7.

22. Sparrow, M. P. and Mitchell, H. W., Modulation by the epithelium of the extent of bronchial narrowing produced by substances perfused through the lumen, *Br. J. Pharmacol.*, 103, 1160, 1991.

23. Small, R. C., Good, D. M., Dixon, J. S., and Kennedy, J., The effect of epithelial removal on the actions of cholinomimetic drugs in open segments and perfused tubular preparations of guinea-pig trachea, *Br. J. Pharmacol.*, 100, 516, 1990.

24. Barnes, P. J., Epithelium acts as a modulator and a diffusion barrier in the responses of canine airway smooth muscle, *J. Appl. Physiol.*, 76, 1841, 1994.

25. Omari, T. I., Mitchell, H.W., and Sparrow, M.P., The epithelial barrier and airway responsiveness, *Can. J. Physiol. Pharmacol.*, 73, 180, 1995.

26. Sparrow, M. P. and Mitchell, H. W., Contraction of smooth muscle of pig airway tissues from before birth to maturity, *J. Appl. Physiol.*, 68, 468, 1990.

27. Okazawa, M., Bai, T. R., Wiggs, B. R., and Pare, P. D., Airway smooth muscle shortening in excised canine lung lobes, *J. Appl. Physiol.*, 74, 1613, 1993.

28. Munakata, M. and Mitzner, W., The protective role of the airway epithelium, in *The Airway Epithelium, Physiology, Pathophysiology, and Pharmacology (Lung Biology in Health and Disease)*, 55, Farmer, S. J. and Hay, D. W., Eds., Marcel Dekker, New York, 1991, 545.

29. Lambert, R. K., Wiggs, B. R., Kuwano, K., Hogg, J. C., and Pare, P. D., Functional significance of increased airway smooth muscle in asthma and COPD, *J. Appl. Physiol.*, 74, 2771, 1993.

30. James, A. L., Hogg, J. C., Dunn, L. A., and Pare, P. D., The use of the internal perimeter to compare airway size and to calculate smooth muscle shortening, *Am. J. Respir. Dis.*, 138, 136, 1988.

31. Okazawa, M., Ishida, K., Road, J., Schellenberg, R. R., and Pare, P. D., *In vivo* and *in vitro* correlation of trachealis muscle contraction in dogs, *J. Appl. Physiol.*, 73, 1486, 1992.

32. James, A. L., Pare, P. D., Moreno, R. H., and Hogg, J. C., Quantitative measurement of smooth muscle shortening in isolated pig trachea, *J. Appl. Physiol.*, 63, 1360, 1987.

33. Shioya, T., Munoz, N. M., and Leff, A. R., Effect of resting smooth muscle length on contractile response in resistance airways, *J. Appl. Physiol.*, 62, 711, 1987.

34. Mitchell, H. W. and Sparrow, M. P., Video-imaging of lumen narrowing: muscle shortening and flow responsiveness in isolated bronchial segments of the pig, *Eur. Respir. J.*, 7, 1317, 1994.

35. Ebina, M., Yaegashi, H., Takashi, T., Motomiya, M., and Tanemura, M., Distribution of smooth muscles along the bronchial tree: a morphometric study of ordinary autopsy lungs, *Am. Rev. Respir. Dis.*, 141, 1322, 1990.

36. Wiggs, B., Moreno, R., James, A. L., Hogg, J. C., and Pare, P. D., A model of the mechanics of airway narrowing in asthma, in *Asthma, Its Pathology and Treatment*, Kaliner, M. A., Barnes, P. J., and Persson, C. G. A., Eds., Marcel Dekker, New York, 1991, 73.
37. Folkow, B., The haemodynamic consequencs of adaptive structural changes of the resistance vessels in hypertension, *Clin. Sci.*, 41, 1, 1971.
38. McFawn, P. K., Sparrow, M. P. and Mitchell, H. W., Measurement of flow through perfused bronchial segments: optimisation of flow head resistance, *Eur. Respir. J.*, 8, 161, 1995.

Chapter 9

# ASSESSMENT OF AIRWAY SMOOTH MUSCLE GROWTH AND DIVISION: *IN VITRO* STUDIES

Stuart J. Hirst

## CONTENTS

0-8493-7813-3/97/$0.00+$.50
© 1997 by CRC Press, Inc.

# I. INTRODUCTION

Asthma is a chronic inflammatory disorder in which many different cell types contribute by releasing proinflammatory mediators, growth factors, and cytokines, which in turn activate several target cells within the airway. In acute and delayed-onset asthma, this cacophony of inflammatory events results in airway narrowing because of bronchoconstriction, microvascular leakage and airway wall oedema, mucus hypersecretion and plugging, basement membrane thickening due to collagen deposition, and stimulation of neural reflexes.[1] Inflammation is also believed to play a central role in the development of persistent nonspecific bronchial hyperresponsiveness[1,2] associated with more chronic and severe forms of asthma, particularly fatal asthma, in which there is also increased airway smooth muscle mass, a key pathological finding contributing to the substantial airway wall thickening found in these patients.[3-6]

Data from clinical studies suggest patients with persistent severe asthma develop irreversible airflow obstruction that is refractory to current bronchodilator and anti-inflammatory strategies.[7,8] This implies a persistent component to the long-term pathology of asthma which may involve remodelling or architectural changes to the airway wall. Recently, Hogg and colleagues[9-11] have hypothesised that nonspecific bronchial hyperresponsiveness can be explained by any process which results in a net geometric thickening of the airway wall. Furthermore, studies using detailed computer models of human airways indicate that increased airway smooth muscle mass is by far the most important abnormality responsible for excessive airway narrowing and compliance of the airway wall in asthma.[12,13] Both hyperplastic (i.e., increases in cell number) and hypertrophic (i.e., increases in cell size) changes contribute to the increased smooth muscle content of the airway wall.[14] The development of suitable methods able to discriminate between these different mechanisms of airway smooth muscle thickening is a prerequisite to understanding the cellular and biochemical events which regulate accelerated growth *and* division of these cells and is fundamental to the design of therapies aimed at preventing or reversing airway wall structural abnormalities contributing to irreversible or poorly reversible airway obstruction. This chapter reviews some of the methods which can be applied to quantitate growth and division of airway smooth muscle *in vitro*. It will focus particularly on methods for the successful maintenance and characterisation of these cells in culture, and also on the techniques which have been used to quantitate growth and division in other cell systems, as well as airway smooth muscle. It is hoped that this critical overview will benefit both new and existing investigators in this rapidly developing area of respiratory research.

# II. AIRWAY SMOOTH MUSCLE THICKENING

Although bronchial smooth muscle thickening is a well-documented pathological feature of the airways of patients with persistent severe asthma, there are only a handful of reports in the literature identifying its anatomic site and the extent to which hyperplasia and hypertrophy contribute to the increase in muscle mass. The techniques available for quantifying this muscle thickening can loosely be divided into *in situ* studies involving morphometric analysis of the bronchial tree from normal and asthmatic patients[3-6] and studies employing cell culture techniques,[15-18] as an *in vitro* model of the smooth muscle present in the airway wall.

## A. MORPHOMETRIC ANALYSIS

Several early studies have quantified bronchial smooth muscle thickening in obstructive airway disease by projecting the image of stained (usually with haematoxylin and eosin), semiserial sections of bronchus onto a screen with a point-counting grid already drawn on it.[3-5] Areas of the image positively identified as smooth muscle were counted, and this process then repeated for each histological section allowing a profile of smooth muscle thickening to be constructed over several hundred serial sections.

The results of these initial studies, however, have done little other than to confirm the existence of smooth muscle thickening in the asthmatic airway, although in one study by Heard and Hossain[4] the nuclei of muscle cells were also counted, and the number was found to correlate well with the increase in muscle area, suggesting that the thickening in asthma was due more to hyperplasia rather than to hypertrophy.

In recent studies using a more refined three-dimensional morphometric approach,[9-11,14] the image was projected onto a computer-assisted graphics tablet or a digital image analyser allowing the bronchial cross-section image to be "stretched" into a uniform circle without changing the overall perimeter of the basement membrane of the section or the overall sectional area of the muscle. This has the advantage, unlike the previous techniques, of standardising the airway, thereby reducing the difficulty in assessing muscle thickening in sections in which the state of muscle contraction is unknown (contracted muscle might show an apparent thickening over relaxed muscle).[6,11,14] Results of these latter studies confirm the presence of airway smooth muscle thickening in asthma, particularly in larger bronchi. Ebina et al.[6] reported initially that asthmatic subjects exhibited thickening throughout the entire range of the bronchial tree including the smaller airways, believed to be the site of immunologically released mediators and growth factors.[1,2,19] In a subsequent study, these authors reported at least two patterns of smooth muscle thickening in asthmatic lung.[14] In "type I" asthma the increase in muscle area was associated with hyperplasia of airway smooth muscle cells and was restricted to the large central airways. No hypertrophy was recorded at any level of the bronchial tree in these patients. In type II asthma however, in addition to the presence of comparatively mild hyperplasia in the larger airways, hypertrophy of airway smooth muscle cells was detected throughout the whole bronchial tree, but was particularly severe in small peripheral airways. These apparently different patterns of airway wall thickening may reflect differing pathogeneses in asthma, but their clinical correlates are unknown. A more detailed account of morphometry and its application to the development of *in vivo* models of airway smooth muscle thickening is discussed in Chapters 1 and 7.

## B. CELL CULTURE

Although morphometric analysis undoubtedly provides valuable information about the anatomic site and severity of airway wall thickening in asthma, it is a cumbersome and labourious technique which makes the direct investigation of controlled exposure of the smooth muscle layers to mitogenic stimuli difficult. Similarly, *ex vivo* airway smooth muscle preparations, which have limited viability under noncultured conditions, make studies of long-term regulation of the airways, such as proliferative changes, extremely difficult to perform. The technique of cell culture, however, offers a more powerful and exacting approach to understanding the cellular and molecular mechanisms of airway smooth muscle growth and division. Indeed, this *in vitro* technique has been exploited heavily in recent years for the study of other proliferative disorders, such as cancer and atherosclerosis. Cell culture has the obvious advantage of allowing longer-term studies on regulation of airway smooth muscle growth and division in response to defined stimuli, which would be otherwise impossible. It can also overcome the problem of obtaining adequate amounts of normal tissue from human airways; the majority of tissue obtained from surgery is often diseased.

## III. AIRWAY SMOOTH MUSCLE IN CULTURE

Despite widespread use of cultured vascular smooth muscle,[20,21] experience in the cultivation of smooth muscle from the airway wall was until recently much more limited. This probably stems from concern about the validity of such a preparation for use in pharmacological studies as a relevant model of the intact tissue[22] and about whether or not the morphological features of such cells in culture are shared with connective tissue cells, such as fibroblasts or other nonmuscle cells.[23] This is compounded by modulations in phenotype which may result in the loss of critical features of the differentiated cell. However, with the increasing realisation of the role of smooth muscle in airway wall thickening and subsequent development of bronchial hyperresponsiveness, various groups have succeeded in culturing airway smooth muscle cells from a number of species, such as canine,[15,16,24,25] bovine,[26-28] rabbit,[29-31] guinea pig,[32,33] sheep,[34] and human.[17,18,35-38] Although many of these initial concerns have been largely overcome, it remains essential to characterise fully the properties of these cells and to make comparisons where possible with the intact tissue.

## A. CULTIVATION

There are essentially three methods which have been employed for successfully establishing and maintaining airway smooth muscle cells in culture.

These are enzymatic dispersion of smooth muscle cells from tracheobronchial muscle, explant culture from cubes of muscle cut from the intact tissue, and subculture passaging.

Enzymatic dispersion is the technique adopted by most investigators to obtain primary cultures of airway smooth muscle cells from a carefully dissected preparation of large or small airway.[15,17] This method is used to obtain isolated smooth muscle cells in a morphologically well-differentiated and contractile state,[20,21] where the immediate cellular environment may be rigorously controlled, especially when determining the effects of soluble or insoluble factors on cellular phenotype (see Section III.C). Alternatively, small explants of dissected smooth muscle can be used to generate primary cultures.[36,37] Cells from explant culture, however, inherently must undergo many more population doublings in order to migrate out from the explant and proliferate throughout the culture dish. Although no systematic study has been carried out, cells from explants may be less contractile, as has been reported for vascular smooth muscle cultures.[21] Whether this makes explant cultures more or less suitable for studies of airway smooth muscle remodelling has not been debated, but considerations such as these may be appropriate when considering the type of study intended. A detailed description of both these protocols for establishing airway smooth muscle cells in primary culture appears in Table 1.

Once the cells are established in culture and have grown to confluence, they can be removed from their growth support, either by scraping or by treatment with trypsin in a low calcium and magnesium ion buffer, reseeded at a subconfluent cell density, and allowed to proliferate once again. This process of subculture passaging can be repeated several times to generate larger numbers of cells, which are often necessary for biochemical assays and molecular biology, over a period of several months. A more detailed account of these culture methods can also be found in Campbell and Campbell.[21]

Success in obtaining viable primary cultures of airway smooth muscle cells is critically dependent on two factors. These are the time elapsed from excision of the tissue to its culture and the care taken in dissection to obtain smooth muscle which is not contaminated by unwanted connective tissue, cartilage, or overlying epithelium and submucosa. Human tissue is available from heart–lung transplant recipients, at post-mortem,[18,36] or at thoracotomy.[17,29,35,38] Transplant tissue probably offers the best, but least accessible, source of human tissue since large amounts of sterile and relatively nonhypoxic smooth muscle can be obtained. The amount of tissue which can be obtained from thoracotomy, however, is often very limited and is usually only available immediately distal to the resection margin, where there is a risk of removing malignant or transformed tissue. Whether or not the patient has been exposed to radiotherapy during treatment should also be considered when obtaining tissue from the operating theatre for culture. Thoracotomy specimens do, however, offer an immediate and relatively frequent source of sterile and nonhypoxic tissue. Tissue obtained at post-mortem is often aseptically compromised and may not

## TABLE 1

**Example of the Methodology Used in Our Laboratory to Establish Human and Rabbit Airway Smooth Muscle Cells in Primary Culture**

Collect tissue (i.e., small ring of human bronchus, 5–10 mm diameter, or rabbit trachea) in sterile Hanks' buffered salt solution (HBSS). Wash tissue 4–5 times in 15–20 ml HBSS containing antibiotics (gentamicin 50 µg/ml, or penicillin G 100 U/ml and streptomycin 100 µg/ml) and an antifungal agent (amphotericin B 1.5 µg/ml). Inclusion of antimicrobial agents is optional at this stage and is dependent on the conditions at tissue collection.

In the laminar flow hood, using sterile instruments and dissecting tray, carefully remove any adherent connective tissue from the adventitial surface. Remove the airway epithelium by firm scraping across the luminal surface with a rounded scalpel blade. Smooth muscle can then be cut away from the remaining cartilage. Dissection under a dissecting microscope is critical to obtaining relatively homogeneous preparations of trachealis or bronchial muscle.

Explant cultures can be established at this stage by placing small cubes (approximately $2 \times 2 \times 2$ mm) of smooth muscle directly into prewetted culture flasks or dishes, and then covering in a minimal volume of Dulbecco's modified Eagle's medium (DMEM) supplemented with foetal calf serum (10% w/v), sodium pyruvate (1 mM), L-glutamate (2 mM), nonessential amino acids (1×) and antimicrobial agents (as above). For the first 3–4 days add sufficient media to just cover the tissue fragments. This ensures their attachment to the growth support.

Alternatively for dissociated cells, dissected smooth muscle can be placed in HBSS containing 10 mg/ml bovine serum albumin and the enzymes collagenase (type XI, 1 mg/ml) and elastase (type I, 3.3 U/ml) at 37°C in 5% $CO_2$/air (i.e., in the incubator) for 30 min, pH 7.4. With the aid of a dissecting microscope, any remaining unwanted connective tissue can be teased away from the smooth muscle. Tissue can then be finely chopped into 1 mm$^2$ fragments and returned to the incubator for 150 min in an identical enzyme solution, except that the elastase content is increased from 3.3 U/ml to 15 U/ml to aid complete dissociation. After centrifugation (100 g, 5 min at 22°C) and washing in DMEM containing 10% FCS, supplemented as above, cells are resuspended at approximately 50,000/dish and returned to a 5% $CO_2$/air humidified incubator, maintained at 37°C. Cells usually adhere to the growth support after 6–18 h. Replace culture medium initially after 4 or 5 days and then every 3 or 4 days. At confluence (usually 5 to 7 days for rabbit and 10 to 14 days for human), cells can be passaged by scraping or by trypsin using standard cell culture techniques.

The purity of primary cultures and subsequent passages should be monitored at increasing confluence under the light microscope and by immunodetection of contractile proteins.

be available until 24 to 48 h after death. Significant autolysis occurs at this time. Given the correct conditions, however, human airway smooth muscle cells can be successfully cultured using tissue from any of these sources.[17,18,29,35,36,38]

The problems most frequently encountered in preparing and maintaining primary cultures of airway smooth muscle cells relate to microbial infection of the tissue prior to culture and contamination of primary cultures with other, nonmuscle cell types. Infection can be overcome by collecting tissue in sterile buffered salt solution containing antimicrobial and antifungal agents, followed by extensive washing in fresh buffer, together with meticulous aseptic technique (see Table 1). Contamination of primary cultures of airway smooth muscle cells by nonmuscle cell types can be more troublesome and should always be borne in mind when interpreting data. The most frequently reported cell contaminants are airway epithelial cells, microvascular and lymphatic endothelial cells, and fibroblasts.[15,16] Epithelial and endothelial cells, both cobblestone in appearance, tend not to survive after a few days in culture and are invariably lost following passaging from primary culture[16] (Hirst, unpublished observations). Fibroblast contamination represents a much more difficult problem since these cells cannot be readily morphologically distinguished from smooth muscle cells, particularly at low cell densities. For this reason, it is essential to assess the morphology, expression of contractile proteins, and pharmacology of airway smooth muscle cells in culture, although this is made more difficult by the phenotype plasticity of these cells.

## B. CHARACTERISTICS IN CULTURE

Airway smooth muscle cells in culture possess a number of specific features recognised as characteristic of smooth muscle cells in general when in culture,[20,21] and which relate them to the intact tissue.[15,16,18,35,39]

### 1. Light Microscopy

Under the light microscope, smooth muscle cells of tracheal or bronchial origin appear flattened and ribbon- or spindle-shaped with phase-dense cytoplasm, central oval nuclei with prominent nucleoli, and dendritic cytoplasmic processes (Figure 1A); thereby displaying features reminiscent of differentiated contractile smooth muscle cells in the intact tissue.[15,16] Confluent airway smooth muscle cells, like those of vascular origin, appear aligned in parallel so that the broad nuclear region of one cell lies adjacent to the thin cytoplasmic area of another, forming a highly contoured architecture of ridges and nodules, giving a characteristic "hill and valley" appearance (Figure 1B), a property not shared by contaminating fibroblasts or other nonmuscle cells.[20,21]

### 2. Electron Microscopy

Ultrastructural examination of near-confluent cultured tracheobronchial smooth muscle cells of either human or animal origin shows that these cells form multiple layers in which the characteristic elongated spindle shape can clearly be seen. The cells appear flattened with numerous cytoplasmic processes and an elongated oval nucleus containing little or no heterochromatin, characteristic of cells during transcription and division, while in the cytoplasm organelles associated with the synthetic phenotype predominate[16,39] (Figure 1C). Examination at higher power confirms the synthetic nature of these cells and reveals detail of the nuclear envelope. The cytoplasm contains mitochondria, highly developed Golgi cisternae, and numerous profiles of rough endoplasmic reticulum (Figure 1C and D), which are frequently associated with dilated cisternae[39] (see Figure 1C). Myofilaments are rarely seen in synthetic smooth muscle cells during proliferation, but are present when the contractile phenotype is expressed.[20,22] Tom-Moy et al.[16] have reported similar observations under the electron microscope in tracheal smooth muscle cells cultured from adult dogs. As in vascular smooth muscle cell culture, the relative quantitative expression of many of these cytoplasmic structures in human

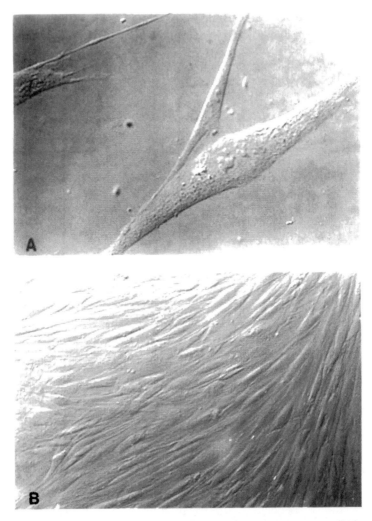

**FIGURE 1**   Typical appearance of (A) subconfluent and (B) confluent human bronchial smooth muscle cells in culture viewed under the light microscope using high (×400) and low (×100) power Nomarski differential interference photomicrography. Central oval nuclei with prominent nucleoli as well as the characteristic hill and valley architecture are clearly visible. Conventional transmission electron micrographs reveal the ultrastructural detail of these cells. Characteristic elongated nuclei (n), as well as cytoplasmic structures, such as mitochondria (m), rough endoplasmic reticulum (rer), and dilated cisternae (c), are all clearly visible in synthetic phenotype proliferating cells at low power (C), bar = 2 μm. At higher power (D) in proliferating cells, details of mitochondria (m), stacked Golgi cisternae (gc), and profiles of rough endoplasmic reticulum (rer) are seen, bar = 1 μm (electron micrographs courtesy of A. Warley). Epifluorescence indirect immunostaining (×150) of smooth muscle–specific contractile proteins reveals the presence of (E) actin- and (F) myosin-reactive longitudinally running parallel fibres in confluent human airway smooth muscle cells. (From Hirst, S. J., *Eur. Resp. J.,* **9,** 808, 1996.)

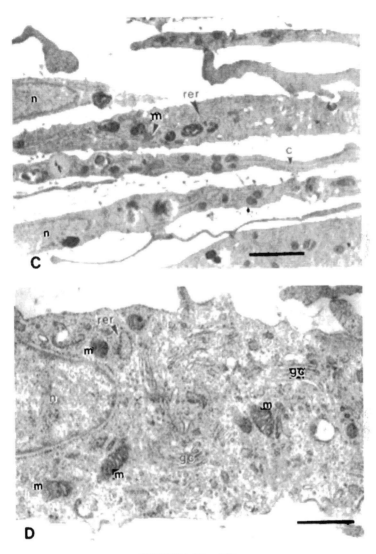

FIGURE 1 (C and D).

and rabbit airway smooth muscle, and probably other species, may be critically dependent upon cell phenotype (see Section III.C) and culture conditions.[40]

## 3. Contractile Protein Staining

Nonmuscle contaminants, such as epithelial or connective tissue cells (usually fibroblasts), can clearly be distinguished from smooth muscle cells using indirect immunofluorescent antibody-staining techniques. Although fibroblasts in culture will weakly stain positively for the contractile protein

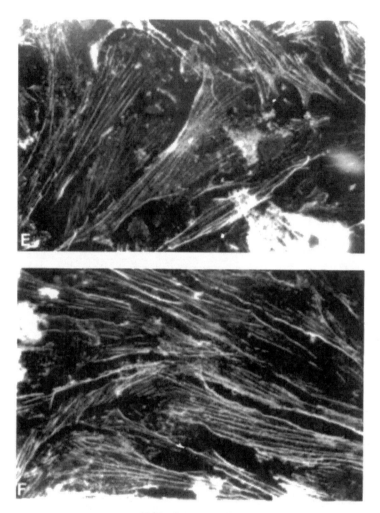

**FIGURE 1 (E and F).**

actin, it is generally accepted that only smooth muscle cells, when quiescent, will stain for *both* actin and myosin using smooth muscle–specific antibodies.[20,21] An example of antiactin and antimyosin immunostaining in confluent human bronchial smooth muscle cells is shown in Figure 1. The pattern of staining in the cytoplasm of cultured airway smooth muscle cells for both actin and myosin reveals filamentous contractile proteins arranged in parallel to the long axis of the cells, resembling the stress fibres occasionally seen by low-power electron microscopy.[20] In fibroblasts, antiactin antibodies often reveal only diffuse cytoplasmic staining.[41] This staining technique alone is particularly useful for screening whole cultures for checks of homogeneity and purity.[16,20] The intensity of contractile protein immunostaining, particularly smooth muscle–specific myosin, declines in late passage[18] (Hirst, unpublished observations), although the total amount of actin and myosin, as in vascular smooth muscle, probably remains relatively unchanged because of the accumulation of nonmuscle isoforms. This phenomenon is well documented in cultured vascular smooth muscle cells[20,21,42] and is discussed in Section III.C.

## 4. Pharmacology

One of the main problems still encountered with culture of airway smooth muscle cells is both a loss of receptors in primary culture and a gradual decline in responses during subsequent passages, due probably to modulations in phenotype during culture.[16,18,20] Twort and van Breemen[17,35] and Panettieri et al.,[18] however, have reported the development of apparently nontransformed lines of human airway smooth muscle cells which are relatively stable in culture over many population doublings. These cells retained smooth muscle–specific contractile protein expression (using indirect immunofluorescent staining) and their physiological responsiveness to agonists implicated in inflammatory airway diseases, such as histamine, leukotrienes, bradykinin, platelet-activating factor, substance P, thromboxane analogues, and carbachol.[18,35] Functional coupling of $\beta_2$-adrenergic receptors has also been demonstrated in explant[36,37] and enzyme-dissociated[38] primary cultures of human airway smooth muscle cells. Recent studies have demonstrated that airway smooth muscle cells cultured from a variety of species in addition to human also retain many other functionally coupled receptors, although there are some differences in the receptors expressed in cultured cells compared with the intact muscle or freshly dispersed cell. Widdop et al.,[43] for example, have recently reported that, although cultured and acutely dissociated human airway smooth muscle cells both express functional $M_2$ and $M_3$ muscarinic cholinergic receptors, expression of $M_3$ receptors is much less in the cultured cells, confirming a preliminary report by Mak et al.[44] Attempts to upregulate this receptor by Widdop et al. were unsuccessful. Other functionally coupled receptors expressed in cultures of airway smooth muscle include histamine $H_1$[45] and $H_2$,[46] bradykinin $B_2$[26,33,47] and $B_3$,[34] endothelin $ET_A$ (Hirst, unpublished),[48,49] 5-hydroxytryptamine 5-$HT_2$,[50] and platelet-derived growth factor type $\alpha$- and $\beta$-receptors.[51] Obviously, cultured airway smooth muscle cells are responsive to many other agonists, but direct evidence implicating the appropriate receptor(s) for each agonist is not always available.

Recent work in our own laboratory and by others suggests that, as well as receptors, smooth muscle cells cultured from rabbit trachealis and human small bronchus also continue to express ion channels, particularly from the voltage-gated potassium channel family.[52] They appear to share many of the biophysical and pharmacological properties of the channels present in acutely dissociated cells from intact tissue and are conserved even during late passage (Snetkov and Hirst, unpublished observations), suggesting that these cells in culture could represent a useful experimental system for examining the expression and behaviour of ion channels in the airways, although the culture conditions should be rigorously defined, since the nature of these channels may be influenced by the proliferative state.[53]

## C. CONTRACTION AND PHENOTYPIC MODULATION
IN CULTURE

The ability of smooth muscle cells in culture to contract or relax in response to specific agonists is well documented.[20,21] Airway smooth muscle cells in culture are no exception to this. Avner et al.[15] reported that subconfluent primary cultures of canine tracheal smooth muscle cells contracted in response to the cholinomimetic carbachol. Contraction, however, in cultured smooth muscle cells is dependent upon a number of carefully defined culture conditions.

Smooth muscle which is enzyme dissociated into single cells and seeded into primary culture attaches and flattens on the culture substratum within 24–48 h, during which the cells closely resemble cells *in situ;*[20] i.e., substantial bundles of thick and thin filaments can easily be recognised using low-power electron microscopy, there is intense immunostaining for smooth muscle–specific contractile proteins,[21,42] and the majority of cells visibly contract in response to spasmogens.[21] Under these conditions, cells are described as being in the *contractile* phenotype. In the continued presence of growth-promoting stimuli, such as fetal calf serum, sparsely seeded contractile smooth muscle cells in culture undergo a number of spontaneous changes in phenotype over a period of a week or so, depending on the species, to what is termed as the *synthetic* phenotype. This is characterised by increased expression of intracellular organelles associated with synthesis, such as Golgi cisternae, ribosomes, and rough endoplasmic reticulum (Figure 1D), and the gap junction protein, connexin43.[54] There is also a simultaneous decrease in the intensity of immunostaining for smooth muscle–specific contractile proteins,[42] although the total amount of actin and myosin remains relatively unaltered because of the accumulation of nonmuscle isoforms.[21,42] At confluence, however, the majority of smooth muscle cells re-express contractile proteins as in the original contractile phenotype. The extent of reversibility of these phenotypic changes at confluence appears to be dependent upon on the initial seeding density.[55] Cells that are seeded at a high density, and thus undergo relatively few population doublings before achieving confluence, re-express the contractile phenotype and are termed *reversibly synthetic*. Sparsely seeded cells, which must undergo more population doublings to reach confluence, are less likely to return to the contractile phenotype and are said to be *irreversibly synthetic*. During increasing passage number, particularly in late passage, smooth muscle cells become increasingly irreversibly synthetic. This may also be related to differences in seeding efficiencies, where low seeding efficiencies at subculture tend to select cells which are able to begin proliferation after a shorter time in culture. Put simply, it may be that synthetic smooth muscle cells adhere more quickly than the contractile phenotype as they contain fewer myofibrils which restrict cell spreading and attachment. Consequently, over successive passages the population of cells will become increasingly noncontractile.[21] Our own studies suggest that in human and rabbit airway smooth muscle cells, even during prolonged culture, marked changes in morphology and in specific intracellular element (phosphorus and potassium) distributions occur in serum-starved, nondividing cells, compared with randomly proliferating cells stimulated by fetal calf serum.[40]

It should not, therefore, be assumed that *all* airway smooth muscle cells are contractile or, indeed, will retain their contractile properties during culture. Similarly, smooth muscle cells either *in situ* or *in vitro* should not be considered exclusively contractile or synthetic. It is more likely that the contractile or synthetic state of any single cell represents a balance of features common to both phenotypes. Thus, some smooth muscle cells, whilst still contractile, will also be capable of dividing.[56] The occurrence of multiple phenotypes of smooth muscle having differing properties or functions within the airway wall *in vivo*, which could be isolated and grown in primary culture and subsequently cloned, has not been investigated, but may have important implications for mechanisms controlling the development of airway wall smooth muscle thickening and bronchial hyperresponsiveness.

## IV. QUANTIFYING GROWTH AND DIVISION

Exposure of an airway smooth muscle cell in culture to an appropriate "growth-promoting" stimulus results either in an increase in size or growth of the cell (hypertrophy) or in its division (hyperplasia) and the generation of diploid progeny cells. Such responses may or may not be mutually exclusive,[57] but may occur simultaneously to a greater or lesser extent.[58] Accurate identification and quantitation of the mode of airway smooth muscle thickening (i.e., hyperplasia vs. hypertrophy) in response to a particular stimulus is a necessary prerequisite to understanding the biologic processes taking place and may ultimately be fundamental to the delineation of the mechanisms of airway wall remodelling and bronchial hyperresponsiveness.

### A. THE CELL CYCLE

Any method of studying growth and division requires a basic understanding of its relationship to the cell cycle. Besides nutritional conditions, many aspects of the cell growth and division process are regulated by production of appropriate growth factors and expression of their receptors. Although cell cycle kinetics have not yet been studied in detail in airway smooth muscle cells, it is clear that proliferation in mammalian cells involves a programmed series of complex genetic and biochemical events which fall into the four distinct phases outlined in Figure 2. The first stage, $G_1$ (further divided into $G_{1A}$ and $G_{1B}$) or post-mitotic "gap," is characterised by a lack of DNA synthesis, where cells contain their normal chromosomal complement (i.e., diploid), but there is elevated synthesis of RNA and protein. The second stage, or S phase, is a period of increased DNA synthesis during which elevated RNA and protein synthesis are maintained and the complete complement of chromosomes is duplicated. In the third stage, the post-synthetic gap or $G_2$ phase, DNA synthesis ceases (cells have two complete sets of chromosomes and, therefore, twice the normal amount of DNA and are termed *tetraploid*) while RNA and

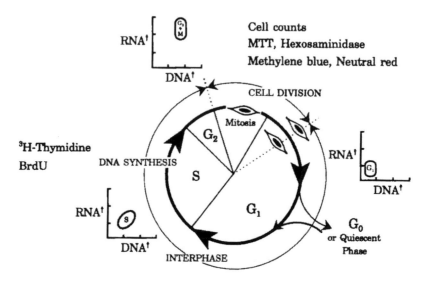

**FIGURE 2** The cell cycle of a typical mammalian cell, showing the phases leading to mitosis (M) and generation of diploid progeny. Schematic histograms indicate the relative DNA and RNA content of exponentially proliferating cells, obtained by multiparameter flow cytometry, at different stages of the cycle. Commonly used cell proliferation assays and their corresponding detection loci in the cycle are also indicated.

protein synthesis continue. This phase often results in cytoplasmic volume expansion. Collectively, $G_1$, S, and $G_2$ constitute the "interphase" which is distinct from the actual cell division, or mitosis, also referred to as mitogenesis or proliferation. Mitosis is the shortest phase of the cell cycle, usually occurring within 60 min. Little or no DNA, RNA, or protein synthesis occurs during this phase.

Recently, a fifth phase called $G_0$ has been proposed in which cells have come to rest and remain viable, but are not traversing the cell cycle. Under conditions when the growth is not irreversible, they can be induced by polypeptide growth factors to reenter the cycle and proliferate. Indeed, it has been standard practice by many investigators when carrying out proliferation experiments to render smooth muscle cells quiescent by incubation for periods of 24–72 h in serum-free culture media supplemented with insulin, ascorbate, and transferrin.[29] This maintains the cells in a viable but nondividing state[59] and has the advantage of synchronising the cell cycle kinetics when in culture. Whether or not this growth-arrested state is positively controlled by the expression of certain inhibitory factors has not been established.

The events that control the ability of a growth-arrested cell to reenter the cell cycle are far from understood, particularly in the airway smooth muscle cell. What is clear, however, is the central role of growth factors which, acting through specific plasma membrane receptors, initiate a complex series of signal transduction events leading to phosphorylation of a large number of target regulatory proteins. These phosphorylated proteins are believed to activate the intracellular processes, including altered gene expression, which culminate in cell growth and division and are discussed in detail in Chapters 10 and 11 of this volume. This chapter, however, is concerned with the detection of the "end response," cell growth and division, which is usually quantified in at least three ways: detecting DNA replication during S phase, observing mitosis, and recording changes in cell volume.

## B. DNA REPLICATION TECHNIQUES

These techniques rely on the cellular uptake and nuclear incorporation of radiolabelled DNA-precursor nucleotides such as tritiated ($^3$H-)thymidine into newly synthesised DNA during S phase of the cell cycle, although the advent of bromodeoxyuridine (BrdU) labelling and its detection by monoclonal antibodies has also allowed the study of S phase by non-radiolabelling techniques. Typically, S phase lasts 6–12 h in mammalian cells, and mitosis is complete within 60 min. The short duration of mitosis as an index of proliferation is, therefore, intrinsically less sensitive than S phase, since the fraction of the cell population which can be detected in mitosis is much smaller than it is in S phase. For this reason, methods such as thymidine and BrdU labelling have continued to be erroneously employed as indices of cell division, when instead their more correct use is as S or $G_2$ phase markers. These and other limitations are discussed below.

### 1. Uptake of $^3$H-Thymidine

The use of this technique requires special interpretation and is reviewed by Maurer.[60] Other potential problems with this assay are due to isotope impurities, the killing of cells by the isotope, and perturbations of cell dynamics, such as blockade of $G_2$ phase by intranuclear radiation. The method also assumes that the rate of DNA synthesis is always constant among cells and that the amount of incorporated precursors is always proportional to the amount of newly synthesised DNA. Varying culture conditions, such as cell density, can also interfere with the assay interpretation, causing thymidine incorporation but no real increase in the individual cell DNA content. Real proliferation, or mitogenesis, as determined by this method, is not necessarily related to $^3$H-thymidine uptake by the culture, stressing the necessity for the development of more-accurate biologic assays to quantitate cell proliferation. This is illustrated in experiments by Neckers et al.,[61] where a significant non-S phase DNA synthesis, nevertheless expressed as $^3$H-thymidine incorporation, was observed with no accompanying cell proliferation. Furthermore, some factors which increase $^3$H-thymidine uptake are unable to support cell growth beyond $G_2$ or even $G_1$ phase of the cell cycle,[62] while preparations containing known growth factors which stimulate cell division give poor thymidine incorporation.[63] In some cell systems, growth factors which stimulate large increases in $^3$H-thymidine uptake fail to stimulate actual cell division, either in the absence or presence of fetal calf serum. The A-chain homodimer of platelet-derived growth factor is a good example of this in rabbit cultured tracheal smooth muscle cells.[51]

## 2. Quantitative Fluorometric Analysis of Nucleic Acids

DNA synthesis measured by flow cytometry is based upon the principle that cells in different stages of the cell cycle have different but predictable amounts of DNA.[64,65] By the use of fluorochromes (e.g., propidium iodide, ethidium bromide, and acridine orange) as nuclear dyes which stoichiometrically bind to DNA, it is possible to distinguish in a single parameter three compartments of the cell cycle based solely on DNA content of exponentially dividing cells. These are the $G_0/G_1$ phase with diploid amounts of DNA, $G_2$ and mitosis with tetraploid quantities of DNA, and S phase with variable intermediate amounts of DNA. A typical DNA distribution of exponentially growing smooth muscle cells is illustrated in Figure 3. Examples of typical DNA distribution profiles at different phases of the cell cycle are shown in Figure 2. A more detailed account of the application of flow cytometry to cell cycle analysis is described elsewhere.[65-67] Clearly, flow cytometry is a very powerful tool which combines detection of DNA synthesis and immunocytochemical markers to provide indices of cell counting, ploidy, and the DNA content in cells.

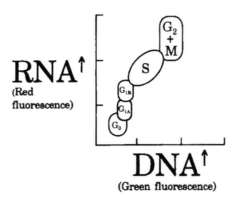

**FIGURE 3** Schematic example of a two-parameter histogram showing the distribution of exponentially proliferating mammalian cells according to their relative DNA and RNA content. At confluence, most cells return to the contractile ($G_{1A}$) or intermediate ($G_{1B}$) phase. Although not yet studied in airway smooth muscle cells, data not dissimilar from this distribution pattern are reported by Yamamoto et al.,[87] where the red to green fluorescence ratio was determined each day until confluence in populations of acridine orange–stained primary cultures of rabbit arterial smooth muscle cells, stimulated by fetal calf serum.

## 3. Quantitative Fluorometric Analysis of Non-Nucleic Acid Cellular Constituents

With the introduction of monoclonal antibodies labelled with fluorescent dyes and the ever-increasing sensitivity of modern flow cytometers, accurate quantitation of cellular components other than nucleic acids and protein synthesis has become feasible. The simultaneous analysis with DNA fluorochromes and cell constituents labelled with antibodies, such as Ki67 (a murine monoclonal antibody directed against a nuclear antigen expressed by all dividing cells except those in $G_0$ and early $G_1$[68]) and PC10 (monoclonal antibody to the proliferating cell nuclear antigen or "PCNA"[69,70]), using multiparameter flow cytometry offers the possibility of correlating the expression of particular cell components with cell cycle progression.[71,72] Of potentially great biologic significance is the application of this technique to the study of cell cycle–related expression of proteins (e.g., proto-oncogenes, elements of intracellular signal transduction pathways, etc.) involved in the control of growth, proliferation, and differentiation. It is with interest that we await the application of this technique to mechanisms of airway smooth muscle growth and division. For more information on flow cytometry and its possible applications to measurements of cell cycle progression, the reader is referred elsewhere.[66,67,73]

## C. POSTMITOTIC TECHNIQUES

A large number of techniques exist to assay actual cell division with varying degrees of direct quantitation. These are divided into noncolourimetric and colourimetric detection systems.

### 1. Noncolourimetric Detection

The most direct and least expensive method for detection of mitotic division is to count the increase in cell number under the light microscope using a haemacytometer. Cells are usually detached from their growth support by brief exposure (2–3 min at 37°C) to a predetermined volume of calcium and magnesium ion-free phosphate buffered saline containing trypsin (0.02% w/v) and EDTA (0.02% w/v). A sample of the cell suspension is mixed with a known volume of a solution of vital dye (e.g., trypan blue) before loading onto the haemacytometer and the number of viable (i.e., those excluding dye) cells counted. Reference to the haemacytometer manufacturers' instructions and a simple calculation allow the number of cells per millilitre or per culture dish to be determined.

Although this is a very simple technique, it is very sensitive to operator error. The subjective nature of cell counting can make it difficult to obtain reproducible counts within the haemacytometer chamber unless a brief "running-in" or learning period is allowed by the operator. Care should also be taken to count only living cells. A minimum of 120–140 viable cells should be counted to limit the statistical error associated with counting. The major disadvantage of this technique, however, is that it is labourious and time-consuming, and only relatively small numbers of samples can easily be processed. Some of these limitations are overcome by electronic cell counting (e.g., with a Coulter counter, Miami, FL, USA), but it is still considerably slower than automated colourimetry and may underestimate some cytotoxic effects because it estimates cell number on the basis of size rather than metabolic activity.

### 2. Automated Colourimetric Detection

Various colourimetric detection assays have been promoted as simple and rapid alternatives to cell counting or DNA-replication assays.[29,74,75] These methods use compounds that stain cells directly (e.g., methylene blue,[75] Coomassie blue,[76] neutral red[77]) or agents that are metabolised into coloured products, (e.g., 3-[4,5-dimethylthiazol]-2-yl-2,5-diphenyl tetrazolium bromide (MTT),[74] *p*-nitrophenol).[78] The intensity of the resulting colour change is quantitated using an automated spectrophotometer and correlated with the number of cells present. These assays have many desirable features, such as the ability to process large numbers of samples *en masse*, but also possess a number of drawbacks. The most obvious is that although colourimetric agents are generally less expensive and less hazardous than radiolabelled compounds, they still offer only an *indirect* measure of increased cell number, in contrast to haemacytometry.

The ideal proliferation assay should be sensitive, simple, rapid, inexpensive, accurate, and reproducible. Several colourimetric assays have shown exceptional promise as indices of proliferation. In our own laboratory, metabolic reduction of the tetrazolium dye MTT has been used with great effect to quantitate fetal calf serum– and growth factor–stimulated proliferation of human[29,79] and rabbit[29] airway smooth muscle cells in culture. The colour development correlated very closely with increasing cell number, determined in parallel experiments by direct cell counting. Similar data were obtained, in these cells, for increasing protein content using the Coomassie blue protein-detection assay.[29]

The MTT assay relies upon the conversion of the soluble yellow tetrazolium dye into insoluble, purple formazan crystals by the action of succinyl dehydrogenase within the mitochondria of living cells.[74] This assay empirically distinguishes between dead and living cells. The time taken to reach equilibrium for the colour reaction, and the sensitivity of the assay for proliferating airway smooth muscle cells, is dependent on both the presence of fetal calf serum in the reaction mixture and on the cell density within the culture dish.[29] Care should, therefore, be taken to choose an optimum incubation time at which the rate of conversion has plateaued at all cell densities present in the culture dish. Typically, this is around 6 h in human bronchial smooth muscle cells and 4 h in smooth muscle cells cultured from rabbit trachealis.[29] The resulting formazan product can then be solubilised and the colour reaction determined by dual wavelength spectrophotometry against a reagent blank.

Other commonly used colourimetric assay systems include the use of (1) *p*-nitrophenol-*N*-acetyl-β-D-glucosaminide as a synthetic substrate for the ubiquitous cytoplasmic enzyme hexosamindase, where the reaction product appears yellow at acidic pH,[78] and (2) neutral red, a weak basic dye which is selectively concentrated in the lysosomes of living cells.[80]

An important limitation of these assay systems is that the colour reaction developed is not only proportional to the cell number, but also to the expression and modulation of the metabolic behaviour exploited by the particular assay. For example, the MTT-reduction assay could give reduced sensitivity compared with cell counts (or ³H-thymidine uptake) in cells of low mitochondrial succinyl dehydrogenase activity or when inhibitors of this enzyme or of mito-chondrial function are used.[81] Preliminary experiments should therefore be performed to discount such limitations.

## D. DETECTION OF CELLULAR HYPERTROPHY

In addition to hyperplasia, the role of cellular enlargement, or hypertrophy, in the pathogenesis of airway wall remodelling in chronic severe asthma,[14] and the subsequent development of bronchial hyperresponsiveness, may be particularly relevant. At the moment, however, almost nothing is known regard-ing the mechanisms that control airway smooth muscle cell size, although interleukin (IL)-1β and IL-6 have recently been reported to promote hyper-trophy as well as hyperplasia of guinea pig tracheal smooth muscle.[82] Of critical importance to such studies is how best to quantitate hypertrophy as distinct from hyperplasia.

Increased protein synthesis, determined by uptake of $^3$H-leucine[24,38,82] or by colourimetric staining with Coomassie blue dye,[29] in the absence of increas-ing cell number (determined by cell counting or by MTT reduction, see Section IV.C.2) may indicate cellular hypertrophy. Care should be taken when interpreting such data to exclude the possibility that increased protein synthesis reflects an increase in cell size, due to increased cellular protein content, rather than increased production and secretion of extracellular matrix proteins (quan-tified directly by incorporation of $^3$H-proline into hydroxyproline[83]), since these methods do not adequately discriminate between these processes. It is possible to overcome this problem by determining either the DNA content per cell or more directly the volume of an individual cell, measured by flow cytometry using a fluorescent-activated cell sorter (FACS). The cell volumes of a population of cells from a single culture dish show a bell-shaped distri-bution. Cellular hypertrophy is quantitated by a shift in the distribution to increasing values for cell volume. In human airway smooth muscle cells the mean cell volume is 4.2 pl/cell.[35] Studies of vascular smooth muscle cells have characterised hypertrophy as enlargement of existing cells with little or no change in cell number. This is accompanied by the development of polyploidy (i.e., increased DNA content per cell) in a large fraction of smooth muscle cells.[84] Development of polyploidy in these cells does not appear to be due to a loss in the capacity of the cells to divide, since tetraploid cells, isolated from the intact tissue and then separated on the basis of DNA content using a FACS (see Section IV.B.2), can be induced to proliferate by fetal calf serum once established in culture.[85] This suggests that smooth muscle growth and division (i.e., hypertrophy and hyperplasia) are a function of the nature of the growth-promoting stimulus. Hypertrophy rather than hyperplasia may result from incomplete growth stimulation, where a cell receives signals for increased cell mass and DNA replication, associated with cell cycle progression, which fail to translate to actual cell division. Alternatively, growth inhibitory factors, such as TGFβ, may alter the pattern of the growth response to mitogens, resulting in incomplete growth stimulation.[86]

# V. CONCLUSION

The maintenance of airway smooth muscle in culture, in which there are only limited changes in expression of key regulatory proteins, undoubtedly represents a useful model for the dissemination of mechanisms, both extracellular and intracellular, implicit in the control of accelerated airway smooth muscle growth *and* division. The validity of this model, however, is critically dependent upon the judicious application of techniques designed to interpret accurately and reliably both hyperplastic *and* hypertrophic changes.[88] The ability to quantitate differentially these changes is therefore a prerequisite to understanding their underlying mechanisms and, ultimately, the extent to which they translate to airway wall thickening and the subsequent development of poorly reversible or irreversible airflow obstruction and bronchial hyperresponsiveness.

# REFERENCES

1. Barnes, P. J., Inflammation, in *Bronchial Asthma*, 3rd ed., Weiss, E. B. and Stein, M., Eds., Little, Brown, Boston, 1993, 80.
2. Chung, K. F., Role of inflammation in the hyperreactivity of the airways in asthma, *Thorax*, 14, 657, 1986.
3. Dunnill, M. S., Masserella, G. R., and Anderson, J. A., A comparison of the quantitative anatomy of the bronchi in normal subjects, in status asthmaticus, in chronic bronchitis and in emphysema, *Thorax*, 24, 176, 1969.
4. Heard, B. E. and Hossain, S., Hyperplasia of bronchial muscle in asthma, *J. Pathol.*, 110, 319, 1973.
5. Hossain, S., Quantitative measurement of bronchial muscle in men with asthma, *Am. Rev. Respir. Dis.*, 107, 99, 1973.
6. Ebina, M., Yaegashi, H., Chibo, R., Takahashi, T., Motomiya, M., and Tanemura, M., Hyperreactive site in the airway tree of asthmatic patients revealed by thickening of bronchial muscles, *Am. Rev. Respir. Dis.*, 141, 1327, 1990.
7. Brown, J. P., Breville, W. H., and Finucane, K. E., Asthma and irreversible airflow obstruction, *Thorax*, 39, 131, 1984.
8. Juniper, E. F., Kline, P. A., Vanieleghem, M. A., Ramsdale, E. H., O'Byrne, P. M., and Hargreave, F. E., Effect of long-term treatment with an inhaled corticosteroid (budesonide) on airway hyperresponsiveness and clinical asthma in non-steroid dependent asthmatics, *Am. Rev. Respir. Dis.*, 142, 832, 1990.
9. James, A. L., Hogg, J. C., Dunn, L. A., and Pare, P. D., The use of internal perimeter to compare airway size and to calculate smooth muscle shortening, *Am. Rev. Respir. Dis.*, 139, 136, 1988.
10. James A. L., Pare, P. D., and Hogg, J. C., The mechanics of airway narrowing in asthma, *Am. Rev. Respir. Dis.*, 139, 242, 1989.
11. Pare, P. D., Wiggs, B. R., Hogg, J. C., and Bosken, C., The comparative mechanics and morphology of airways in asthma and in chronic obstructive pulmonary disease, *Am. Rev. Respir. Dis.*, 143, 1189, 1991.
12. Lambert, R. K., Wiggs, B. R., Kuwano, K., Hogg, J. C., and Pare, P. D., Functional significance of increased airway smooth muscle in asthma and COPD, *J. Appl. Physiol.*, 74, 2771, 1993.

13. Bramley, A. M., Thomson, R. J., Roberts, C. R., and Schellenberg, R. R., Excessive bronchoconstriction in asthma is due to decreased airway elastance, *Eur. Respir. J.*, 7, 337, 1994.

14. Ebina, M., Takahashi, T., Chiba, T., and Motomiya, M., Cellular hypertrophy and hyperplasia of airway smooth muscle underlying bronchial asthma, *Am. Rev. Respir. Dis.*, 148, 720, 1993.

15. Avner, B. P., DeLongo, J., Wilson, S., and Ladman, A. J., A method for culturing canine tracheal smooth muscle cells *in vitro*: Morphological and pharmacological observations, *Anat. Rec.*, 200, 357, 1981.

16. Tom-Moy, M., Madison, J. M., Jones, C. A., DeLanerolle, P., and Brown, J. K., Morphological characterisation of cultured smooth muscle cells isolated from the tracheas of adult dogs, *Anat. Rec.*, 218, 313, 1987.

17. Twort, C. H. C. and van Breemen, C., Human airway smooth muscle in culture, *Tissue Cell*, 20, 339, 1988.

18. Panettieri, R. A., Murray, R. K., DePalo, L. R., Yadvish, P. A., and Kotlikoff, M. I., A Human airway smooth muscle cell line that retains physiological responsiveness, *Am. J. Physiol.*, 256, C329, 1989.

19. Holgate, S., Mediator and cytokine mechanisms in asthma, *Thorax*, 48, 103, 1993.

20. Chamley-Campbell, J., Campbell, J., and Ross, R., The smooth muscle cell in culture, *Physiol. Rev.*, 59, 1, 1979.

21. Campbell, J. H. and Campbell, G. R., Culture techniques and their applications to studies of vascular smooth muscle, *Clin. Sci.*, 85, 501, 1993.

22. Thyberg, J., Nilsson, J., and Palmberg, L., Adult human arterial smooth muscle cells in primary culture, *Cell Tissue Res.*, 239, 69, 1985.

23. Gabella, G., Structure of smooth muscles, in *Smooth Muscle: An Assessment of Current Knowledge*, Bulbring, E., Brading, A. F., Jones, A. W., and Tomita, T., Eds., University of Texas Press, Austin, 1981, 1.

24. Panettieri, R. A., Yadvish, P. A., Kelly, A. M., Rubinstein, N. A., and Kotlikoff, M. I., Histamine stimulates proliferation of airway smooth muscle and induces c-*fos* expression, *Am. J. Physiol.*, 259, L365, 1990.

25. Yang, C. M. and Chou, S.-P., Primary culture of canine tracheal smooth muscle cells in serum-free medium: effects of insulin-like growth factor-1 and insulin, *J. Receptor Res.*, 13, 943, 1993.

26. Marsh, K. A. and Hill, S. J., Bradykinin $B_2$ receptor-mediated phosphoinositide hydrolysis in bovine cultured tracheal smooth muscle cells, *Br. J. Pharmacol.*, 107, 443, 1992.

27. Lew, D. B., Nebigil, C., and Malik, K. U., Dual regulation of cAMP of β-hexosaminidase-induced mitogenesis in bovine tracheal myocytes, *Am. J. Respir. Cell Mol. Biol.*, 7, 614, 1992.

28. Delamere, F., Holland, E., Patel, S., Bennett, J., Pavord, I., and Knox, A., Production of $PGE_2$ by bovine cultured airway smooth muscle cells and its inhibition by cyclooxygenase, *Br. J. Pharmacol.*, 111, 983, 1994.

29. Hirst, S. J., Barnes, P. J., and Twort, C. H. C., Quantifying proliferation of cultured human and rabbit airway smooth muscle in response to serum and platelet-derived growth factor, *Am. J. Respir. Cell Mol. Biol.*, 7, 574, 1992.

30. Noveral, J. P., Rosenberg, S. M., Anbar, R. A., Pawlowski, N. A., and Grunstein, M. M., Role of endothelin-1 in regulating proliferation of cultured rabbit airway smooth muscle cells, *Am. J. Physiol.*, 263, L317, 1992.

31. Noveral, J. P. and Grunstein, M. M., Role and mechanism of thromboxane-induced proliferation of cultured airway smooth muscle cells, *Am. J. Physiol.*, 263, L555, 1992.

32. De, S., Zelazny, E. T., Souhrada, J. F., and Souhrada, M., Interleukin-1β stimulates the proliferation of cultured airway smooth muscle cells via platelet-derived growth factor, *Am. J. Respir. Cell Mol. Biol.*, 9, 645, 1993.

33. Pyne, S. and Pyne, N. J., Bradykinin stimulates phospholipase D in primary cultures of guinea-pig tracheal smooth muscle, *Biochem. Pharmacol.*, 45, 595, 1993.

34. Farmer, S. G., Ensore, J. E., and Burch, R. M., Evidence that cultured airway smooth muscle cells contain bradykinin $B_2$ and $B_3$ receptors, *Am. J. Respir. Cell Mol. Biol.*, 4, 273, 1991.

35. Twort, C. H. C. and van Breemen, C., Human airway smooth muscle in culture: control of the intracellular calcium store, *Pulm. Pharmacol.*, 2, 45, 1989.

36. Hall, I. P., Widdop, S., Townsend, P., and Daykin, K., Control of cyclic AMP content in primary cultures of human airway smooth muscle cells, *Br. J. Pharmacol.*, 107, 422, 1992.

37. Hall, I. P., Daykin, K., and Widdop, S., $\beta_2$-Adrenoceptor desensitisation in cultured human airway smooth muscle, *Clin. Sci.*, 84, 151, 1993.

38. Tomlinson, P. R., Wilson, J. W., and Stewart, A. G., Inhibition by salbutamol of the proliferation of human airway smooth muscle cells grown in culture, *Br. J. Pharmacol.*, 111, 641, 1994.

39. Warley, A., Cracknell, K. P. B., Cammish, H. B., Twort, C. H. C., Ward, J. P. T., and Hirst, S. J., Preparation of cultured airway smooth muscle cells for study of intracellular element concentrations by x-ray microanalysis: comparison of whole cell mounts with cryosections, *J. Microsc.*, 175, 143, 1994.

40. Warley, A., Hirst, S. J., Twort, C. H. C., and Ward, J. P. T., Changes in element content and morphology of rabbit cultured tracheal smooth muscle cells after stimulation with fetal calf serum, *Am. J. Respir. Crit. Care Med.*, 149, A302, 1994.

41. Gown, A. M., Vogel, A. N., Gordon, D., and Lu, P. L., A smooth muscle-specific monoclonal antibody recognises smooth muscle actin isozymes, *J. Cell Biol.*, 100, 807, 1985.

42. Owens, G. K., Loeb, A., Gordon, D., and Thompson, M. M., Expression of smooth muscle-specific $\alpha$-isoactin in cultured vascular smooth muscle cells: a relationship between growth and cytodifferentiation, *J. Cell Biol.*, 102, 343, 1986.

43. Widdop, S., Daykin, K., and Hall, I. P., Expression of muscarinic $M_2$ receptors in cultured human airway smooth muscle cells, *Am. J. Respir. Cell Mol. Biol.*, 9, 541, 1993.

44. Mak, J. C., Baraniuk, J. N., and Barnes, P. J., Localisation of muscarinic receptor subtype mRNAs in human lung, *Am. J. Respir. Cell Mol. Biol.*, 7, 344, 1992.

45. Daykin, K., Widdop, S., and Hall, I. P., Control of histamine-induced inositol phospholipid hydrolysis in human tracheal smooth muscle cells, *Eur. J. Pharmacol.*, 246, 135, 1993.

46. Florio, C., Flezar, M., Martin, J. G., and Heisler, S., Identification of adenylate cyclase-coupled histamine $H_2$ receptors in guinea-pig tracheal smooth muscle cells in culture and the effect of dexamethasone, *Am. J. Respir. Cell Mol. Biol.*, 7, 582, 1992.

47. Yang, C. M., Hsai, H.-C., Chou, S.-P., Ong, R., and Luo, S.-F., Bradykinin-stimulated phosphoinositide metabolism in cultured canine tracheal smooth muscle cells, *Br. J. Pharmacol.*, 111, 21, 1994.

48. Yang, C. M., Yo, Y.-L., Ong, R., and Hsai, H.-C., Endothelin- and sarafotoxin-induced phosphoinositide hydrolysis in cultured canine tracheal smooth muscle cells, *J. Neurochem.*, 62, 1440, 1994.

49. Stewart, A. G., Tomlinson, P. R., and Wilson, J., Airway wall remodelling in asthma: a novel therapeutic target for the development of anti-asthma drugs, *Trends Pharmacol. Sci.*, 14, 275, 1993.

50. Yang, C. M., Yo, Y.-L., Hsai, H.-C., and Ong, R., 5-Hydroxytryptamine receptor-mediated phosphoinositide hydrolysis in canine cultured tracheal smooth muscle cells, *Br. J. Pharmacol.*, 111, 777, 1994.

51. Hirst, S. J., Barnes, P. J., and Twort, C. H. C., Proliferation of human and rabbit airway smooth muscle cells in culture by platelet-derived growth factor isoforms, *Am. J. Respir. Crit. Care Med.*, 149, A302, 1994.

52. Snetkov, V. A., Hirst, S. J., Twort, C. H. C., and Ward, J. P. T., Potassium currents in human bronchial and rabbit tracheal smooth muscle cells in culture, *Am. J. Respir. Crit. Care Med.*, 149, A1082, 1994.

53. Snetkov, V. A., Hirst, S. J., Twort, C. H. C., and Ward, J. P. T., Alterations to large conductance $K^+$ currents during proliferation in human bronchial smooth muscle cells, *Am. J. Respir. Crit. Care Med.*, 151, A49, 1995.

54. Rennick, R. E., Connat, J.-L., Burnstock, G., Rothery, S., Severs, N. J., and Green, C. R., Expression of connexin43 gap junctions between cultured vascular smooth muscle cells is dependent upon phenotype, *Cell Tissue Res.*, 271, 323, 1993.

55. Campbell, J. H., Kocher, O., Skalli, O., Gabbiani, G., and Campbell, G. R., Cytodifferentiation and expression of alpha-smooth muscle actin mRNA and protein during primary culture of aortic smooth muscle cells. Correlation with cell density and proliferative state, *Arteriosclerosis*, 9, 633, 1989.

56. Campbell, J. H. and Campbell, G. R., Mitosis of contractile smooth muscle cells in tissue culture, *Exp. Cell Res.*, 84, 105, 1974.

57. Geisterfer, A. A. T., Peach, M. J., and Owens, G. K., Angiotensin II induces hypertrophy not hyperplasia of cultured rat aortic smooth muscle cells, *Circ. Res.*, 62, 749, 1988.

58. Lee, S.-L., Wang, W. W., Lanzillo, J. J., and Fanburg, B. L., Serotonin produces both hyperplasia and hypertrophy of bovine pulmonary artery smooth muscle cells in culture, *Am. J. Physiol.*, 266, L46, 1994.

59. Libby, P. and O'Brien, K. V., Culture of quiescent arterial smooth muscle cells in a defined serum-free medium, *J. Cell. Physiol.*, 115, 217, 1983.

60. Maurer, H. R., Potential pitfalls of $^3$H-thymidine techniques to measure cell proliferation, *Cell Tissue Kinet.*, 14, 111, 1981.

61. Neckers, L. M., Funkhouser, W., Trepal, J., Cossman, J., and Gratzner, H. G., Significant non-S phase DNA synthesis visualised by flow cytometry in activated and malignant human lymphoid cells, *Exp. Cell Res.*, 156, 429, 1985.

62. Bagby, S. P., O'Reilly, M. M., Kirk, E. A., Mitchel, L. H., Stenberg, P. E., Makler, M. T., and Bakke, A. C., EGF is incomplete mitogen in porcine aortic smooth muscle cells: DNA synthesis without cell division, *Am. J. Physiol.*, 262, C578, 1992.

63. Grimm, E. A. and Rosenberg, S. A., Production and properties of human IL-2, in *Isolation, Characterisation and Utilisation of T-Lymphocyte Clones*, Fathman, G. and Fitch, F., Eds., Academic Press, New York, 1982, 57.

64. Lovett, E. J., Schnitzer, B., Keran, D. F., Flint, A., Hudson, J. L., and McClatchey, K. D., Application of flow cytometry to diagnostic pathology, *Lab. Invest.*, 50, 115, 1984.

65. Lavergne, J. A. and del Llano, A. M., Assessment of cellular activation by flow cytometric methods, *Pathobiology*, 58, 107, 1990.

66. Jacob, M. C., Favre, M., and Bensa, J.-C., Membrane cell permeabilisation with saponin and multiparametric analysis by flow cytometry, *Cytometry*, 12, 550, 1991.

67. Pollice, A. A., McCoy, J. P., Shackney, S. E., Smith, C. A., Agarwal, J., Burholt, D. R., Janocko, L. E., Hornicek, F. J., Singh, S. G., and Hartsock, R. J., Sequential paraformaldehyde and methanol fixation for simultaneous flow cytometric analysis of DNA, cell surface proteins, and intracellular proteins, *Cytometry*, 13, 432, 1992.

68. Gerdes, J., Lemke, H., Baisch, H., Wacker, H. H., Schwab, V., and Stein, H., Cell cycle analysis of a cell proliferation-associated nuclear antigen defined by the monoclonal antibody Ki67, *J. Immunol.*, 133, 1710, 1984.

69. Waseem, N. H. and Lane, D. P., Monoclonal antibody analysis of the proliferating cell nuclear antigen (PCNA): structural conservation and the detection of a nucleolar form, *J. Cell Sci.*, 96, 121, 1990.

70. Landberg, G. and Roos, G., Antibodies to proliferating cell nuclear antigen (PCNA) as S phase probes in flow cytometric cell cycle analysis, *Cancer Res.*, 51, 4570, 1991.

71. Czerniak, B., Herz, F., Wersto, R. P., and Koss, L. G., Expression of Ha-*ras* oncogene p21 protein in relation to the cell cycle of cultured human tumor cells, *Am. J. Pathol.*, 126, 411, 1987.

72. Czerniak, B., Herz, F., Wersto, R. P., and Koss, L. G., Modulation of Ha-*ras* oncogene p21 expression and cell cycle progression in the human colonic cancer cell line HT-29, *Cancer Res.*, 47, 2826, 1987.

73. Koss, L. G., Czerniak, C., Herz, F., and Wersto, R. P., Flow cytometric measurements of DNA and other cell components in human tumors: a critical appraisal, *Human Pathol.*, 20, 528, 1989.

74. Denziot, F. and Lang, R., Rapid colourimetric assay for cell growth and survival, *J. Immunol. Methods*, 89, 271, 1986.

75. Oliver, M. H., Harrison, N. K., Bishop, J. E., Cole, P. J., and Laurent, G. J., A rapid and convenient assay for counting cells cultured in microwell plates: application for assessment of growth factors, *J. Cell Sci.*, 92, 513, 1989.

76. Baumgarten, H., A simple microplate assay for the determination of cellular protein, *J. Immunol. Methods*, 82, 25, 1985.

77. Fiennes, A., Walton, J., Winterbourne, D., McGlashan, D., and Hermon-Taylor, J., Quantitative correlation of neutral red dye uptake with cell number in human cancer cell cultures, *Cell Biol. Int. Rep.*, 11, 373, 1987.

78. Landegren, U., Measurement of cell numbers by means of the endogenous enzyme hexosaminidase: applications to detection of lymphokines and cell surface antigens, *J. Immunol. Methods*, 67, 379, 1984.

79. Johnson, P. R. A., Armour, C. L., Carey, D., and Black, J. L., The effect of heparin on human airway smooth muscle growth in culture, *Am. J. Respir. Crit. Care Med.*, 149, A300, 1994.

80. Bulychev, A., Trouet, A., and Tulkens, P., Uptake and intracellular distribution of neutral red in cultured fibroblasts, *Exp. Cell Res.*, 115, 343, 1978.

81. Berridge, M. V. and Tan, A. S., The protein kinase C inhibitor, calphostin C, inhibits succinate-dependent mitochondrial reduction of MTT by a mechanism that does not involve protein kinase C, *Biochem. Biophys. Res. Commun.*, 185, 806, 1992.

82. De, S., Zelazny, E. T., Souhrada, J. F., and Souhrada, M., Interleukin-1β and interleukin-6 induce both hyperplasia and hypertrophy of cultured guinea-pig airway smooth muscle cells, *J. Appl. Physiol.*, 78, 1555, 1995.

83. Ang, A. H., Tachas, G., Campbell, J. H., Bateman, J. F., and Campbell, G. R., Collagen synthesis by cultured rabbit aortic smooth muscle cells: alteration with phenotype, *Biochem. J.*, 265, 461, 1990.

84. Owens, G., Rabinovitch, P., and Schwartz, S., Smooth muscle cell hypertrophy vs. hyperplasia in hypertension, *Proc. Natl. Acad. Sci. U.S.A.*, 78, 7759, 1981.

85. Goldberg, I., Rosen, E., Shapiro, H., Zoller, L., Kmyrick, K., Levinson, S., and Christenson, L., Isolation and culture of a tetraploid subpopulation of smooth muscle cells from the normal rat aorta, *Science*, 226, 559, 1984.

86. Owens, G. K., Geisterfer, A. A. T., Yang, Y. W.-H., and Komoriya, A., Transforming growth factor-β-induced growth inhibition and cellular hypertrophy in cultured vascular smooth muscle cells, *J. Cell Biol.*, 107, 771, 1988.

87. Yamamoto, M., Fujita, K., Shinkai, T., Yamamoto, K., and Noumura, T., Identification of the phenotypic modulation of rabbit arterial smooth muscle cells in primary culture by flow cytometry, *Exp. Cell Res.*, 198, 43, 1992.

88. Boulton, R. A. and Hodgson, H. J. F., Assessing cell proliferation: a methodological review, *Clin. Sci.*, 88, 119, 1995.

Chapter 10

# REGULATION OF GROWTH OF AIRWAY SMOOTH MUSCLE BY SECOND MESSENGER SYSTEMS

Reynold A. Panettieri, Jr.

## CONTENTS

## I. INTRODUCTION

Asthma, a common cause of pulmonary impairment, is a chronic disease characterized by airway hyperreactivity and airflow obstruction. Despite considerable research effort, asthma mortality rates continue to rise and the primary

0-8493-7813-3/97/$0.00+$.50
© 1997 by CRC Press, Inc.

defects that underlie airway hyperreactivity remain unknown, although an intrinsic abnormality of airway smooth muscle has been postulated.[1-4]

Although asthma typically induces reversible airway obstruction, in some patients with asthma airflow obstruction can become irreversible.[5-7] Such obstruction may be a consequence of persistent structural changes in the airway wall due to the frequent stimulation of airway smooth muscle (ASM) by contractile agonists, inflammatory mediators, and growth factors. Increased smooth muscle mass, which has been attributed to increases in myocyte number, is a well-documented pathological finding in the airways of patients with chronic severe asthma.[8-12] Little information is available, however, with respect to factors that promote ASM cell proliferation or the cellular mechanisms that regulate airway myocyte growth.

Many studies have characterized the stimulation of smooth muscle growth in response to mitogenic agents, such as polypeptide growth factors,[13-17] inflammatory mediators,[18] and cytokines.[19] Other trophic factors, such as alterations in extracellular matrix and mechanical stress, have also been identified.[20] In recent studies, the important observations that contractile agonists induce smooth muscle proliferation may be a critical link between the chronic stimulation of muscle contraction and myocyte proliferation.[21-23] Although the mechanisms by which agonists induce cell proliferation are unknown, similarities exist between signal transduction processes activated by these agents and those of known growth factors. Interestingly, growth factors also stimulate smooth muscle contraction.[24,25] These diverse extracellular stimuli induce cell growth, in part, by activating common intracellular signal-transduction pathways. The identification of critical regulatory sites in these pathways may provide new therapeutic approaches to alter airway remodeling seen in patients with chronic severe asthma.

This chapter will review current knowledge of the second messenger pathways that modulate ASM cell proliferation and will address whether or not these pathways are necessary and sufficient to induce cell growth. Specifically, the role that inositol lipids, intracellular calcium, and cyclic nucleotides play in modulating airway myocyte growth will be examined.

## II. EXTRACELLULAR STIMULI TRANSDUCE GROWTH SIGNALS BY ACTIVATING RECEPTORS COUPLED TO SECOND MESSENGER SYSTEMS

### A. OVERVIEW

The binding of mitogens to their receptors promotes the generation of early signals in the membrane, cytosol, and the nucleus that lead to cell growth. Since the initiation of DNA synthesis occurs 10–15 h after the addition of the mitogens, it is expected that knowledge of these early events will provide clues to primary regulatory mechanisms.

Smooth muscle cell proliferation is stimulated by mitogens that fall into two broad categories: (1) those that activate receptors with intrinsic tyrosine kinase activity (RTK) or (2) those that mediate their effects through receptors coupled to heterotrimeric GTP-binding proteins (G proteins) and activate non-receptor-linked tyrosine kinases found in the cytoplasm (Figure 1). Although both pathways increase cytosolic calcium through activation of phospholipase C (PLC), different PLC isoenzymes appear to be involved. Activated PLC hydrolyzes phosphatidylinositol bisphosphate (PIP$_2$) to phosphatidylinositol trisphosphate (IP$_3$) and diacylglycerol (DAG).[26] These second messengers activate other cytosolic tyrosine kinases as well as serine and threonine kinases — protein kinase C (PKC) and A — that have pleotrophic effects including the activation of proto-oncogenes.[27,28] Proto-oncogenes, which are a family of cellular genes (c-*onc*) that control normal cellular growth and differentiation, were characterized initially from viral genes (v-*onc*) that induced cellular transformation in eukaryotic cells. The protein products of proto-oncogenes play a critical role in transducing growth signals from the cell surface to the nucleus and in regulating gene transcription.

## B. INOSITOL LIPIDS IN THE REGULATION OF CELL PROLIFERATION

### 1. Phospholipase C Activation and Inositol Trisphosphate

The recognition of PIP$_2$ hydrolysis as a ubiquitous receptor-activated signaling mechanism in eukaryotic cells was one of the major achievements of the 1980s. Recent studies have focussed on other aspects of phospholipid metabolism in signaling cell growth — candidates include phosphatidylinositol 3,4,5-trisphosphate (PtdIns 3,4,5-P$_3$) formation by inositol lipid 3-kinases and phospholipase D-catalyzed phosphotidylcholine hydrolysis. Although there is little doubt that inositol lipids are important in cell signaling, the precise mechanism by which these molecules modulate cell proliferation remains unknown.

To date, two phosphoinositide (PI) pathways have been characterized. In the canonical PI pathway, activation of phosphatidylinositol-specific PLC hydrolyzes PIP$_2$ to IP$_3$ and DAG. In the 3-phosphoinositide pathway, activation of phosphatidylinositol 3-kinase (PtdIns 3-kinase), which may be regulated by protein tyrosine kinase activation, phosphorylates phosphatidylinositides at the D3 position of the inositol ring and leads to the formation of phosphatidylinositol 3-phosphate, phosphatidylinositol 3,4-bisphosphate and PtdIns 3,4,5-P$_3$ (Figure 2).[29-32]

Receptors with intrinsic tyrosine kinase activity and those coupled to G proteins both activate specific PLC isoforms. These phosphoinositidases are the critical regulatory enzymes in activation of the PI pathway. The γ family of PLC contains src-homology (SH)-2 and SH-3 domains and are regulated by tyrosine phosphorylation. The other PLC isoforms are controlled by G proteins and/or Ca$^{2+}$.

The regulation of the PLC-γ$_1$ family has been elucidated in considerable detail. Kim et al.[33] have determined the relative contributions made to PLC-γ$_1$ activation by three tyrosine residues that are phosphorylated when PLC-γ$_1$

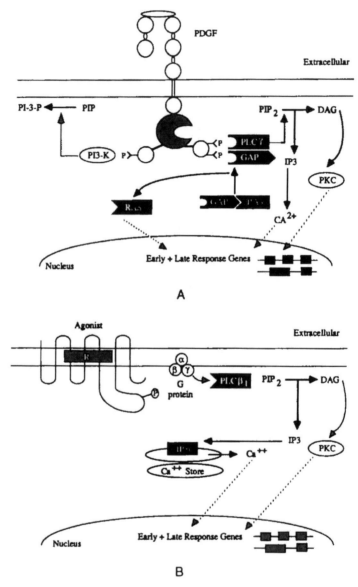

**FIGURE 1**  Characterization of smooth muscle cell mitogens: an overview. A. Some growth factors stimulate cell surface receptors with RTK. B. Others activate receptors coupled to heterotrimeric G proteins. Activation of either receptor increases cytosolic calcium through activation of specific PLC isozymes that hydrolyze $PIP_2$ to $IP_3$ and DAG. These second messengers then activate other cytosolic tyrosine kinases as well as serine and threonine kinases such as PKC. Stimulation of RTK-dependent receptors also activates phosphatidylinositol 3-phosphate kinase (PI 3-kinase); however, the role of 3'-inositol phosphates in signaling smooth muscle cell growth remains unknown. (From Panettieri, R. A., in *Airways Smooth Muscle: Development and Regulation of Contractility*, Raeburn, D. and Giembycz, M. A., Eds., Birkhauser Verlag, Basel, Switzerland, 1994. With permission.)

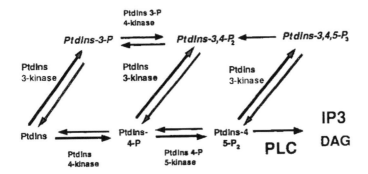

FIGURE 2  Synthesis of phosphoinositides. The lipid products generated by the 3-phosphoinositide pathway are shown in *italics* to differentiate those involved in the canonical PI turnover pathway. The solid arrows indicate pathways known to occur *in vivo*. PLC, PtdIns-specific phospholipase C; DAG, diacylglycerol. (Modified from Kapeller, R. and Cantley, L. C., *BioEssays*, 16, 565, 1994. With permission.)

associates with the PDGF receptor in 3T3 cells. Substitution of Tyr771 with phenylalanine slightly enhanced the activation, but a similar substitution of Tyr1254 markedly decreased the extent to which the enzyme was activated by the PDGF receptor in these cells.[33] An even stronger attenuation was caused by substituting Tyr783 with phenylalanine; the PLC-$\gamma_1$ Tyr783Phe could associate with the PDGF receptor and was serine phosphorylated as a consequence, although no activation occurred. Thus, tyrosine residues 783 and, to a lesser degree, 1254 are those that contribute to the control of the activity of PLC-$\gamma_1$ in intact cells.[33] Interestingly, others have shown that mutant EGF and PDGF receptors, which fail to activate PLC-$\gamma_1$ and to increase cytosolic calcium *in vivo*, effectively induced gene expression and mitogenesis.[34] Taken together, these studies suggest that formation of receptor–SH-2 complexes are important in some, but not all, responses of cells to growth factors, and other parallel signaling pathways apart from PLC-$\gamma_1$ activation may be necessary to mediate growth factor–induced mitogenesis.

In ASM cells, some growth factors, which activate receptors with intrinsic RTKs, have been identified. PDGF and EGF in human ASM cells[35-37] and IGF-1 in bovine and rabbit ASM cells[38-40] have been shown to induce myocyte proliferation. However, the role of PLC-$\gamma_1$ activation in modulating ASM cell growth remains unknown.

In recent years, our understanding of the regulation of PLC by G proteins has grown remarkably. Although the role of PLC activation in mediating G protein–dependent cell growth is complex, G protein activation is critically important in transducing contractile agonist-induced cell growth. G proteins are composed of three distinct subunits, $\alpha$, $\beta$, $\gamma$, the latter two existing as a tightly associated complex (see Reference 41 for review). Although $\alpha$ subunits were considered to be the functional components important in downstream signaling events, recent evidence suggests that $\beta\gamma$ subunits also play a critical role in modulating cell function.[42] To date, there exists a total of approximately 15 distinct genes that encode mammalian $G\alpha$ subunits grouped into four classes ($G_s$, $G_i$, $G_q$, and $G_{i2}$) based on their amino acid sequence.[43] On the basis of the ADP-ribosylation of certain $\alpha$ subunits by pertussis toxin (PTX), G proteins may also be classified as PTX sensitive and as PTX insensitive. The subunits $G_{i\alpha1}, G_{i\alpha2}, G_{i\alpha3}, G_{o\alpha1}$, and $G_{o\alpha2}$ are PTX sensitive; all other $\alpha$ subunits are PTX insensitive.

Advances in single cell microinjection techniques in combination with the development of neutralizing antibodies to specific $G\alpha$ subunits have enabled investigators to characterize the role of G protein activation in cell proliferation. Using these techniques, studies with 3T3 fibroblasts have determined that while both thrombin and bradykinin required Gq activation to mobilize cytosolic calcium, to generate $IP_3$, and to induce mitogenesis, thrombin but not bradykinin appeared also to require $G_{i2}$ in addition to $G_q$ to stimulate cell growth.[44] These studies determined that a single mitogen may require functional coupling to distinct subtypes of G proteins in order to stimulate cell growth. This also provides a mechanism to explain why some, but not all, agonists induce cell proliferation while mobilizing comparable levels of cytosolic calcium.

Recently, the role of PLC activation and inositol trisphosphate in mediating contractile agonist-induced ASM cell growth has been explored. Several contractile agonists, which mediate their effects through G protein-coupled receptors, induce ASM cell proliferation. Studies have determined that histamine[45] and serotonin[46] induce canine and porcine ASM cell proliferation. Endothelin-1, leukotriene (LT) $D_4$, and U-46619, a thromboxane $A_2$ mimetic, induce rabbit ASM cell growth,[47,48] and thrombin induces mitogenesis in human ASM cells.[35,37] Although the mechanisms that mediate these effects are unknown, agonist-induced cell growth probably is modulated by activation of G proteins in a similar manner as that described in vascular smooth muscle.

Using human ASM cells, Panettieri et al.[37] recently examined whether or not contractile agonist-induced human ASM cell growth was dependent on PLC activation and inositol trisphosphate formation.[37] These investigators examined the relative effects of bradykinin and thrombin on myocyte proliferation and PI turnover. Thrombin, but not bradykinin, stimulated ASM cell proliferation despite a fivefold greater increase in [$^3$H]-inositol phosphate formation in cells treated with bradykinin as compared with those treated with thrombin. These investigators also determined that inhibition of PLC activation with U-73122 had no effect on thrombin- or EGF-induced myocyte proliferation. In addition, PTX completely inhibited thrombin-induced ASM cell growth, but had no effect on PI turnover induced by either thrombin or bradykinin.[37] Taken together, these studies suggest that thrombin induced human ASM cell growth by activation of a pathway that was PTX sensitive and independent of PLC activation or PI turnover.

In comparison to RTK-dependent growth factors, contractile agonists, with the exception of thrombin, appear to be less-effective human ASM mitogens.[49] In cultured human ASM cells, 100 µM histamine or serotonin induces two- to threefold increases in [³H]-thymidine incorporation as compared with that obtained from unstimulated cells. EGF, serum, or phorbol esters, which directly activate PKC, induce 20- to 30-fold increases in [³H]-thymidine incorporation.[46,50,51] Interestingly, histamine is as effective as serum in stimulating cell growth and c-*fos* expression in canine ASM cells.[45] In rabbit ASM cells, endothelin-1 induces cell proliferation by activating phospholipase $A_2$ and by generating thromboxane $A_2$ and $LTD_4$.[47,48] In human ASM cells, however, endothelin-1, thromboxane $A_2$, and $LTD_4$ appear to have little effect on ASM cell proliferation despite these agonists inducing increases in cytosolic calcium.[37,50,52] Clearly, interspecies variability exists with regard to contractile agonist-induced cell proliferation. These models, however, may prove useful in dissecting downstream signaling events that modulate the differential effects of contractile agonists on ASM cell proliferation.

## 2. 3-Phosphorylated Inositol Lipids

Recently, these phospholipids have been recognized as a new class of second messengers.[30,53,154] Based on a number of studies, PtdIns 3,4,5-$P_3$ appears to be the critical signaling 3-phospholipid (see Figure 2). This assumption is supported by the time course of accumulation and the subsequent metabolism of the individual 3-phosphoinositides following agonist stimulation.[32,54] Although the routes of metabolism of these lipids are poorly understood when compared with those of the canonical PIs, some important features have emerged. The 3-phosphoinositides are not substrates for any known PLC,[30-32] are not components of the canonical PI turnover pathway, and their rapid increase upon growth factor stimulation suggests that the lipids themselves may act as second messengers mediating PtdIns 3-kinase mitogenic signals.[29] The recent identification that 3-phosphoinositides directly activate the $\zeta$ isoform of PKC may have important implications in understanding mechanisms that induce smooth muscle cell proliferation, since myocyte growth is thought to be PKC dependent.[55]

Compelling evidence suggests a role for PtdIns 3-kinase and its lipid products in regulating various cellular functions that include mitogenesis.[29] PtdIns 3-kinase, which consists of an 85-kDa regulatory subunit (p85) and a 110-kDa catalytic subunit (p110), is required for DNA synthesis induced by some, but not all, growth factors.[56] In 3T3 fibroblasts, microinjection of cells with a neutralizing antibody to the p110 catalytic subunit of PtdIns 3-kinase completely inhibited PDGF- and EGF-induced mitogenesis.[56] The role of PtdIns 3-kinase activation in modulating cell proliferation is cell-type specific. In some cells, bombesin and LPA, which induce cell proliferation by activating receptors coupled to G proteins, stimulated cell growth in the absence of PtdIns 3-kinase activity.[29,56] Taken together, these studies suggest that mitogens may activate different intracellular signaling pathways in a cell-specific manner.

Few investigators have examined the role of PtdIns 3-kinase activation in modulating human ASM cell proliferation. A recent study examined whether PtdIns 3-kinase mediated ASM cell growth or modulated calcium transients

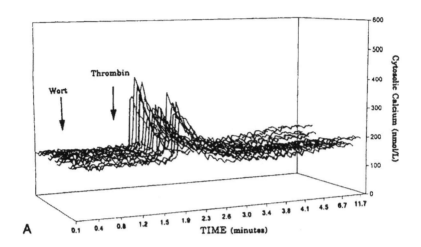

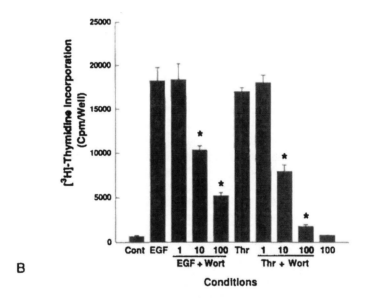

**FIGURE 3** Effects of PtdIns 3-kinase on cytosolic calcium mobilization and [3H]-thymidine incorporation in ASM cells. A. PtdIns 3-kinase inhibition does not modulate agonist-induced calcium transients. Monolayers were pretreated for 10 min with 100 nM wortmannin (Wort) and then stimulated with 0.3 U/ml thrombin. The experiment is representative of five with similar results. B. Inhibition of PtdIns 3-kinase abolishes DNA synthesis induced by agonists and growth factors in ASM cells. Confluent, growth-arrested ASM cells were pretreated with 1.0, 10, or 100 nM wortmannin (Wort) for 10 min and then stimulated with either 1 U/ml thrombin, 100 ng/ml EGF, or diluent. [3H]-Thymidine incorporation was then measured and compared with that obtained in cells treated with either thrombin (Thr), EGF, 100 nM wortmannin, or diluent (Cont) alone. Data represent means ± SEM from six experiments, each containing four replicates for each condition (*P < 0.01). (Data from Panettieri, R. A., Chilvers, E. R., Al-Hafidh, J., Eszterhas, A., and Murray, R. K., *J. Allergy Clin. Immunol.*, in press. With permission.)

induced by contractile agonists. Thrombin-induced increases in cytosolic calcium were examined in fura-2-loaded cells pretreated with wortmannin, a PtdIns 3-kinase inhibitor.[57] As shown in Figure 3A, inhibition of PtdIns 3-kinase did not alter calcium transients induced by thrombin.[57] In parallel experiments, confluent ASM cells that were growth arrested for 24 h were pretreated with wortmannin and then stimulated with thrombin or EGF. DNA synthesis was then measured by [³H]-thymidine incorporation. In a dose-dependent manner, wortmannin inhibited thrombin and EGF-induced DNA synthesis as shown in Figure 3B. Wortmannin had no effect on basal levels of [³H]-thymidine incorporation as compared with cells treated with diluent alone. If wortmannin was added 6 h after the cells were stimulated with mitogens, then wortmannin did not inhibit cell proliferation. These data suggest that PtdIns 3-kinase may mediate early signaling events that modulate myocyte growth. Taken together, these studies indicate that PtdIns 3-kinase activation may play an important role in modulating ASM cell proliferation induced by growth factors and contractile agonists.

## 3. Diacylglycerol Synthesis from PI- and PC-PLC Activation

Although the hydrolysis of polyphosphoinositides, especially $PIP_2$, to DAG is critically important in agonist-induced activation of PKC, recent evidence suggests that phosphatidylcholine (PC) hydrolysis is also a major source of DAG and may be as important in regulating PKC activation (Figure 4). PC hydrolysis produces a prolonged increase in cellular DAG, which has been hypothesized to induce sustained activation of PKC. The experimental evidence to support the role of agonist-induced PC hydrolysis in DAG synthesis is derived from two observations: (1) The time course and magnitude of increases in DAG levels with receptor stimulation differ from those of $IP_3$ levels[58-61] and (2) the fatty acid composition of DAG often differs from the mass of DAG and/or phosphatidic acid that is produced and markedly exceeds the decrease in the mass of inositol phospholipids.[59-65] Since increases in DAG activate PKC, the regulation of DAG formation is likely to play an important role in the regulation of cell proliferation.

The role of DAG formation in mediating mitogenesis has been supported by studies in 3T3 cells[66-68] and hematopoietic cell lines[69] stimulated with permeable DAG analogues. Other investigators, using 3T3 cells transfected with vectors that express the entire Ha-ras oncogene p21 protein or infected with Kirsten sarcoma virus, have observed that these cells underwent cellular transformation and have sustained increases in DAG, PC, and phosphatidylethanolamine, but unchanged PI levels.[70] Increases in DAG levels with agonist stimulation may result not only from newly synthesized DAG, but also from decreased degradation. Diacylglycerol kinase (DGK), which rapidly converts DAG to phosphatidic acid, plays a central role in the degradation of DAG.[71-73] To date, studies have only characterized the regulatory role of this pathway in

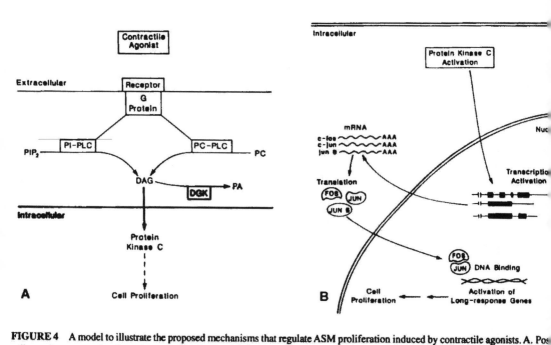

**FIGURE 4** A model to illustrate the proposed mechanisms that regulate ASM proliferation induced by contractile agonists. A. Pos cell membrane–associated regulatory events. B. Possible nuclear regulatory events. Abbreviations are: G proteins, guanine nucle binding regulatory protein; PIP$_2$, phosphatidylinositol 4,5 bisphosphate; DAG, 1,2-diacylglycerol; PC, phosphatidylcholine; PI-phosphoinositol-specific phospholipase C; PC-PLC, phosphatidylcholine-specific phospholipase C; DGK, diacylglycerol kinase phosphatidic acid. For ease of presentation, the receptor is linked to one G protein; however, it is possible that different G protein involved. (Modified from Panettieri, R. A., in *Airways Smooth Muscle: Development and Regulation of Contractility*, Raeburn, D Giembycz, M. A., Eds., Birkhauser Verlag, Basel, Switzerland, 1994. With permission.)

cells undergoing malignant transformation.[74] Alteration in the activity of this kinase may also affect PKC activation and, potentially, cell growth.

In vascular smooth muscle studies, investigators have determined that vasopressin, a vascular smooth muscle mitogen, and phorbol esters appear to induce a sustained elevation of DAG, derived primarily from PC hydrolysis or from phospholipase D activation.[65,75] This sustained elevation in DAG may then induce prolonged activation of PKC and stimulate cell proliferation. Most investigators of airway smooth muscle have not resolved the individual contribution of PI and PC hydrolysis to DAG synthesis.

### 4. Nuclear Inositides

There exists indirect evidence that polyphosphoinositides are found in the nucleus. These studies also suggest that stimulation of a nuclear phosphoinositidase C, which increases DAG formation in the nucleus, may induce PKC translocation from the cytosol to the nucleus. In 3T3 cells, IGF-1 stimulates a decrease in nuclear $PIP_2$ and PIP with an increase in DAG suggesting activation of a PLC.[76,77] The specificity of this response was determined in 3T3 cells stimulated with bombesin, which induced a marked increase in cytosolic $IP_3$ and DAG, but did not increase nuclear DAG levels. Interestingly, in cells treated with bombesin, PKC translocated to the plasma membrane, while in cells treated with IGF-1, PKC translocated to the nucleus.[78,79] Since both bombesin and IGF-1 stimulate mitogenesis in 3T3 cells, the significance of nuclear inositide formation in regulating cell proliferation remains unknown. These recent studies, however, suggest that the function of inositides appears to be increasingly complex.

### C. INTRACELLULAR CALCIUM MODULATES MITOGEN-INDUCED CELL PROLIFERATION

To a large extent, cellular processes regulated by alterations in the cytoplasmic concentration of ionized calcium are initiated by the release of this ion from sequestered intracellular stores. The most well-studied example is the release mediated by $IP_3$ gating of its receptor/ion channel. Compelling evidence, however, suggests that there are more calcium storage pools and release mechanisms than can be explained by the action of $IP_3$ alone. The exact nature of these pools and how they interact is an intensely investigated topic, which has been extensively reviewed.[80-82] In this section, the role of intracellular calcium signaling in regulating cell proliferation will be discussed as it pertains to smooth muscle cell growth.

Numerous studies have postulated the involvement of intracellular calcium signals in growth.[83] Studies using the $Ca^{2+}$ ionophore A23187 have determined that increases in cytosolic calcium induce proto-oncogene expression and cell proliferation.[84,85] The interpretation of these experiments, however, remains difficult since this molecule has pleiotrophic effects.[86,87] Despite these drawbacks, much evidence supports the role of growth factor–induced cytosolic

$Ca^{2+}$ signals as being necessary for activation of $G_o$ to $G_1$ transition and mitogenesis in some cell types.[88,89]

More recent studies suggest that the levels of $Ca^{2+}$ remaining in $Ca^{2+}$-accumulating organelles may also have important consequences for signaling and growth regulation.[90,91] Depletion of calcium stores within the endoplasmic reticulum by thapsigargin markedly inhibited growth factor–induced mitogenesis in a transformed smooth muscle cell line.[90] Such effects may result from either an altered ability of the endoplasmic reticulum to generate specific $Ca^{2+}$ signals necessary for cell growth or a modulation of key endoplasmic reticulum functions that are dependent on intraluminal $Ca^{2+}$ to induce mitogenesis. Interestingly, the effects of thapsigargin on cell growth were independent of any observed effects on PKC activation.[90] Taken together, current evidence suggests that cytosolic $Ca^{2+}$ mobilization or depletion of $Ca^{2+}$ stores in response to growth factors may be critical to modulate cell proliferation in some cells.

Although both growth factors and contractile agonists evoke calcium transients by stimulation of PLC in smooth muscle cells, the role of $Ca^{2+}$ in regulating smooth muscle cell growth remains controversial. Contractile agonists that both induce cell proliferation and contraction appear to do so by receptors coupled to different G proteins.[21,23,37,92,93] Some, but not all, contractile agonists stimulate ASM cell proliferation, despite the fact that most of these agonists induce comparable levels of polyphosphoinositide hydrolysis, cytosolic calcium transients, and c-fos mRNA expression.[28,46,50,94] Despite bradykinin and thrombin evoking comparable levels of cytosolic calcium in human ASM cells, thrombin, but not bradykinin, induced DNA synthesis in these cells.[37] In other studies, Stewart et al.[35] determined that EGF stimulated guinea pig ASM cell proliferation at concentrations that were markedly less than those necessary to evoke calcium transients. These studies suggest that other regulatory components apart from calcium mobilization are important in mediating smooth muscle cell proliferation.

## D. CYCLIC NUCLEOTIDES AND SMOOTH MUSCLE CELL GROWTH

Recognition that vascular smooth muscle proliferation is important in the pathogenesis of atherosclerosis has focussed attention on identifying cellular and molecular mechanisms that inhibit smooth muscle cell growth. An understanding of these mechanisms is not only critical in preventing cell growth but also in addressing whether or not the loss of inhibitory signals may induce myocyte proliferation.

Activation of cAMP-dependent kinase (A-kinase) or cGMP-dependent kinase (G-kinase) and alterations in extracellular matrix proteins have been reported to inhibit myocyte proliferation.[95] To date, several studies have determined that similar mechanisms inhibit ASM cell growth.[45,49,51,96,97]

### 1. cAMP and Cell Proliferation

New insights into the mechanisms by which cAMP-dependent pathways inhibit cell growth have recently been described. The activation of A-kinase results in the inhibition of Raf-1 activation in mammalian cells.[98,99] Raf-1, a serine/threonine protein kinase, is an effector for Ras-GTP, and the interaction of Raf-1 with Ras-GTP induces Raf activation. Activation of Raf-1 phosphorylates and activates other serine/threonine kinases, which ultimately activates the mitogen-activated protein kinase (MAPK) pathway. This pathway is thought to be critically important in modulating mitogen-induced cell proliferation of some cell types.

A-kinase is capable of phosphorylating Raf-1 at Ser43 in the amino-terminal regulatory domain of the kinase.[99] Inhibition of Raf-1 activation by A-kinase was independent of Ras-GTP loading stimulated by growth factors, PtdIns 3-kinase activation, or PLC-$\gamma_1$ activity. A-kinase, therefore, selectively inhibited Raf activation, but not activation of other components of the signal-transduction pathway required for mitogenesis in 3T3 cells. It remains unclear whether or not this phosphorylation site is responsible for uncoupling Raf-1 from Ras-GTP-dependent activation. Despite these advances in our knowledge concerning A-kinase effects on cell growth, mitogenesis of some cell types appears to be independent of Raf-1 inhibition, suggesting substantial redundancy in signal-transduction pathways that induce cell proliferation.[100,101]

In vascular smooth muscle as well as in ASM cells, activation of receptors coupled to Gs, which increases cytosolic cAMP levels and activates A-kinase, inhibits cell growth induced by growth factors.[49,51,102-105] A-kinase activation, however, appears to selectively inhibit mitogens that induce ASM cell growth through PI-PLC- and PKC-dependent pathways.[105] Alternatively, mitogens that stimulate cell proliferation through activation of RTKs are less sensitive to this inhibition.[51,105] Interestingly, these mitogens stimulate growth, in part, through PKC-independent mechanisms. In smooth muscle, "cross talk" between intracellular kinases appears crucial in coordinating cell proliferation.

In other cell lines, these distinctions have been questioned.[106] Growth inhibition by protein kinase activation is markedly cell specific. While elevations of intracellular cAMP inhibit cell growth in a wide variety of cell types,[103,104,107,108] it acts as a potent mitogen in other cells, such as 3T3 cells or PC12 cells.[109,110] Investigators using bovine ASM cells have reported that β-hexosaminidase, which transiently increases cytosolic cAMP levels, induces cell growth.[111,112] In these studies, however, sustained increases in cytosolic cAMP levels also inhibited myocyte proliferation induced by β-hexosaminidase.[112]

Using a human ASM cell line that retains a coupled β-adrenergic receptor–adenylate cyclase system, investigators have determined the role of A-kinase activation in modulating ASM cell proliferation induced by phorbol ester, EGF,[105] or thrombin.[113] Confluent growth-arrested cells were pretreated with forskolin, which directly activates adenylate cyclase, and were then stimulated with PMA or EGF. Forskolin pretreatment inhibited PMA-induced DNA synthesis by $70 \pm 3.2\%$ and that induced with EGF by $23 \pm 5\%$.[49,105] Receptor specificity was confirmed by pretreating cells with either isoproterenol or isoproterenol and propranolol, and DNA synthesis was measured after stimulating the cells with PMA. In a receptor-specific manner, isoproterenol completely abolished PKC-dependent DNA synthesis.[105] Similarly, PGE$_2$, which also induces increases in cAMP levels and activates A-kinase, inhibited PMA- and EGF-induced DNA synthesis (Panettieri, unpublished observations). In rabbit ASM cells[96] and in guinea pig ASM,[97] activation of cAMP-dependent pathways also inhibited mitogen-induced ASM cell growth. Taken together, these studies suggest that DNA synthesis induced by growth factors or agonists is inhibited by pathways that activate A-kinase.

Identifying cellular mechanisms that inhibit ASM cell growth may be relevant not only with regard to preventing ASM cell proliferation, but also in terms of understanding the full spectrum of pathways that regulate cell growth. For example, further studies may clarify whether or not myocyte proliferation results from a loss of tonic inhibitory effects of A-kinase. Such studies may have important implications concerning the chronic use of therapeutic agents that manipulate these signal-transduction pathways.

## 2. Role of cGMP in Modulating Smooth Muscle Cell Growth

Atrial naturetic factor, sodium nitroprusside, and nitric oxide are potent vasodilators that mediate their effects by increasing cytosolic cGMP levels and activating G-kinase. Recently, investigators have reported that vascular smooth muscle cell proliferation induced by serum or by serotonin is inhibited by pretreating cells with atrial naturetic peptide or with permeant cGMP analogues.[114-116] In a preliminary study using guinea pig ASM cells, nitroprusside and dibutyryl cGMP, a permeable cGMP analogue, also inhibited serum-induced cell proliferation.[117] However, the downstream signaling events that mediate G-kinase inhibition of cell growth remain unknown.

In some cell types, cGMP may enhance the formation of cyclic adenosine diphosphate ribose (cADPR), a metabolite of NAD that can release Ca$^{2+}$ by acting on the ryanodine receptor.[118-120] In these cells, increases in cGMP induced cell proliferation. Clearly, further studies are needed to define the role of cGMP in modulating cell proliferation.

## III. SECOND MESSENGERS MODULATE SMOOTH MUSCLE CELL GROWTH BY ACTIVATION OF DOWNSTREAM EFFECTORS

The above discussion has focussed on the second messenger systems that modulate ASM cell proliferation. An exhaustive review of the sequential protein kinase cascades activated by mitogens was beyond the scope of this chapter. However, it is important to review some recent advances in our understanding of downstream effector molecules that are activated by second messengers and that may play critical roles in transducing growth signals in smooth muscle cells.

## A. ACTIVATION OF RAS

The proteins encoded by *ras* genes serve as essential transducers of diverse physiological signals, and ras proteins, which are mutationally altered, can induce cell transformation. Although the *ras* gene was first identified in transforming retroviruses (v-ras), the identification that retroviral oncogenes (v-*ras)* were derived from normal cellular genes (c-*ras*) has led to the recognition that Ras activation plays a critical role in mediating normal cell growth and differentiation.[121,122]

Ras, which migrates as a 21-kDa protein (p21^ras), has served as a prototype for the superfamily of Ras-related proteins, a group of guanine nucleotide–binding proteins that share structural homology.[121-123] The discovery that Ras proteins bind guanine nucleotides (GTP and GDP) with high affinity and possess intrinsic GTPase activity suggested a mechanism by which Ras activity is regulated. Ligand-bound receptors induce the active GTP-bound form of Ras by enhancing the ability of guanine nucleotide-exchange factors to accelerate the replacement of bound GDP with GTP. Ras proteins are then deactivated by interaction with GTPase-activating proteins (GAPs) that promote GTP hydrolysis by Ras (see Figure 1). In some cell types, active Ras promotes cell proliferation; in others, it arrests cell division and induces the expression of differentiated phenotypes.[121] The role of Ras activation in mediating mitogen-induced smooth muscle cell proliferation remains unknown.

Recent studies have identified that activated Ras interacts with both Raf kinase and PtdIns 3-kinase, two important Ras effector proteins that modulate growth factor–induced proliferation of 3T3 and Rat-1 fibroblasts.[122,124] The initial step in Ras activation of Raf involves the binding of active GTP-Ras to Raf kinase.[122] Ras binding alone does not activate the intrinsic kinase activity of Raf; rather, it localizes Raf to the plasma membrane where Raf is activated. Activated Raf then stimulates a cascade of other kinases, including MAPK, whose activation, in some cells, is necessary to induce cell proliferation. A parallel pathway, however, by which activated Ras may induce cell growth involves PtdIns 3-kinase activation.[124] Evidence suggests that Ras binds to PtsIns 3-kinase *in vitro* only when Ras is in the active state and the level of PtdIns 3-kinase generated *in vivo* can be increased or decreased depending on whether activated or dominant negative Ras mutants are expressed.[121,122,124] Interestingly, Raf activation does not alter the level of these molecules, suggesting that PtdIns 3-kinase may be one component of a distinct parallel downstream pathway from Ras. To date, investigators of ASM have not addressed the role that Ras activation may play in regulating mitogen-induced ASM proliferation.

## B. PROTEIN KINASE C ACTIVATION

Activation of PKC, either directly by phorbol esters or indirectly by mitogens, is an important signaling event for the proliferation of many cells,[27,66,125-127] including smooth muscle.[128] Activated PKC in conjunction with increased cytosolic calcium induces intracellular alkalinization by promoting

Na⁺/H⁺ exchange and by phosphorylating specific substrates that have been associated with cell proliferation. PKC, a family of protein kinases activated by calcium and DAG, induces protein phosphorylation of serine and threonine residues of many proteins. One such protein with a molecular weight of 76,000 (p76) has been well characterized and its phosphorylation associated with mitogenesis.[125,128,129,130-132] Cloning and molecular biology studies have revealed the existence of multiple isotypes of PKC. To date, at least four calcium- and phosphatidyl serine-dependent PKC isotypes (α, βI-, βII-, γ-PKC) and four calcium-independent isotypes (δ-, ε-, ζ-, and η-PKC) have been identified.[133-137] A recent study has determined that most of the above PKC isotypes are found in canine ASM except for PKC-η which was not present.[138] Currently, there is little evidence to designate specific functions for each PKC isotype; however, their distribution appears to be tissue specific.

The role of PKC activation in fibroblast and smooth muscle cell proliferation induced by contractile agonists has been demonstrated by down regulation of PKC following prolonged pretreatment with phorbol esters. In these cells, pretreatment diminished phorbol ester–induced p76 phosphorylation by 80–90%, abolished phorbol ester stimulation of cell proliferation in 3T3 cells[129,139] and vascular smooth muscle cells,[128] as well as markedly attenuating phorbol ester-induced c-fos expression.[94] However, the mitogenic responses of PKC-deficient 3T3 cells to PDGF,[140] EGF,[141] and FGF[142] were not attenuated. Other studies have demonstrated that rabbit ASM cell proliferation induced by serum was inhibited by selective PKC inhibitors, RO-318220 and RO-317549.[143] Taken together, these data suggest that PKC activation is necessary in transducing growth signals from receptors coupled to G proteins and from RTK in some cell types.

The dependence of receptor-activated mitogenesis on PKC appears to be growth factor and cell specific. For example, EGF- or IGF-1-induced proliferation of 3T3 cells was PKC-independent,[141] while PKC activation of human fibroblasts actually inhibited EGF-induced cell proliferation.[142] Further, some but not all contractile agonists that activate PKC induce vascular smooth muscle cell proliferation.[94,144] These data suggest that PKC activation may be necessary but not sufficient to induce G protein–dependent cell growth and other signaling pathways must modulate the proliferative response.

## C.  MITOGEN-ACTIVATED PROTEIN KINASES

MAPKs, which constitute a family of 40–46 kDa serine/threonine kinases, are activated early in response to extracellular signals and appear to play an integral role in the signaling cascade initiated by diverse stimuli. A variety of mitogens activate MAPK *in vivo,* including PDGF,[153] EGF,[145] and nerve growth factor,[146] all of which induce autophosphorylation of their receptors on tyrosine residues. Evidence also suggests that MAPK activation occurs in response to stimulation of receptors coupled to heterotrimeric G proteins.[40,152] Although the precise signaling events that modulate MAPK activation remain unknown, a major pathway requires the sequential activation of Ras, Raf, and

MAPK/Erk-activating kinase, also known as MAPK kinase (MAPKK). MAPKK has been shown to directly phosphorylate MAPK on both tyrosine and threonine residues.[147,148] The phosphorylation of both these residues is required for maximal enzymatic activation of MAPK.[147,148] Subsequently, the activated MAPK, which translocates from the cytoplasm to the nucleus,[147] induces expression of the proto-oncogenes, c-jun and c-myc, which are necessary for cell proliferation.[149,150] In Chinese hamster fibroblasts, transient expression of p44[mapk] antisense RNA or a p44[mapk] kinase-deficient mutant abolished growth factor–stimulated c-fos and c-jun expression as well as cell proliferation.[151] The integration of signal events activated by tyrosine and serine/threonine phosphorylation at the level of MAPK suggests that MAPK plays a central role in the downstream regulation of cell proliferation.

Recent studies have revealed that growth factors that stimulate RTK and those that stimulate receptors coupled to G proteins activate MAPK in bovine ASM cells.[40,152] The investigators suggested that sustained activation of MAPK correlated with the proliferative response of bovine ASM cells to the putative mitogen. Others have also suggested that prolonged activation of MAPK is necessary to induce cell proliferation of CCL 39 cells stimulated with thrombin.[147] Despite these studies, the role of MAPK in regulating cell proliferation remains controversial. It is likely that the role of MAPK activation as a requirement for growth factor–stimulated DNA synthesis will vary among different cell types, and more studies are needed to determine whether MAPK activation is necessary and sufficient to induce ASM cell growth.

## ACKNOWLEDGMENT

Source(s) of support: National Institutes of Health, HL02647; National Aeronautics and Space Administration.

## REFERENCES

1. NHLBI Workshop on Airway Smooth Muscle, *Am. Rev. Respir. Dis.*, 131, 159, 1985.
2. Boushey, H. A., Holtzman, M. J., Sheller, J. R., and Nadel, J. A., State of the art: bronchial hyperreactivity, *Am. Rev. Respir. Dis.*, 121, 389, 1980.
3. Andersson, K.-E., Airway hyperreactivity, smooth muscle and calcium, *Eur. J. Respir. Dis.*, 131, 49, 1983.
4. Leff, A. R., State of the art: Endogenous regulation of bronchomotor tone, *Am. Rev. Respir. Dis.*, 137, 1198, 1988.
5. Barnes, P. J., Inflammation, in *Bronchial Asthma*, Weiss, E. B., and Stein, M., Eds., Little, Brown, Boston, 1993, 80.
6. Brown, J. P., Breville, W. H., and Finucane, K. E., Asthma and irreversible airflow obstruction, *Thorax*, 39, 131, 1984.
7. Peat, J. K., Woolcock, A. J., and Cullen, K., Rate of decline of lung function in subjects with asthma, *Eur. J. Respir. Dis.*, 70, 171, 1987.

8. Woolcock, A. J., Asthma — what are the important experiments? State of the art/conference summary, *Am. Rev. Respir. Dis.*, 138, 730, 1988.

9. Dunnill, M. S., Massarella, G. R., and Anderson, J. A., A comparison of the quantitative anatomy of the bronchi in normal subjects, in status asthmaticus, in chronic bronchitis and in emphysema, *Thorax*, 24, 176, 1969.

10. Hossain, S., Quantitative measurement of bronchial muscle in asthma, *Am. Rev. Respir. Dis.*, 107, 99, 1973.

11. Huber, H. L. and Koessler, K. K., The pathology of bronchial asthma, *Arch. Intern. Med.*, 30, 690, 1922.

12. Heard, B. E. and Hossain, S., Hyperplasia of bronchial muscle in asthma, *J. Pathol.*, 110, 319, 1973.

13. Bobik, A., Grooms, A., Millar, J. A., Mitchell, A., and Grinpukel, S., Growth factor activity of endothelin on vascular smooth muscle, *Am. J. Physiol.*, 258 (*Cell Physiol.* 27), C408, 1990.

14. Taubman, M. B., Berk, B. C., Izumo, S., Tsuda, T., Alexander, R. W., and Nadal Ginard, B., Angiotensin II induces c-*fos* mRNA in aortic smooth muscle. Role of $Ca^{2+}$ mobilization and protein kinase C activation, *J. Biol. Chem.*, 264, 526, 1989.

15. Berk, B. C., Brock, T. A., Webb, R. C., Taubman, M. B., Atkinson, W. J., Gimbrone, M. A., Jr., and Alexander, R. W., Epidermal growth factor, a vascular smooth muscle mitogen, induces rat aortic contraction, *J. Clin. Invest.*, 75, 1083, 1985.

16. Berk, B. C., Alexander, R. W., Brock, T. A., Gimbrone, M., and Webb, R., Vasoconstriction: a new activity for platelet-derived growth factor, *Science*, 232, 87, 1986.

17. Glenn, K., Bowen-Pope, D. F., and Ross, R., Platelet-derived growth factor. III. Identification of a platelet-derived growth factor receptor by affinity labeling, *J. Biol. Chem.*, 257, 5172, 1982.

18. Rozengurt, E., Early signals in the mitogenic response, *Science*, 234, 161, 1986.

19. Sporn, M. B. and Roberts, A. B., Peptide growth factors and inflammation, tissue repair, and cancer, *J. Clin. Invest.*, 78, 329, 1986.

20. Clowes, A. W., Clowes, M. M., Kocher, O., Ropraz, P., Chaponnier, C., and Gabbiani, G., Arterial smooth muscle cells in vivo: relationship between actin isoform expression and mitogenesis and their modulation by heparin, *J. Cell Biol.*, 107, 1939, 1988.

21. Panettieri, R. A., Goldie, R. G., Rigby, P., Eszterhas, A. J., Hay, D. W. P., Endothelin-1-induced potentiation of human airway smooth muscle proliferation: An $ET_A$ receptor-mediated phenomenon, *Br. J. Pharmacol.*, 118, 191, 1996.

22. Nemecek, G. M., Coughlin, S. R., Handley, D. A., and Moskowitz, M. A., Stimulation of aortic smooth muscle cell mitogenesis by serotonin, *Proc. Natl. Acad. Sci. U.S.A.*, 83, 674, 1986.

23. Kavanaugh, W. M., Williams, L. T., Ives, H. E., and Coughlin, S. R., Serotonin-induced deoxyribonucleic acid synthesis in vascular smooth muscle cells involves a novel, pertussis toxin-sensitive pathway, *Mol. Endocrinol.*, 123, 599, 1988.

24. Fabisiak, J. P., Kelley, J., Platelet-derived growth factor, in *Cytokines of the Lung*, Kelley, J., Ed., Marcel Dekker, New York, NY, 1993, p. 3.

25. Raines, E. W., Bowen-Pope, D. F., Ross, R., Platelet-derived growth factor, in *Peptide Growth Factors and Their Receptors*, Part I, Sporn, M. B., Roberts, A. B., Eds., Springer-Verlag, New York, 1991, p. 173.

26. Nishizuka, Y., Turnover of inositol phospholipids and signal transduction, *Science*, 225, 1365, 1984.

27. Nishizuka, Y., The role of protein kinase C in cell surface signal transduction and tumour promotion, *Nature (London)*, 308, 693, 1984.

28. Nambi, P., Watt, R., Whitman, M., Aiyar, N., Moore, J. P., Evan, G. I., and Crooke, S., Induction of c-*fos* protein by activation of vasopressin receptors in smooth muscle cells, *FEB*, 245, 61, 1989.

29. Kapeller, R. and Cantley, L. C., Phosphatidylinositol 3-kinase, *BioEssays*, 16, 565, 1994.

30. Stephens, L. T., Jackson, T., and Hawkins, P., Agonist stimulated synthesis of phosphatidylinositol (3,4,5)-trisphosphate: a new intracellular signalling system?, *Biochim. Biophys. Acta*, 1179, 27, 1993.

31. Varticovski, L., Harrison-Findik, D., Keeler, M. L., and Susa, M., Role of PI 3-kinase in mitogenesis, *Biochim. Biophys. Acta*, 1226, 1, 1994.

32. Fry, M. J., Structure, regulation and function of phosphoinositide 3-kinases, *Biochim. Biophys. Acta*, 1226, 237, 1994.

33. Kim, H. K., Kim, J. W., Zilberstein, A., Margolis, B., et al., PDGF stimulation of inositol phospholipid hydrolysis requires PLC-γ1 phosphorylation on tyrosine residues 783 and 1254, *Cell*, 65, 435, 1991.

34. Chen, W. S., Lazar, C. S., Lund, K. A., Welsh, J. B., et al., Functional independence of the epidermal growth factor receptor from a domain required for ligand-induced internalization and calcium regulation, *Cell*, 59, 33, 1989.

35. Stewart, A. G., Grigoriadis, G., and Harris, T., Mitogenic actions of endothelin-1 and epidermal growth factor in cultured airway smooth muscle, *Clin. Exp. Pharmacol. Physiol.*, 21, 277, 1994.

36. Hirst, S. I., Barnes, P.J., and Twort, C.H.C., Quantifying the proliferative response in cultured human and rabbit airway smooth muscle, *Am. Rev. Respir. Dis.*, 7, 544, 1992.

37. Panettieri, R. A., Hall, I. P., Maki, C. S., and Murray, R. K., α-Thrombin increases cytosolic calcium and induces human airway smooth muscle cell proliferation, *Am. J. Respir. Cell Mol. Biol.*, 13, 205, 1995.

38. Cohen, P., Noveral, J. P., Bhala, A., Nunn, S. E., Herrick, D. J., and Grunstein, M. M., Leukotriene D₄ facilitates airway smooth muscle cell proliferation via modulation of the IGF axis, *Am. J. Physiol.* 269 (*Lung Cell. Mol. Physiol.* 13), L151, 1995.

39. Noveral, J. P., Bhala, A., Grunstein, M., and Cohen, P., The insulin-like growth factor axis in airway smooth muscle cells, *Am. J. Physiol.* 267 (*Lung Cell. Mol. Physiol.* 11), L761, 1994.

40. Kelleher, M. D., Abe, M. K., Chao, T.-S. O., Jain, M., Green, J. M., Solway, J., Rosner, M. R., and Hershenson, M. B., Role of MAP kinase activation in bovine tracheal smooth muscle mitogenesis, *Am. J. Physiol.* 268 (*Lung Cell. Mol. Physiol.* 12), L894, 1995.

41. Hepler, J. R. and Gilman, A. G., G proteins, *Trends Biochem. Sci.*, 17, 383, 1992.

42. Sternweis, P. C., The active role of βγ in signal transduction, *Curr. Opin. Cell Biol.*, 6, 198, 1994.

43. Simon, M. I., Strathmann, M. P., and Gautam, M., Diversity of G proteins in signal transduction, *Science*, 252, 802, 1991.

44. Lamorte, V. J., Harootunian, A. T., Spiegel, A. M., Tsien, R. Y., and Feransisco, J. R., Mediation of growth factor induced DNA synthesis and calcium mobilization by Gq and G₁₂, *J. Cell Biol.*, 121, 91, 1993.

45. Panettieri, R. A., Yadvish, P. A., Kelly, A. M., Rubinstein, N. A., and Kotlikoff, M. I., Histamine stimulates proliferation of airway smooth muscle and induces c-*fos* expression, *Am. J. Physiol.* 259 (*Lung Cell. Mol. Physiol.* 3), L365, 1990.

46. Panettieri, R. A., Eszterhas, A., and Murray, R. K., Agonist-induced proliferation of airway smooth muscle cells is mediated by alteration in cytosolic calcium, *Am. Rev. Respir. Dis.*, 145, A15, 1992.

47. Noveral, J. P., Rosenberg, S. M., Anbar, R. A., Pawlowski, N. A., and Grunstein, M. M., Role of endothelin-1 in regulating proliferation of cultured rabbit airway smooth muscle cells, *Am. J. Physiol.* 263 (*Lung Cell. Mol. Physiol.* 7), L317, 1992.

48. Noveral, J. P. and Grunstein, M. M., Role and mechanism of thromboxane-induced proliferation of cultured airway smooth muscle cells, *Am. J. Physiol.* 263 (*Lung Cell. Mol. Physiol.* 7), L555, 1992.

49. Panettieri, R. A., Airways smooth muscle cell growth and proliferation, in *Airways Smooth Muscle: Development and Regulation of Contractility*, Raeburn, D. and Giembycz, M. A., Eds., Birkhauser Verlag, Basel, Switzerland, 1994, 41.

50. Panettieri, R. A., Rubinstein, N. A., Kelly, A. M., and Kotlikoff, M. I., The specificity of c-*fos* expression in the induction of airway smooth muscle proliferation by contractile agonists, *Am. Rev. Respir. Dis.*, 143, A934, 1991.

51. Panettieri, R. A., Cohen, M. D., and Bilgen, G., Airway smooth muscle cell proliferation is inhibited by microinjection of the catalytic subunit of cAMP dependent kinase, *Am. Rev. Respir. Dis.*, 147, A252, 1993.

52. Panettieri, R. A., Murray, R. K., DePalo L. R., Yadvish, P. A., and Kotlikoff, M., A human airway smooth muscle cell line that retains physiological responsiveness. *Am. J. Physiol.* 256 (*Cell Physiol.* 25), C329, 1989.

53. Stephens, L., Cooke, F. T., Walters, R., Jackson, T., Volinia, S., Gout, I., Waterfield, M. D., and Hawkins, P. T., Characterization of a phosphatidylinositol-specific phosphoinositide 3-kinase from mammalian cells, *Curr. Biol.*, 4, 203, 1994.

54. Irvine, R. F., Inositol lipids in cell signalling, *Curr. Opin. Cell Biol.*, 4, 212, 1992.

55. Nakarish, H., Brewer, K. A., and Exton, J. H., Activation of the zeta isoenzyme of protein kinase C by phosphotidylinositol 3,4,5-trisphosphate, *J. Biol. Chem.*, 268, 13, 1993.

56. Roche, S., Koeg, M., and Courtneidge, S. A., The phosphatidylinositol 3-kinase is required for DNA synthesis induced by some, but not all, growth factors, *Proc. Natl. Acad. Sci. U.S.A.*, 91, 9185, 1994.

57. Panettieri, R. A., Chilvers, E. R., Al-Hafidh, J., Eszterhas, A., and Murray, R. K., Thrombin induces human airway smooth muscle (ASM) cell proliferation by activation of a novel signaling pathway, *J. Allergy Clin. Immunol.*, in press.

58. Exton, J. H., Mechanisms of alpha-1-adrenergic and related responses: roles of calcium, phosphoinositides, calmodulin and guanine nucleotides and changes in protein phosphorylation, in *Cell Membranes: Methods and Reviews*, Vol. 3, Elson, E. L., Frazier, W. A., and Glaser, L., Eds., Plenum, New York, 1987, 113.

59. Bocckino, S. B., Blackmore, P. F., Wilson, P. B., and Exton, J. H., Phosphatidate accumulation in hormone-treated hepatocytes via a phospholipase D mechanism, *J. Biol. Chem.*, 262, 15309, 1987.

60. Bocckino, S. B., Blackmore, P. F., and Exton J. H., Stimulation of 1,2-diacylglycerol accumulation in hepatocytes by vasopressin, epinephrine, and angiotensin II, *J. Biol. Chem.*, 260, 14201, 1985.

61. Exton, J. H., Mechanisms of action of calcium-mobilizing agonists: some variations on a young theme, *FASEB J.*, 2, 2670, 1988.

62. Grillone, L. R., Clark, M. A., Godfrey, R. W., Stassen, F., and Crooke, S.T., Vasopressin induces $V_1$ receptors to activate phosphatidylinositol- and phosphatidylcholine-specific phospholipase C and stimulates the release of arachidonic acid by at least two pathways in the smooth muscle cell line, A-10, *J. Biol. Chem.*, 263, 2658, 1988.

63. Takuwa, N., Takuwa, Y., and Rasmussen, H., A tumour promoter, 12-*O*-tetradecanoylphorbol 13-acetate, increases cellular 1,2-diacylglycerol content through a mechanism other than phosphoinositide hydrolysis in Swiss-mouse 3T3 fibroblasts, *Biochem. J.*, 243, 647, 1987.

64. Daniel, L.W., Waite, M., and Wykle, R. L., A novel mechanism of diglyceride formation. 12-*O*-tetradecanoylphorbol-13-acetate stimulates the cyclic breakdown and resynthesis of phosphatidylcholine, *J. Biol. Chem.*, 261, 9128, 1986.

65. Griendling, K. K., Rittenhouse, S. E., Brock, T. A., Ekstein, L. S., Gimbrone, M. A., Jr., and Alexander, R. W., Sustained diacylglycerol formation from inositol phospholipids in angiotensin II-stimulated vascular smooth muscle cells, *J. Biol. Chem.*, 261, 5901, 1986.

66. Rozengurt, E., Rodriguez-Pena, A., Coombs, M., and Sinnett-Smith, J., Diacylglycerol stimulates DNA synthesis and cell division in mouse 3T3 cells: role of $Ca^{2+}$-sensitive phospholipid-dependent protein kinase, *Proc. Natl. Acad. Sci. U.S.A.*, 81, 5748, 1984.

67. Kishimoto, A., Takai, Y., Mori, T., Kikkawa, U., and Nishizuka, Y., Activation of calcium and phospholipid-dependent protein kinase by diacylglycerol, its possible relation to phosphatidylinositol turnover, *J. Biol. Chem.*, 255, 2273, 1980.

68. Davis, R. J., Ganong, B. R., Bell, R. M., and Czech, M. P. *sn*-1,2-Dioctanoylglycerol. A cell-permeable diacylglycerol that mimics phorbol diester action on the epidermal growth factor receptor and mitogenesis, *J. Biol. Chem.*, 260, 1562, 1985.

69. Pai, J.-K. and Siegel, M. I., Activation of phospholipase D by chemotactic peptide in HL-60 granulocytes, *Biochem. Biophys. Res. Commun.*, 150, 355, 1988.

70. Lacal, J. C., Moscat, J., and Aaronson, S. A., Novel source of 1,2-diacylglycerol elevated in cells transformed by Ha-*ras* oncogene, *Nature (London)*, 330, 269, 1987.

71. Hokin, M. R. and Hokin, L. E., The synthesis of phosphatidic acid from diglyceride and adenosine triphosphate in extracts of brain microsomes, *J. Biol. Chem.*, 234, 1381, 1959.

72. Michell, R. H., Inositol lipids and their role in receptor function: history and general principles, in *Phosphoinositides and Receptor Mechanisms*, Putney, J. W., Jr., Ed., Alan R. Liss, New York, 1986, 1.

73. Irving, H. R. and Exton, J. H., Phosphatidylcholine breakdown in rat liver plasma membranes. Roles of guanine nucleotides and $P_2$-purinergic agonists, *J. Biol. Chem.*, 262, 3440, 1987.

74. Huang, M., Chida, K., Kamata, N., Nose, K., Kato, M., Homma, Y., Takenawa, T., and Kuroki, T., Enhancement of inositol phospholipid metabolism and activation of protein kinase C in *ras*-transformed rat fibroblasts, *J. Biol. Chem.*, 263, 17975, 1988.

75. Konishi, F., Kondo, T., and Inapami, T., Phospholipase D in cultured rat vascular smooth muscle cells and its activation by phorbol ester, *Biochem. Biophys. Res. Commun.*, 179, 1070, 1991.

76. Cocco, L., Gilmour, R. S., Ognibene, A., Letcher, A. J., Manzou, F. A., and Irvine, R. F., Synthesis of polyphosphoinositides metabolism inside the nucleus which changes with cell differentiation, *Biochem. J.*, 248, 765, 1987.

77. Leach, K., Powers, E. A., Ruff, V. A., Jaker, S., Kaufmann, S., Type 3 protein kinase C localisation to the nuclear envelope of phorbol ester-treated NIH 3T3 cells, *J. Cell Biol.*, 109, 685, 1989.

78. Hocevar, B. A. and Fields, A. P., Selective translocatioin of $\beta_{11}$-protein kinase C to the nucleus of human promyelocytic (HL60) leukemia cells, *J. Biol. Chem.*, 266, 28, 1991.

79. Divecha, N., Banfic, H., and Irvine, R. F., The polyphosphoinositide cycle exists in the nuclei of Swiss 3T3 cells under the control of a receptor (for IGF-I) in the plasma membrane, and stimulation of the cycle increases nuclear diacylglycerol and apparently induces translocation of protein kinase C to the nucleus, *EMBO J.*, 10, 3207, 1991.

80. Cheek, T. R., Calcium regulation and homeostasis, *Curr. Opin. Cell Biol.*, 3, 199, 1991.

81. Tsien, R. W. and Tsien, R. Y., Calcium channels, stores and oscillations, *Annu. Rev. Cell Biol.*, 6, 715, 1990.

82. Burgoyne, R. D. and Cheek, T. R., Locating intracellular calcium stores, *Trends Biochem. Sci.*, 16, 319, 1991.

83. Whitaker, M. and Patel, R., Calcium and cell cycle control, *Development*, 108, 525, 1990.

84. Büscher, M., Rahmsdorf, H. J., Litfin, M., Karin, M., and Herrlich, P., Activation of the c-*fos* gene by UV and phorbol ester: different signal transduction pathways converge to the same enhancer element, *Oncogene*, 3, 301, 1988.

85. Fisch, T. M., Prywes, R., and Roeder, R. G., c-*fos* sequences necessary for basal expression and induction by epidermal growth factor, 12-*O*-tetradecanoyl phorbol-13-acetate, and the calcium ionophore, *Mol. Cell. Biol.*, 7, 3490, 1987.

86. Smith, P. L. and McCabe, R. D., A23187-induced changes in colonic K and Cl transport are mediated by separate mechanisms, *Am. J. Physiol.*, 247 (*Gastrointest. Liver Physiol.* 10), G695, 1984.

87. Erlij, D., Gersten, L., Sterba, G., and Schoen, H. F., Role of prostaglandin release in the response of tight epithelia to $Ca^{2+}$ ionophores, *Am. J. Physiol.*, 250 (*Cell Physiol.* 19), C629, 1986.

88. Rozengurt, E., Growth factors and cell proliferation, *Curr. Opin. Cell Biol.*, 4, 161, 1992.

89. Lopez-Rivas, A., Mendoza, S. A., Nanberg, E., Sinnett-Smith, J., and Rozengurt, E., $Ca^{2+}$-mobilizing actions of platelet-derived growth factor differ from those of bombesin and vasopressin in Swiss 3T3 mouse cells, *Proc. Natl. Acad. Sci. U.S.A.*, 84, 5768, 1987.

90. Ghosh, T. K., Bian, J., Short, A. D., Rybak, S. L., and Gill, D. L., Persistent intracellular calcium pool depletion by thapsigargin and its influence on cell growth, *J. Biol. Chem.*, 266, 24690, 1991.

91. Schönthal, A., Sugarman, J., Brown, J. H., Hanley, M. R., and Feramisco, J. R., Regulation of c-*fos* and c-*jun* protooncogene expression by the Ca²⁺-ATPase inhibitor thapsigargin, *Proc. Natl. Acad. Sci. U.S.A.*, 88, 7096, 1991.

92. Chambard, J. C., Paris, S., L'Allemain, G., and Pouyssegur, J., Two growth factor signaling pathways in fibroblasts distinguished by pertussis toxin, *Nature (London)*, 326, 800, 1987.

93. Vicentini, L. M. and Villereal, M. L., Serum, bradykinin and vasopressin stimulate release of inositol phosphates from human fibroblasts, *Biochem. Biophys. Res. Commun.*, 123, 663, 1984.

94. Block, L. H., Emmons, L. R., Vogt, E., Sachinidis, A., Vetter, W., Hoppe, J., Ca²⁺-channel blockers inhibit the action of recombinant platelet-derived growth factor in vascular smooth muscle cells, *Proc. Natl. Acad. Sci. U.S.A.*, 85, 2388, 1989.

95. Pastan, I. H., Johnson, G. S., and Anderson, W. B., Role of cyclic nucleotides in growth control, *Annu. Rev. Biochem.*, 44, 491, 1975.

96. Noveral, J. P. and Grunstein, M. M., Adrenergic receptor-mediated regulation of cultured rabbit airway smooth muscle cell proliferation, *Am. J. Physiol.* 267 (*Lung Cell. Mol. Physiol.* 11), L291, 1994.

97. Florio, C., Martin, J. G., Styhler, A., and Heisler, S., Antiproliferative effect of prostaglandin E₂ in cultured guinea pig tracheal smooth muscle cells, *Am. J. Physiol.* 266 (*Lung Cell. Mol. Physiol.* 10), L131, 1994.

98. Sevetson, B. R., Kong, X., and Lawrence, J. C., Jr., Increasing cAMP attenuates activation of mitogen-activated protein kinase, *Proc. Natl. Acad. Sci. U.S.A.*, 90, 10305, 1993.

99. Wu, J., Dent, P., Jelinek, T., Wolfman, A., Weber, M. J., and Sturgill, T. W., Inhibition of the EGF-activated MAP kinase signaling pathway by adenosine 3,5-monophosphate, *Science*, 262, 1065, 1993.

100. Thomas, S. M., DeMarco, M., D'Arcangelo, G., Halegoua, S., and Brugge, J. S., Ras is essential for nerve growth factor- and phorbol ester-induced tyrosine phosphorylation of MAP kinases, *Cell*, 68, 1031, 1992.

101. Rekenstein, A., Rydel, R. E., and Greene, L.A., Multiple agents rescue PC12 cells from serum-free cell death by translation- and transcription-independent mechanisms, *J. Neurosci.*, 11, 2552, 1991.

102. Jonzon, B., Nilsson, J., and Fredholm, B. B., Adenosine receptor-mediated changes in cyclic AMP production and DNA synthesis in cultured arterial smooth muscle cells, *J. Cell. Physiol.*, 124, 451, 1985.

103. Loesberg, C., Van Wijk, R., Zandbergen, J., Van Aken, W. G., Van Mourik, J. A., and De Groot, P. G., Cell cycle-dependent inhibition of human vascular smooth muscle cell proliferation by prostaglandin E₁, *Exp. Cell Res.*, 160, 117, 1985.

104. Nilsson, J. and Olsson, A. G., Prostaglandin E₁ inhibits DNA synthesis in arterial smooth muscle cells stimulated with platelet-derived growth factor. *Atherosclerosis*, 53, 77, 1984.

105. Panettieri, R. A., Rubenstein, N. A., Feurstein, B., and Kotlikoff, M. I., Beta-adrenergic inhibition of airway smooth muscle proliferation, *Am. Rev. Respir. Dis.*, 143, A608, 1991.

106. Magnaldo, I., Pouyssegur, J., and Paris, S., Cyclic AMP inhibits mitogen-induced DNA synthesis in hamster fibroblasts, regardless of the signaling pathway involved, *FEB*, 245, 65, 1989.

107. Rozengurt, E., Cyclic AMP: a growth-promoting signal for mouse 3T3 cells, *Adv. Cyclic Nucleotide Res.*, 14, 429, 1981.

108. Speir, E. S. and Epstein, S. E., Inhibition of smooth muscle cell proliferation by antisense oligodeoxynucleotide targeting the messenger RNA encoding proliferating cell nuclear antigen, *Circulation*, 86, 538, 1992.

109. Rozengurt, E., Legg, A., Strang, G., and Courtenay-Luck, N., Cyclic AMP: a mitogenic signal for Swiss 3T3 cells, *Proc. Natl. Acad. Sci. U.S.A.*, 78, 4392, 1981.

110. Deuel, T. F., Polypeptide growth factors: roles in normal and abnormal cell growth, *Annu. Rev. Cell Biol.*, 3, 443, 1987.

111. Lew, D. B. and Prattazzi, M. C., Mitogenic effect of lysosomal hydrolases on bovine tracheal myocytes in culture, *J. Clin. Invest.*, 88, 1969, 1991.

112. Lew, D. B., Nebigil, C., and Malik, K. U., Dual regulation by cAMP of β-hexosaminidase-induced mitogenesis in bovine tracheal myocytes, *Am. J. Respir. Cell Mol. Biol.*, 7, 614, 1992.

113. Tomlinson, P. R., Wilson, J. W., and Stewart, A. G., Inhibition by salbutamol of the proliferation of human airway smooth muscle cells grown in culture, *Br. J. Pharmacol.*, 111, 641, 1994.

114. Garg, V. C. and Hassid, A., Nitric oxide-generating vasodilators and 8-bromo-cyclic guanosine monophosphate inhibit mitogenesis and proliferation of cultured rat smooth muscle cells, *J. Clin. Invest.*, 83, 1771, 1989.

115. Itoh, H., Pratt, R. E., and Dzau, V. J., Atrial naturetic polypeptide inhibits hypertrophy of vascular smooth muscle cells, *J. Clin. Invest.*, 86, 1690, 1990.

116. Assender, J. W., Southgate, K. M., Hallet, M. B., and Newby, A. C., Inhibition of proliferation, but not of Ca²⁺ mobilization, by cyclic AMP and GMP in rabbit aortic smooth muscle cells, *Biochem. J.*, 288, 527, 1992.

117. De, S., Zelazny, E., Souhrada, J. F., and Souhrada, M., Nitric oxide has an inhibitory effect on growth of airway smooth muscle (ASM) cells, *Am. J. Respir. Crit. Care Med.*, 151, A49, 1995.

118. Galione, A., White, A., Willmott, N., Turner, M., Potter, B. V. L., and Watson, S. P., cGMP mobilizes intracellular Ca²⁺ in sea urchin eggs by stimulating cyclic ADP-ribose synthesis, *Nature (London)*, 365, 456, 1993.

119. Galione, A., McDougall, A., Busa, W. B., Willmott, N., Gillot, I., and Whitaker, M., Redundant mechanisms of calcium-induced calcium release underlying calcium waves during fertilization of sea urchin eggs, *Science*, 261, 348, 1993.

120. Lee, H. C., Aarhus, R., and Walseth, T. F., Calcium mobilization by dual receptors during fertilization of sea urchin eggs, *Science*, 261, 352, 1993.

121. Lowy, D. R. and Willumsen, B. M., Function and regulation of ras, *Annu. Rev. Biochem.*, 62, 851, 1993.

122. Feig, L. A. and Schaffhausen, B., The hunt for ras targets, *Nature (London)*, 370, 508, 1994.

123. Monia, B. P., Johnston, J. F., Ecker, D. J., Zounes, M. A., Lima, W. F., and Freier, S. M., Selective inhibition of mutant Ha-ras mRNA expression by antisense oligonucleotides, *J. Biol. Chem.*, 267, 19954, 1992.

124. Rodriguez-Viciana, P., Warne, P. H., Dhand, R., Vanhaesebroeck, B., Gout, I., Fry, M. J., Waterfield, M. D., and Downward, J., Phosphatidylinositol-3-OH kinase as a direct target of ras, *Nature (London)*, 370, 527, 1994.

125. Isacke, C. M., Meisenhelder, J., Brown, K. D., Gould, K. L., Gould, S. J., and Hunter, T., Early phosphorylation events following the treatment of Swiss 3T3 cells with bombesin and the mammalian bombesin-related peptide, gastrin-releasing peptide, *EMBO J.*, 5, 2889, 1986.

126. Heldin, C.-H. and Westermark, B., Growth factors: Mechanism of action and relation to oncogenes, *Cell*, 37, 9, 1984.

127. Chen, L. B. and Buchanan, J. M., Mitogenic activity of blood components. I. Thrombin and prothrombin, *Proc. Natl. Acad. Sci. U.S.A.*, 72, 131, 1975.

128. Kariya, K., Kawahara, Y., Tsuda, T., Fukuzaki, H., and Takai, Y., Possible involvement of protein kinase C in platelet-derived growth factor-stimulated DNA synthesis in vascular smooth muscle cells, *Atherosclerosis*, 63, 251, 1987.

129. Rozengurt, E., Rodriguez-Pena, M., and Smith, K. A., Phorbol esters, phospholipase C, and growth factors rapidly stimulate the phosphorylation of a $M_r$ 80,000 protein in intact quiescent 3T3 cells, *Proc. Natl. Acad. Sci. U.S.A.*, 80, 7244, 1983.

130. Albert, K. A., Walaas, S. I., Wang, J. K.-T., and Greengard, P., Widespread occurrence of "87 kDa," a major specific substrate for protein kinase C, *Proc. Natl. Acad. Sci. U.S.A.*, 83, 2822, 1986.

131. Blackshear, P. J., Wen, L., Glynn, B. P., and Witters, L. A., Protein kinase C-stimulated phosphorylation *in vitro* of a M, 80,000 protein phosphorylated in response to phorbol esters and growth factors in intact fibroblasts. Distinction from protein kinase C and prominence in brain, *J. Biol. Chem.*, 261, 1459, 1986.
132. Blackshear, P. J., Witters, L. A., Girard, P. R., Kuo, J. F., and Quamo, S. N., Growth factor-stimulated protein phosphorylation in 3T3-L1 cells. Evidence for protein kinase C-dependent and -independent pathways, *J. Biol. Chem.*, 260, 13304, 1985.
133. Sekiguchi, K., Tsukuda, M., Ogita, K., Kikkawa, U., and Nishizuka, Y., Three distinct forms of rat brain protein kinase C: differential response to unsaturated fatty acids, *Biochem. Biophys. Res. Commun.*, 145, 797, 1987.
134. Todo, T., Nakamura, H., Mobuyuki, S., et al. Personal communication, 1990.
135. Sekiguchi, K., Tsukuda, M., Ase, K., Kikkawa, U., and Nishizuka, Y., Mode of activation and kinetic properties of three distinct forms of protein kinase C from rat brain, *J. Biochem. (Tokyo)*, 103, 759, 1988.
136. Jones, S. D., Hall, D. J., Rollins, B. J., and Stiles, C. D., Platelet-derived growth factor generates at least two distinct intracellular signals that modulate gene expression, *Cold Spring Harbor Symp. Quant. Biol.*, 53, 531, 1988.
137. Majundar, S., Kane, L. H., Rossi, M. W., et al., Protein kinase C isotypes and signal transduction in human neutrophils: selective substrate specificity of calcium-dependent β PKC and novel calcium-independent η PKC, *Biochim. Biophys. Acta*, 1176, 276, 1993.
138. Donnelly, R., Yang, K., Omary, M. B., Azhar, S., and Black, J. L., Expression of multiple isoenzymes of protein kinase C in airway smooth muscle, *Am. J. Respir. Cell Mol. Biol.*, 13, 253, 1995.
139. Greenberg, M. E., Hermanowski, A. L., and Ziff, E. B., Effect of protein synthesis inhibitors on growth factor activation of c-*fos* and c-*myc* and actin gene transcription, *Mol. Cell. Biol.*, 6, 1050, 1986.
140. Castellot, J., Wong, K., Herman, B., Hoover, R., Abberini, D., et al., Binding and internalization of heparin by vascular smooth muscle cells, *J. Cell. Physiol.*, 124, 13, 1985.
141. Dicker, P. and Rozengurt, E., Phorbol esters and vasopressin stimulate DNA synthesis by a common mechanism, *Nature (London)*, 287, 607, 1980.
142. Decker, S. J., Effects of epidermal growth factor and 12-*O*-tetradecanoylphorbol-13-acetate on metabolism of the epidermal growth factor receptor in normal human fibroblasts, *Mol. Cell. Biol.*, 4, 1718, 1984.
143. Hirst, S. J., Webb, B. L. J., Giembycz, M. A., Barnes, P. J., and Twort, C. H. C., Inhibition of fetal calf serum-stimulated proliferation of rabbit cultured tracheal smooth muscle cells by selective inhibitors of protein kinase C and protein tyrosinekinase, *Am. J. Respir. Cell Mol. Biol.*, 12, 149, 1995.
144. Berk, B. C., Aronov, M. S., Brock, T. A., Cragoe, E., Gimbrone, M. A., and Alexander, R. W., Angiotensin II stimulates $Na^+/H^+$ exchange in cultured vascular smooth muscle cells. Evidence for protein kinase C-dependent and -independent pathways, *J. Biol. Chem.*, 262, 5057, 1988.
145. Ahn, N. G., Seger, R., Bratlien, R. L., Diltz, C. D., Tonks, N. K., and Krebs, E. G., Multiple components in an epidermal growth factor-stimulated protein kinase cascade: in vitro activation of a myelin basic protein/microtubule-associated protein 2 kinase, *J. Biol. Chem.*, 266, 4220, 1991.
146. Gotoh, Y., Nishida, E., Yamashita, T., Hoshi, M., Kawakami, M., and Sakai, H., Microtubule-associated-protein (MAP) kinase activated by nerve growth factor and epidermal growth factor in PC12 cells: identity with mitogen-activated MAP kinase of fibroblastic cells, *Eur. J. Biochem.*, 193, 661, 1990.
147. Blenis, J., Signal transduction via the MAP kinases: proceed at your own RSK. *Proc. Natl. Acad. Sci. U.S.A.*, 90, 5889, 1993.
148. Vouret-Craviari, V., Van Obberghen-Schilling, E., Rasmussen, U. B., Pavirani, A., Lecocq, J.-P., and Pouyssegur, J., Synthetic α-thrombin receptor peptides activate G protein-coupled signaling pathways but are unable to induce mitogenesis, *Mol. Biol. Cell*, 3, 95, 1992.

149. Alvarez, E., Northwood, I. C., Gonzalez, F. A., Latour, D. A., Seth, A., Abate, C., Curran, T., and Davis, R. J., Pro-Leu-Ser/Thr-Pro is a consensus primary sequence for substrate protein phosphorylation: characterization of the phosphorylation of c-myc and c-jun proteins by an epidermal growth factor receptor threonine 669 protein kinase, *J. Biol. Chem.*, 266, 15277, 1991.
150. Pulverer, B. J., Kyriakis, J. M., Avruch J., Nikolakaki, E., and Woodgett, J. R., Phosphorylation of c-jun mediated by MAP kinases, *Nature (London)*, 353, 670, 1991.
151. Pages, G., Lenormand, P., L'Allemain, G. L., Chambard, J.-C., Meloche, S., and Pouyssegur, J., Mitogen-activated protein kinases p42^mapk and p44^mapk are required for fibroblast proliferation, *Proc. Natl. Acad. Sci. U.S.A.*, 90, 8319, 1993.
152. Abe, M., Chao, T.-S. O., Solway, J., Rosner, M. R., and Hershenson, M., Hydrogen peroxide stimulates MAP kinase activation in bovine tracheal myocytes: implications for human airway disease, *Am. J. Respir. Cell Mol. Biol.*, 11, 577, 1994.
153. L'Allemain, G., Sturgill, T. W., and Weber, M. J., Defective regulation of mitogen-activated protein kinase activity in a 3T3 cell variant mitogenically nonresponsive to tetradecanoyl phorbol acetate, *Mol. Cell. Biol.*, 11, 1002, 1991.
154. Stephens, L., Smrcka, A., Cooke, F. T., Jackson, T. R., Sternweis, P. C., and Hawkins, P. T., A novel phosphoinositide 3-kinase activity in myeloid-derived cells is activated by G protein βγ subunits, *Cell*, 77, 83, 1994.

Chapter 11

# REGULATION OF AIRWAY SMOOTH MUSCLE PROLIFERATION BY β₂-ADRENOCEPTOR AGONISTS

Alastair G. Stewart, Paul R. Tomlinson, and Leslie Schachte

## CONTENTS

# I. INTRODUCTION

Inhaled $\beta_2$-adrenoceptor agonists remain the most important bronchodilator therapy for acute exacerbation of asthma. The recent introduction of long-acting $\beta_2$-adrenoceptor agonists such as salmeterol and formoterol has led to an increase in the chronic usage of bronchodilator therapy at a time when the possibility of a causal link between excessive usage of $\beta_2$-adrenoceptor agonists and increases in asthma-related morbidity and mortality has yet to be fully resolved.[1,2] Nevertheless, the available data suggest that control of asthma symptoms with long-acting $\beta$-agonists may be superior to that achieved with short-acting agents used on demand or regularly.[3] In addition, the long-standing interest in the possible relationship between defects in endogenous $\beta_2$-adrenoceptor mechanisms and airway hyperresponsiveness (AHR)[4] has been reignited by recent molecular biology studies of genetic polymorphisms in $\beta_2$-adrenoceptors in asthma of varying severity.[5]

AHR is clearly associated with the severity of asthma in most, if not all, patients. AHR may be considered to comprise a fixed component and a more variable component which is exacerbated by allergen inhalation[6] and partially resolved by treatment with anti-inflammatory steroids.[7] Mathematical modelling studies using morphometric observations on post-mortem airways from asthmatic and normal specimens suggest that airway wall thickening, including an increase in the volume of airway smooth muscle, accounts for a large part of the AHR in asthma[8] and, presumably, represents the relatively fixed component of AHR. Airway wall thickening is an established feature of asthma that is due in part to airway smooth muscle hyperplasia.[9-11] The cause of this airway wall remodelling has yet to be identified, and the impact of anti-asthma medications on the various processes subserving the remodelling (cell proliferation, extracellular matrix deposition) have not been extensively examined.

It is not established whether or not the remodelling is reversible, either spontaneously or upon drug treatment. One long-term study of patients receiving inhaled steroids indicated that epithelial abnormalities could resolve at least in part,[12] but the depth of biopsy limits information to the mucosa.

In view of the renewed interest in the effects of β-agonists on AHR, cultured airway smooth muscle has been used to examine interactions between mitogens and these anti-asthma drugs.[13] In this chapter, the regulation of $\beta_2$-adrenoceptors in asthma and the effects of $\beta_2$-adrenoceptor agonists on airway smooth muscle proliferation are reviewed. In addition, the interaction between cyclic AMP (cAMP)-dependent protein kinase (PKA) and the cascade of intracellular signalling events which accompany the progression of cells through the cell cycle are examined, with particular emphasis on events occurring hours rather than minutes after mitogen addition.

## II. THE $\beta_2$-ADRENOCEPTOR AND ASTHMA

Szentivanyi[4] hypothesised that the underlying mechanism of asthma was an imbalance in autonomic control of airway smooth muscle. This theory was derived from observations in animal models of asthma involving innoculation with *Bordetella pertussis* and from the results of $\beta_2$-adrenoceptor blockade in experimental animals and in human subjects.

### A. β-ADRENOCEPTOR BLOCKERS AND
### AIRWAY RESPONSIVENESS

Antagonism of $\beta_2$-adrenoceptors in guinea pigs increased airway reactivity to antigen challenge[14] or to specific bronchoconstrictors such as histamine.[15,16] In asthmatic subjects, β-adrenoceptor blockade exacerbated the disease, causing rapid and prolonged falls in forced expired volume in 1 s ($FEV_1$),[17] increased airway responsiveness to methacholine,[18] and increased airway reactivity to inhaled allergens.[19] In nonasthmatic patients with seasonal allergic rhinitis, increases in airway reactivity to inhaled methacholine following β-adrenoceptor blockade were observed.[20] In healthy subjects, β-adrenoceptor blockade caused up to a doubling of airway resistance,[21] and, at higher doses, an acute airway obstruction of similar intensity to that in asthmatic subjects was observed.[20] Although the β-adrenoceptor theory of bronchial asthma is supported by the bronchoconstrictor-enhancing effect of pharmacological blockade of β-adrenoceptors, these observations could be explained by asthmatic airways being more dependent on β-adrenoceptor activation for protection against bronchospasm, rather than by a specific defect in β-adrenoceptors.

### B. β-ADRENOCEPTOR RESPONSES IN ISOLATED
### HUMAN LEUKOCYTES, LYMPHOCYTES,
### AND MACROPHAGES

The proposal of defective β-adrenoceptors in patients with asthma (see Table 1) was based on observations of decreased isoprenaline-stimulated cAMP accumulation in lymphocytes isolated from peripheral blood of asthmatic subjects.[22] In asthmatic patients not using β-adrenoceptor agonists, lymphocyte β-adrenoceptor numbers were decreased to a degree that correlated with disease severity.[23-25] In a further study, leukocytes from asthmatic subjects not being treated with β-adrenoceptor agonists showed reduced responsiveness to isoprenaline and an increased respiratory burst, both of which correlated with the degree of airway responsiveness to methacholine.[26] These latter observations appear to be incompatible with the suggestion that diminished β-adrenoceptor responsiveness was merely due to tachyphylaxis resulting from drug treatment.[25,27,28] In contrast to observations on leukocyte membranes from human asthmatic subjects, β-adrenoceptor numbers and affinities on leukocytes from hyperresponsive basenji-greyhound were not significantly different from those of nonhyperresponsive control dogs. However, isoprenaline-stimulated adenylate cyclase activity was reduced, whereas responses to prostaglandin $E_2$, NaF, or forskolin were unaffected.[29] These findings suggest a specific defect in the coupling between $\beta_2$-adrenoceptors and adenylate cyclase in this species.

Meurs and co-workers[30] demonstrated that house-dust mite challenge of asthmatic patients resulted in a reduction in β-adrenoceptor number and adenylate cyclase activity in lymphocytes, whereas the prechallenge levels were not significantly different from those of nonasthmatic subjects. Thus, reduced β-adrenoceptor responsiveness may not be an intrinsic component of allergic asthma, but rather a consequence of an active disease state.[30] Alveolar macrophages isolated from the bronchoalveolar lavage (BAL) fluids of asthmatic patients showed less accumulation of cAMP compared with nonasthmatic subjects when incubated with the nonspecific phosphodiesterase inhibitor isobutyl-methylxanthine, salbutamol, or prostaglandin $E_2$. Thus, the reduction of adenylate cyclase activity in this cell type does not appear to be related to specific β-adrenoceptor desensitisation.[31]

## C. β-ADRENOCEPTOR NUMBERS AND RESPONSES IN AIRWAYS OF EXPERIMENTAL ANIMALS

In lung homogenates from ovalbumin-sensitised and challenged guinea pigs, β-adrenoceptor number decreased, whereas α-adrenoceptor number increased.[32-34] In a similar study it was observed that β-adrenoceptor density decreased and there was an exaggerated airway responsiveness to histamine at 24 h after the antigen challenge, but no increase in $\alpha_1$-adrenoceptor numbers.[35] In nonchallenged, ovalbumin-sensitised guinea pigs decreases in β-adrenoceptor numbers were noted in alveolar and conducting airway epithelium and in bronchial and vascular smooth muscle.[36] Immunological sensitisation also decreased isoprenaline-stimulated adenylate cyclase activity in guinea pig lung homogenates and increased phospholipase $A_2$ ($PLA_2$) activity.[37] Moreover, activation of $PLA_2$ in fresh lung homogenates decreased $\beta_2$-adrenoceptor number, indicating that these effects may be causally linked.[37]

## TABLE 1
### Changes in β₂-Adrenoceptor Function/Number

| | Cell type (species) | Ref. |
|---|---|---|
| Decreased β-adrenoceptor number | Lymphocytes (asthmatics) | 22–25 |
| Decreased β-adrenoceptor responsiveness | Leukocytes (untreated asthmatics) | 26 |
| Decreased β-adrenoceptor number and adenylate cyclase activity | Lymphocytes (asthmatics — after allergen challenge) | 30 |
| Decreased adenylate cyclase activity | Alveolar macrophages (asthmatics) | 31 |
| Decreased β-adrenoceptor number | Lymphocytes (asthmatics — treatment related) | 27, 28, 31 |
| Unchanged β-adrenoceptor density | Bronchial smooth muscle (asthmatics) | 54 |
| Increased β-adrenoceptor number | Lung (asthmatics) | 49, 56 |
| Unchanged relaxation induced by β-agonists | Bronchial smooth muscle (asthmatics) | 60 |
| Decreased relaxation induced by β-agonists | Bronchial smooth muscle (asthmatics) | 49, 61–63 |
| Decreased β-adrenoceptor number | Pulmonary membranes exposed to PAF, LTB₄, or LTC₄ (human — nonasthmatic) | 47 |
| No change in β-adrenoceptor number, uncoupling of receptor from adenylate cyclase | Isolated leukocytes (hyperresponsive basenji-greyhounds) | 29 |
| Increased β-adrenoceptor number, decrease binding and responsiveness | Tracheal muscle (hyperresponsive basenji-greyhounds) | 43 |
| Normal β-adrenoceptor function | Cultured tracheal muscle (hyperresponsive basenji-greyhounds) | 44 |
| Decreased β-adrenoceptor number, increased α-adrenoceptor number | Lung homogenates (ovalbumin-sensitised guinea pigs) | 32–34 |
| Decreased β-adrenoceptor number, no change in α-adrenoceptor number | Lung homogenates (ovalbumin-sensitised guinea pigs) | 35 |
| β-adrenoceptor numbers unchanged, decreased β-agonist stimulation of adenylate cyclase | Influenza vaccinated (murine lung) | 38 |
| Attenuated β₂-adrenoceptor | Isolated tracheal muscle exposed to TNFα or IL-1β (guinea pig) | 46 |

In a murine model of airway disease produced by vaccination with the influenza virus, β-adrenoceptor agonist stimulation of adenylate cyclase was decreased, but β-adrenoceptor numbers were unchanged in the lung.[38] In experiments of a similar design in guinea pigs, β-adrenoceptor numbers were increased in the trachea, primarily because of changes in the epithelium rather than the airway smooth muscle.[39] In contrast, in another study of vaccinated guinea pigs there was no change in β-adrenoceptor density on either the airway smooth muscle or trachea, although there were decreases in β-adrenoceptor numbers in the peripheral lung, alveolar septa, endothelial cells, and vascular smooth muscle.[40] Hyperresponsiveness to contractile muscarinic agonists and hyporesponsiveness to β-adrenoceptor agonists in a guinea pig model of asthma, in the absence of changes in levels of either receptor type or of $G_s\alpha$

protein, have been ascribed to an increase in the expression of $G_{i2}\alpha$ and $G_q\alpha$ proteins which could alter coupling of receptors to effector systems.[41]

In basenji-greyhounds with naturally occurring AHR, bronchoconstrictor responses to methacholine are resistant to inhibition by β-adrenoceptor agonists.[42] Decreased cAMP generation in response to isoprenaline in the trachealis muscle was observed, whereas functional and biochemical responses to forskolin, NaF, prostaglandin $E_2$, and dibutyryl cAMP in basenji-greyhound and control dogs were similar.[43] Interestingly, β-adrenoceptor receptor numbers were increased in the tracheal muscle membranes of basenji-greyhound dogs, with a decreased affinity for the β-adrenoceptor ligand [125]I-cyanopindolol, compared with control dogs. There was a similar quantity of $G_s\alpha$ protein detected in trachealis muscle membranes of both groups. Thus, the reduced responsiveness to isoprenaline in basenji-greyhounds may be due to a defect in ligand binding to the β-adrenoceptor or in receptor–G protein coupling.[43] The impaired β-adrenoceptor function observed in isolated tracheal muscle from basenji-greyhounds was not observed when these cells were cultured, possibly because of the absence in cell cultures of the proinflammatory cytokines present in the asthmatic lung.[44]

## D. INFLAMMATORY CYTOKINES AND β-ADRENOCEPTOR FUNCTION

In antigen-challenged guinea pigs, the development of reduced β-adrenoceptor-mediated relaxation of isolated trachea was paralleled by a progressive infiltration of inflammatory cells in the airways *in vivo*, consistent with a role for inflammatory mediators in the β-adrenoceptor dysfunction.[45] *In vitro* incubation of guinea pig trachea with either of the proinflammatory cytokines TNFα or IL-1β resulted in diminished $\beta_2$-adrenoceptor-mediated relaxation.[46] Incubation of human pulmonary membranes with mediators of inflammation including PAF, $LTB_4$, or $LTC_4$ caused decreases in β-adrenoceptor density and in agonist-stimulated cAMP synthesis in lymphocytes.[47]

# III. ADRENOCEPTORS IN HUMAN AIRWAYS

## A. RECEPTOR SUBTYPES AND DISTRIBUTION

Autoradiographic studies indicate that the majority of adrenoceptors in the lung are of the $\beta_2$-adrenoceptor subtype, with greater than 90% of the total number localised to the alveolar wall. $\beta_2$-Adrenoceptors are also widely distributed in airway epithelium and submucosal glands of conducting airways. There is a lower density of β-adrenoceptors over vascular and airway smooth muscle which are of the $\beta_2$-adrenoceptor subtype [48,49]. The density of $\alpha_1$-adrenoceptors in the human lung is low,[50,51] and the α-adrenoceptor agonist phenylephrine failed to induce significant increases in tone of isolated bronchi from either nondiseased or asthmatic lung.[50] The $\beta_3$-adrenoceptor agonist BRL 37344 does not induce relaxaton of human, sheep, or guinea pig airway smooth muscle,[52] although in isolated canine bronchial segments an increase in cAMP and relaxation responses have been observed.[53] Data concerning the density of β-adrenoceptor on the bronchial muscle of patients with severe asthma[54] and those with chronic airflow obstruction[55] indicate either no change or an increase in receptor density in the asthmatic lung compared with nonasthmatic preparations.[49,56]

The *in vivo* autonomic responses of asthmatic subjects to adrenoceptor agonists indicated a reduced β-adrenoceptor responsiveness, consistent with the hypothesis of β-adrenoceptor deficiency in bronchial asthma, and an increase in sensitivity to α-adrenoceptor.[57,58] Neither of these studies examined bronchomotor responses to adrenoceptor agonists. The α-adrenoceptor agonist has been shown to provoke bronchoconstriction in asthmatic, but not in non-asthmatic individuals.[59]

## B. ISOLATED AIRWAY RESPONSIVENESS

Relaxation induced by β-adrenoceptor agonists of bronchial smooth muscle derived from patients with severe asthma is reported to be either normal[60] or decreased[49,61-63] compared with preparations from nonasthmatic subjects. Furthermore, a correlation between the degree of $β_2$-adrenoceptor hypofunction in isolated airway smooth muscle and the hyperresponsiveness to histamine has been reported.[64]

There is an apparent contradiction between the finding of increased $β_2$-adrenoceptor number in asthmatic airways and decreased responsiveness of smooth muscle to the relaxant actions of β-agonists. One explanation of these observations is that there may be uncoupling at some point in the cascade of events between receptor binding, the signalling mechanism, and the subsequent relaxation. Increases in $β_2$-adrenoceptor number may be a result of a homeostatic or compensatory mechanism.[56]

## C. AUTOANTIBODIES TO β-ADRENOCEPTORS

The existence of β-blocking autoantibodies has been reported, with a higher incidence being observed in asthmatic individuals having reduced endocrine and autonomic responses to β-adrenoceptor agonists.[57] Sera from approximately 5% of a juvenile population of asthmatic subjects had antibodies that inhibited the binding of the β-adrenoceptor antagonist iodohydroxybenzylpindolol to canine lung-plasma membrane β-adrenoceptors.[65] In contrast, in adult asthmatic subjects, sera had no effect on the binding of $^{125}$I-cyanopindolol to cloned human $β_2$-adrenoceptors or on isoprenaline-stimulated cAMP increases.[66]

# IV. $β_2$-ADRENOCEPTOR AGONISTS AND EXACERBATION OF ASTHMA

It is important to consider the actions of both the short- and the long-acting β-agonists in the context of the ongoing debate over the potential relationship between the pattern of use of these compounds and increases in morbidity and mortality of asthma.

Acutely, inhalation of $\beta_2$-adrenoceptor agonists reduces AHR by functionally antagonising the actions of constrictors on airway smooth muscle. However, some studies suggest that, following chronic use of these agents, an increase in the underlying AHR is observed after an appropriate $\beta$-agonist-free period. Over the last decade a series of studies has identified an association between the use of $\beta_2$-adrenoceptor agonists and both excerbations of asthma and increased AHR. Notwithstanding all the possible confounding influences, such as asthma severity, on the interpretation of this association, it has given rise to serious concern over both the pattern and the amount of $\beta$-agonist usage.[1]

In a double-blind, randomised, placebo-controlled crossover study of 1 year duration, the regular use of fenoterol led to significant decreases in $FEV_1$ and vital capacity, increased airway responsiveness, and more exacerbations of asthma, compared with its symptomatic use.[67] Importantly, the apparent deleterious effect of regular $\beta$-adrenoceptor use was not prevented by the concurrent use of inhaled corticosteriods.[67] The use of bronchodilators alone (either salbutamol or ipratropium bromide) for symptomatic relief of episodes of asthma was associated with an accelerated decline in lung function, prompting the recommendation that anti-inflammatory treatment be used concurrently with bronchodilators.[68] More recently, a medium-term study provided evidence that lung function was better maintained with inhaled budesonide than with inhaled terbutaline in newly diagnosed asthmatic patients.[69] In New Zealand, analysis of case control studies indicated that there was an association between the use of inhaled fenoterol and mortality.[70] The existence of the association between the risk of a fatal asthma attack and number of prescriptions for cannisters of $\beta$-agonist aerosols (either fenoterol or salbutamol) filled per month was supported by the larger Saskatchewan asthma epidemiology project, which was initially carried out in a nested, case-control study.[71] Attempts to adjust for clinical markers of severity did not remove the increased risk,[72] and later analysis of the whole cohort (12,301 asthmatic subjects) led to the conclusion that the increase in mortality was restricted to asthma-related deaths and was particularly associated with usage of $\beta$-agonists in excess of the recommended maximum amounts.[73]

## A. POSSIBLE SIGNIFICANCE OF THE PATTERN OF $\beta$-AGONIST USAGE

Regular, as opposed to symptomatic, use of short-acting $\beta_2$-adrenoceptor agonists has specifically been associated with a deterioration in control of asthma symptoms. Although regular use of short-acting $\beta_2$-agonists may be considered to be similar to twice daily inhalation of long-acting compounds, a significant period during the early-morning hours would be free of stimulation by short-acting $\beta_2$-agonists, but the effects of long-acting compounds would persist throughout sleep.[74] Evidence indicating possible adverse effects of regular usage of $\beta_2$-agonists is much more abundant than that for the long-acting agents on which fewer studies have been carried out.[75,76] These clinical findings raise the question of whether or not the duration of $\beta_2$-adrenoceptor stimulation is important in association with exacerbation of asthma. Three patterns of usage of $\beta_2$-adrenoceptors are evident: (1) short-acting agents used symptomatically activate $\beta_2$-receptors for brief periods with dose intervals ranging from hours to weeks, but they are presumably used only when airway muscle spasm is perceived. (2) Short-acting $\beta_2$-adrenoceptors used regularly are administered at 4-6-hour intervals daily during consciousness and, therefore, act on smooth muscle and inflammatory cells that may or may not be under the influence of inflammatory mediators. Moreover, there would be an obligatory period during sleep in most individuals in which levels of $\beta_2$-agonists would fall below active concentrations. (3) Long-acting agents would produce stimulation of similar intensity throughout the day and night.

These issues of duration of action have some importance for the design of laboratory-based studies which address possible adverse effects of chronic $\beta_2$-agonists usage. This is well illustrated by our investigations of the effects of $\beta_2$-agonists on proliferative responses of human cultured airway smooth muscle. Initial investigations indicated that continuous stimulation of $\beta_2$-adrenoceptors decreased DNA synthesis and cell division.[77] However, when shorter periods (0.5–2 h) of receptor activation were examined, inhibition of DNA synthesis was not observed. Even 8 h of receptor stimulation delayed rather than prevented cell division.[78] We concluded from these observations that the pharmacokinetic properties of $\beta$-agonists are an important consideration in the design and interpretation of both *in vivo* and *in vitro* studies when the duration of the study extends beyond the duration of action of the agents being examined.

## B. EFFECTS OF ACUTE AND CHRONIC ADMINISTRATION OF $\beta$-AGONISTS ON AIRWAY RESPONSIVENESS IN EXPERIMENTAL ANIMALS

Chronic fenoterol exposure in guinea pigs increased airway responsiveness *in vivo* and contractility of isolated tracheal smooth muscle.[79] This increase in contractility was not due to increase in smooth muscle mass, and there was no evidence of long-term $\beta_2$-adrenoceptor desensitisation. A similar effect in human asthmatic subjects may explain the adverse effects observed during prolonged treatment with $\beta_2$-adrenoceptor agonists, but the authors[79] were cautious in reaching this conclusion, since the dose of fenoterol was higher than that used by most asthmatic patients. It is clearly of importance to confirm the findings of this study.

# V. BIOCHEMICAL AND STRUCTURAL ASPECTS OF THE $\beta_2$-ADRENOCEPTOR

## A. LIGAND BINDING OF THE $\beta_2$-ADRENOCEPTOR

The human $\beta_2$-adrenoceptor is encoded by an intronless gene located at q31-q32 on chromosome 5.[80] The deduced amino acid sequence of 413 residues

## TABLE 2
### Structure/Function of the $\beta_2$-Adrenoceptor

| Structural alterations | Consequences | Ref. |
|---|---|---|
| Asp[79] to Ala[79] (2nd transmembrane domain) | Decreased agonist affinity | 220 |
| Asp[113] to Asn[113] (3rd transmembrane domain) | Decreased agonist affinity | 220 |
| Asn[318] to Lys[318] (7th transmembrane domain) | Decreased agonist affinity | 220 |
| Ser[204] to Ala[204] (5th transmembrane domain) | Decreased agonist affinity | 221 |
| Pro[323] to Ser[323] (7th transmembrane domain) improperly processed receptor (nonglycosylated or partially glycosylated) | No ligand binding | 220 |
| Asp[130] to Asn[130] (3rd transmembrane domain) | Uncoupling of adenylate cyclase | 222 |
| Substitution or deletions in C terminal area of third cytoplasmic loop and N terminal of cytoplasmic tail | Uncoupling of receptor from G-protein | 82, 83, 223, 224 |
| Substitution or deletions in C terminal area of third cytoplasmic loop and N terminal of cytoplasmic tail | Impaired G-protein coupling but normal sequestration; reduced downregulation | 86 |
| Deletions in phosphorylation sites for PKA or βARK | Lack of attenuation of adenylate cyclase activity | 84 |
| Cys[184] to Val[184] (2nd extracellular loop) leads to enhanced agonist induced phosphorylation | Enhanced sequestration but partially uncoupled from adenylate cyclase | 88 |
| Deletion of sequences phosphorylated by PKA (increased levels of intracellular cAMP produce downregulation in these mutants) | Decreased sequestration; no effect on downregulation | 92 |
| Substitution of four serine and threonine residues in C terminal of cytoplasmic tail (βARK phosphorylation sites) | Decreased sequestration; no effect on downregulation | 89 |

corresponds to a seven membrane-spanning domain protein with an extracellular N terminus and contains two putative sites for asparagine-linked glycosylation and an intracellular C terminus.[80] Much of the information on the functional domains of the $\beta_2$-adrenoceptor has been derived from studies using site-directed mutagenesis (Table 2).

The fourth transmembrane domain is largely responsible for determining $\beta_1$- vs. $\beta_2$-agonist-binding properties (adrenaline and noradrenaline relative affinities), and transmembrane regions 5 and 7 play an important role in determining the binding of $\beta_1$- vs. $\beta_2$-antagonists.[80,81] Construction of receptor protein mutants has revealed that the C terminal portion of the third cytoplasmic loop and the N terminal segment of the cytoplasmic tail appear to be critical for receptor coupling to G proteins.[82,83]

## B. MOLECULAR MECHANISMS CONTROLLING $\beta_2$-ADRENOCEPTOR NUMBERS

Short-term exposure to $\beta_2$-adrenoceptor agonists leads to a rapid desensitisation involving receptor sequestration. Longer-term exposure causes a decrease in receptor expression, referred to as downregulation, resulting from a decrease in the total amount of receptor protein.

## 1. β₂-Adrenoceptor Desensitisation

The β₂-adrenoceptor-linked adenylate cyclase undergoes desensitisation upon agonist exposure, causing an uncoupling from G proteins and diminished capacity to stimulate increases in cAMP. Phosphorylation of the receptor by PKA and the β-adrenoceptor kinase (βARK) both play a role in this phenomenon. Mutant forms of the human β₂-adrenoceptor that lack target amino acids for phosphorylation by PKA (serines 261, 262, 345, 346 substituted with alanines) or putative βARK phosphorylation sites (11 serines and threonines at the carboxy terminus of the protein substituted with alanines or glycines) exhibit the same initial rate of cAMP generation as wild-type receptors. However, none of the mutant forms of the receptor undergoes desensitisation to the extent observed upon stimulation of the wild-type receptors.[84] Desensitisation has also been demonstrated in human cultured airway smooth muscle.[85]

## 2. Sequestration of the β₂-Adrenoceptor Receptor

The rapid desensitisation of the β₂-adrenoceptor response is linked to its sequestration into the cell. In the hamster β₂-adrenoceptor, the deletion of residues 222–229 results in inability to couple to G protein, as well as loss of agonist-mediated sequestration. However, human β₂-adrenoceptor mutants with impaired coupling to $G_s$ are able to be sequestered normally.[86,87] Receptor mutants (valine for cysteine at 184), which undergo an enhanced desensitisation, are partially uncoupled from adenylate cyclase activation and have an impaired ability to form high-affinity agonist–receptor–G protein complexes, but display an increased agonist-stimulated receptor phosphorylation.[88] Substitution of the four serine and threonine residues located in a 10-amino acid segment of the carboxy terminal this domain prevented the phosphorylation, sequestration, and, thus, rapid desensitisation of the β₂-adrenoceptor.[89] The sequestration of the receptor appears to play a physiological role in dephosphorylation and resensitisation, since, upon removal of the β-agonist from cultures of the A431 cell line, the β₂-adrenoceptor is rapidly recycled to the cell surface in a nonphosphorylated form.[90]

## 3. Downregulation of the β₂-Adrenoceptor Receptor

In Chinese hamster fibroblast cells transfected with the wild-type human β₂-adrenoceptor, treatment with the cAMP analogue dibutyryl cAMP induced phosphorylation of membrane-associated β₂-adrenoceptors, a time-dependent reduction in β₂-adrenoceptor number, and a decline in the steady-state level of β₂-adrenoceptor mRNA. Thus, downregulation is achieved through both an increased rate of receptor degradation and a decreased rate of synthesis.[91] Increased levels of cAMP cause a decrease in β₂-adrenoceptor number through both cAMP-dependent and -independent mechanisms.[92]

In asthmatic patients, receptor numbers are either unchanged or increased despite the expectation that increased agonist exposure would activate mechanisms which reduce $\beta_2$-adrenoceptor. In studies of cell lines transfected with $\beta_2$-adrenoceptors, as $\beta$-adrenoceptor numbers increased, the efficacy of isoprenaline in stimulating adenylate cyclase also increased,[93,94] suggesting that the concentration of receptors was the limiting factor for adenylate cyclase activity and not $G_s\alpha$. Therefore, an increase in $\beta$-adrenoceptor number should lead to an increase in the maximal adenylate cyclase activity. The extensive evidence that stimulated adenylate cyclase activity is impaired in asthmatic patients suggests the presence of an as yet undescribed overriding influence on $\beta_2$-adrenoceptor-signalling mechanisms in these patients.

## C. POLYMORPHISMS IN HUMAN $\beta$-ADRENOCEPTORS

The production of mutants of the $\beta_2$-adrenoceptor which have different binding affinities for agonists, variable ability to couple to G proteins, differing rates of sequestration and downregulation leads to the search for polymorphisms in the population which could predispose to asthma. Polymorphisms in the $\beta_2$-adrenoceptor occur predominantly adjacent to glycosylation sites of the N terminus of the receptor.[95] However, the frequency and distribution of polymorphisms of the receptor are no higher in patients with asthma than those in subjects without chronic obstructive pulmonary disease, suggesting that asthma is not primarily caused by a genetic defect in the $\beta_2$-adrenoceptor receptor. However, within the asthma group one mutation (Arg16 to Gly) identified a subset of patients who were more likely to be steroid dependent and to require immunisation therapy as compared with those without this polymorphism receptor.[95] Further investigations of this polymorphism have revealed that it is present in higher frequency in patients suffering nocturnal asthma as compared with those without marked exacerbation of asthma during sleep,[5] although this may simply reflect the more severe asthma in the nocturnal asthma group. One consequence of this polymorphism is an increase in the extent of receptor downregulation as determined by isoprenaline exposure of airway smooth muscle cultured from post-mortem asthmatic bronchial specimens.[96] Interest in these polymorphisms is further stimulated by the recent linkage between chromosome 5q, where the gene for the $\beta_2$-adrenoceptor is located, and both AHR and atopy.[97]

## D. POTASSIUM CHANNELS AND
## $\beta_2$-ADRENOCEPTOR AGONISTS

The relaxant effects of $\beta_2$-adrenoceptor agonists have, until the last 5 years, been thought to be fully explained by PKA-dependent phosphorylation of proteins associated with intracellular regulation of calcium levels, including inhibition of inositol phosphate hydrolysis following phospholipase C activation, increased sodium/calcium exchange, and increased calcium reuptake (Figure 1). Inhibition of myosin light chain kinase activity is an additional site of action of PKA.[98]

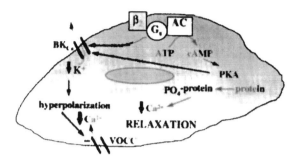

**FIGURE 1** Mechanisms for the relaxant response of airway smooth muscle to $\beta_2$-adrenoceptor agonists. Receptor activation results in activation of the GTP-binding protein ($G_s$) with consequent activation of adenylate cyclase (AC). cAMP-dependent PKA phosphorylates a number of proteins, which then reduce the level of intracellular calcium causing relaxation. Recent studies also suggest that the $\alpha$ subunit of Gs activates the large conductance ($BK_{Ca}$) channel, causing a PKA-independent membrane hyperpolarisation which reduces entry of $Ca^{2+}$ through voltage-operated calcium channels (VOCC).

There is now evidence from a number of studies which indicates that $K^+$ channel activation plays a role in the relaxant effects of $\beta$-agonists, but the relative importance of this mechanism is yet to be clearly established. The presence of several types of potassium channels on airway smooth muscle has been established by electrophysiological techniques: large conductance, calcium-activated potassium channels ($K_{Ca}$);[99] voltage-dependent potassium channels ($K_V$);[100] and ATP-sensitive potassium channels ($K_{ATP}$).[101] The relaxant action of potassium channel–opening drugs such as cromakalim has been demonstrated on airway smooth muscle of a number of species including guinea pig[102,103] and human.[104] $K_{Ca}$ channels are implicated as important target proteins for $\beta_2$-adrenoceptor agonist-induced relaxation.[105-108] These channels are densely distributed in the cell membranes of airway smooth muscle in humans,[109] dogs,[99] rabbits,[105] pigs,[110] and guinea pigs[111] and are selectively inhibited by charybdotoxin,[112,113] which attenuates the relaxant responses of isoprenaline and salbutamol.[106] Opening of $K_{Ca}$ channels induced by $\beta_2$-adrenoceptor agonists occurs via two distinct mechanisms. One mechanism, involving a PKA-activated $K_{Ca}$ channel, was originally described in cultured aortic smooth muscle.[114] Using the patch-clamp technique, Kume and coworkers[105] confirmed the existence of a similar mechanism in isoprenaline-stimulated rabbit tracheal smooth muscle cells. The open-state probability of $K_{Ca}$ channels increased with the extracellular application of isoprenaline, the intracellular application of cAMP and PKA together, or the application of catalytic subunit of PKA alone. Furthermore, neither the holoenzyme nor the catalytic subunit of PKA had any effect on channel activity in the absence of ATP, suggesting that the activation of $K_{Ca}$ channels by $\beta_2$-adrenoceptor agonists was mediated by protein phosphorylation.[105] The other mechanism involves a G protein–dependent, PKA-independent stimulation of $K_{Ca}$ activity,[115,116] which appears to occur through the release of the $\alpha$ subunit of the stimulatory G protein of adenylate cyclase ($G_s$) and can be inhibited by methacholine acting via a pertussis toxin–sensitive G protein ($G_i$).[108] Recently, Kume and colleagues[117] provided further, more direct evidence of dual mechanisms of regulation of $K_{Ca}$ channels by $\beta_2$-adrenoceptor receptor agonists. The application of PKA stimulated channel activity in a concentration-dependent manner. At maximal stimulation of $K_{Ca}$ channel activity elicited by PKA, it was possible to further increase channel activity by the application of $\alpha_s$. PKA and $\alpha_s$ also have distinct effects on channel open-time kinetics, suggesting independent mechanisms of channel stimulation. The observation that equivalent levels of relaxation induced by isoprenaline and forskolin in precontracted muscle were associated with dissimilar levels of intracellular cAMP is also consistent with the possibility that cAMP-independent mechanisms contribute to the relaxant response.[117]

There is evidence against an important contribution of K channel opening in the relaxant effects of $\beta_2$-adrenoceptor agonists on airway smooth muscle. Agonists with low efficacy, such as salmeterol, fail to activate K channels in the smooth muscle cells.[118,119] It is potentially significant that many of the studies of the importance of K channels in the relaxant effects of $\beta_2$-adrenoceptor agonists have used the high-efficacy agonist, isoprenaline (see, for example, References 107 and 117). In addition, large reductions in the hyperpolarisation induced by isoprenaline in the guinea pig trachea have no effect on the relaxant actions of this agonist.[118]

## VI. PHOSPHODIESTERASE INHIBITORS AND AIRWAY SMOOTH MUSCLE

Human airway smooth muscle expresses phosphodiesterase (PDE) types I, II, III, IV, and V,[120-123] which are now recognised to represent families of isoenzymes.[124] Sensitivity of airway smooth muscle cAMP levels to inhibition by the type IV selective PDE inhibitor rolipram[125] identified the type IV enzyme as the major PDE which preferentially hydrolyses cAMP.[121] In addition, while rolipram did not induce relaxation of spontaneous muscle tone, it did relax muscle strips precontracted with methacholine,[121] suggesting that prevention of cAMP hydrolysis is sufficent to elicit relaxation in contracted smooth muscle. The papaverine-derived bronchodilator AH 21-132, which selectively inhibits type IV PDE, has also been shown to increase cAMP content and relax precontracted muscle strips in bovine airway smooth muscle.[126] There are species differences in the expression of PDE subtypes in airway smooth muscle with the pattern of bovine smooth muscle resembling that observed in human airway smooth muscle.[127] There is an interaction between type III and type IV PDE inhibitors, with the combination of rolipram and siguazodan producing a greater relaxation of small or large human bronchi than either agent alone.[123] The nonselective PDE inhibitor isobutyl methylxanthine inhibits airway smooth muscle proliferation and enhances the inhibitory effect of salbutamol,[77] but there is little known about the antiproliferative effects of selective PDE isoenzyme inhibitors.

# VII. AIRWAY SMOOTH MUSCLE PROLIFERATION AND ADRENOCEPTORS

The regulation of cultured airway smooth muscle proliferation by β-adrenoceptor agonists has been described in several species including human,[77,128] canine,[129] bovine,[130] and guinea pig.[131] Noveral and Grunstein[132] observed that the $\alpha_1$-adrenoceptor agonists phenylephrine and methoxamine and the $\alpha_2$-selective agonist clonidine stimulated rabbit cultured airway smooth muscle proliferation. However, as there are few α-adrenoceptors in the human airways,[50,51] this may be of little consequence in the pathophysiology of human asthma. Indeed, studies in human airway smooth muscle indicated that α-adrenoceptor stimulation has no effect on DNA synthesis (Harris and Stewart, unpublished observations).

## A. IMPORTANCE OF DURATION AND TIMING OF EXPOSURE FOR THE INHIBITORY EFFECTS OF $\beta_2$-ADRENOCEPTOR AGONISTS

The duration of exposure to $\beta_2$-adrenoceptor agonists may be important in determining whether or not these agonists exert an antiproliferative effect. Short-term exposure to agonists that increase intracellular cAMP (30 min to less than 6 h) stimulated proliferation of bovine airway smooth muscle. However, longer exposure periods were inhibitory to airway smooth muscle proliferation.[133] Observations made in other cell types suggest that cAMP elevation has different effects at different points in the cell cycle.[134] Thus, in addition to duration, the timing of addition of salbutamol relative to that of the mitogen exposure could also be significant. Since salbutamol is a short-acting bronchodilator,[74] the investigation of periods of exposure of cultured cells to this agonist that match the duration of its clinical effectiveness may indicate whether this $\beta_2$-adrenoceptor agonist has a direct proliferative or antiproliferative effect *in vivo*. Preliminary studies of the effects of short durations of exposure to salbutamol indicate that its antiproliferative effects are greatly reduced compared with those of continuous exposure.[78] However, further studies that also examine the effects of repeated exposures are required to provide data of greater relevance to the clinical usage of salbutamol.

## B. MECHANISM OF ACTION OF $\beta_2$-ADRENOCEPTOR AGONISTS IN INHIBITION OF CELL PROLIFERATION

Continuous exposure of human cultured airway smooth muscle to β-adrenoceptor agonists inhibits mitogen-induced proliferation (Figure 2) by a mechanism which is mediated in part by an increase in intracellular cAMP.[128] Initially, cAMP modulation of intracellular calcium increases was considered likely to explain the inhibition of DNA synthesis since (1) inhibition of calcium

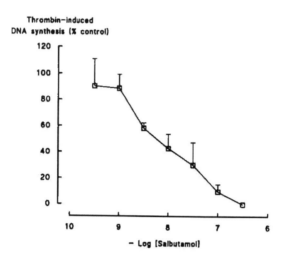

**FIGURE 2**  Pretreatment of airway smooth muscle for 30 min before exposure to thrombin concentration dependently reduces mitogen-induced DNA synthesis.

rise is inhibitory to growth of other cell types;[135] (2) most mitogens have the capacity to stimulate a rise in intracellular calcium; and (3) modulation of increased calcium by $\beta_2$-adrenoceptor agonists is believed to underlie their relaxant actions.[136] The inhibitory effect of salbutamol is associated with an increase in cAMP, but thrombin-induced elevation of intracellular calcium concentrations is not affected by either salbutamol or 8bromo-cAMP.[128] These observations are consistent with the antiproliferative effect of cAMP on rabbit aortic smooth muscle, which is also independent of inhibition of calcium mobilisation.[137] However, studies in freshly obtained bovine tracheal muscle indicate that salbutamol reduces histamine-induced inositol phospholipid hydrolysis and presumably, therefore, histamine-induced calcium mobilisation.[138] This contrasting observation may be explained by species differences or changes upon culture of smooth muscle. Furthermore, in guinea pig cultured tracheal smooth muscle there is a clear dissociation between the mitogenic actions of endothelin-1 and epidermal growth factor (EGF) and their capacity to elevate intracellular calcium.[139]

The membrane-permeable analogue of cAMP, 8bromo-cAMP, mimics the action of salbutamol, as does inhibition of cyclic nucleotide PDEs with the nonselective inhibitor, isobutyl-methylxanthine.[77] Other agents that elevate cAMP, including prostaglandin $E_2$,[128,140] forskolin,[128,133] cholera toxin,[133] and vasoactive intestinal peptide,[141] are also inhibitors of smooth muscle proliferation. Microinjection of the catalytic subunit of PKA into the cytoplasm has an inhibitory effect on airway smooth muscle proliferation,[142] and the use of a cAMP antagonist, Rp-8-Br-cAMPS, reduces the antiproliferative effect of the $\beta_2$-adrenoceptor agonist salbutamol on mitogen-induced proliferation.[128]

Further investigations into the mechanism of this antiproliferative effect have indicated that it does not involve activation of potassium channels, since blockers of these channels do not influence the antiproliferative effect and potassium channel openers, such as cromakalim, are also without effect on airway smooth muscle proliferation (Gillzan and Stewart, unpublished observations).

### 1. The Mitogen-Activated Protein Kinase Pathway

Over the last 5 years the importance of the link between growth factor receptors and Ras protein activation of the mitogen-activated protein kinases (MAPKs) has become increasingly clear.[143] In this pathway, binding of growth factor results in receptor dimerisation and autophosphorylation which provides docking sites for binding of adaptor proteins, Grb2/SOS. These adaptor proteins bind and activate Ras protein, initiating a cascade of kinase activity including Raf kinase, MAPKK, and MAPK. MAPK phosphorylates Jun and fos which form AP-1 complexes in the nucleus initiating the transcription of *myc* and, in turn, cyclin D[144] (Figure 3). Elevation of cAMP in the fibroblast rat1 cell line has no effect on the assembly of adaptor proteins or activation of ras,[145] but the affinity of Raf kinase for Ras is reduced by PKA-dependent phosphorylation.[146] Ultimately, reduction in Raf activation would decrease the level of cyclin D synthesis (Figure 4). Our recent experiments in human cultured airway smooth muscle indicate that the inhibitory effects of salbutamol may be explained by a similar mechanism, since salbutamol reduced thrombin-stimulated cyclin D synthesis (Figure 5). The potential role of other cAMP-sensitive cell cycle regulatory proteins and the importance of cyclins are discussed in later sections (VII.B.3).

### 2. CREB Protein and Cell Proliferation

A number of genes contain sequences in the promoter regions called cAMP response elements (CREs) which are activated by CRE-binding protein (CREB). Increases in cAMP may cause activation and nuclear translocation of PKA, which is then able to phosphorylate CREB, increasing its transcriptional activity.[147] CREB binds to a nuclear protein called CREB-binding protein (CBP)[148] which is also bound by the phosphorylated (active) form of Jun. It has been suggested that limiting levels of CBP may cause competition between CREB and Jun, resulting in mutual inhibition.[149] Given the importance of Jun in activating mitogen-sensitive genes (see Figure 4), it is plausible that cAMP could inhibit cell proliferation by phosphorylated CREB sequestering the available CBP and, therefore, inhibiting the transcriptional activity of Jun complexes.

### 3. Cell Cycle Progression

Airway smooth muscle cells *in situ* in a normal airway are in a nonproliferative or quiescent, state. In cultures of airway smooth muscle entry into the cell cycle (G0 to G1 transition) can be stimulated by a wide range of growth factors and certain bronchoconstrictors.[13] The early events following growth

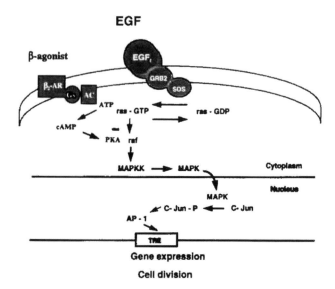

**FIGURE 3**   Interaction between β-agonists and Ras/MAPK cascade. Ligand binding of growth factor receptors (exemplified by EGF) causes Ras activation leading to the translocation of MAPK, phosphorylation and activation of the transactivating activity of Jun (homo- or heterodimers) and cell cycle progression. cAMP-dependent PKA inhibits the cascade by phosphorylating Raf and thereby reducing its affinity for Ras.

factor–stimulated entry of cells into G1 are discussed by Reynold Panettieri in Chapter 10 of this volume. The potential modulation of these early events by elevated cAMP has been discussed in the preceding section. Many pathways appear to converge, late in G1, on a common biochemical pathway that integrates signals and determines whether the cell progresses to a round of DNA synthesis. The inhibition of thrombin-stimulated DNA synthesis when smooth muscle is exposed to salbutamol 18 h after thrombin addition,[78] corresponding to 4 h before entry into S phase,[150] is consistent with an action of salbutamol on the passage of cells through the so-called restriction point.

### a. G1 Restriction Point

In mammalian cells there is a point in late G1 after which the cell cycle proceeds to DNA synthesis without the requirement of the continued presence of mitogenic stimulation or despite the addition of certain inhibitors of mitogenesis. The molecular gate that constitutes the restriction point is believed to be underphosphorylated retinoblastoma protein (Rb). Mitogenic stimulation activates the transcription of cyclins and cyclin-dependent kinases (Cdks). Cyclins and Cdks form complexes which are then phosphorylated by a cyclin-activating kinase (CAK). Activated cyclin–Cdk complexes appear in mid G1 and are responsible for the phosphorylation of the tumor suppressor gene product, Rb. Hypophosphorylated Rb is normally bound to the transcription factor E2F, inhibiting transcriptional activity. Phosphorylation of Rb by

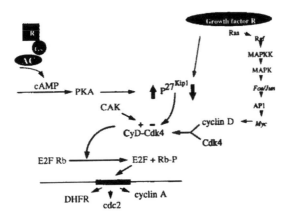

**FIGURE 4** PKA has two potential sites at which it regulates the transcriptional activity of E2F. However, both these sites are in the upstream signalling pathways activated by growth factor receptor occupation. Phosphorylation of raf may reduce the level of cyclin D synthesis which is essential to activate Cdk4 and, hence, Retinoblastoma (Rb) protein. Since hyperphosphorylated Rb does not bind and inhibit E2F, the transcriptional activity of the latter is derepressed allowing the synthesis of a number of gene products that are essential for cell passage through S phase, including cyclin A, cdc2, and dihydrofolate reductase (DHFR). The second mechanism for regulating Rb phosphorylation involves PKA-dependent generation of p27$^{Kip1}$, which competes with cyclin-activating kinase (CAK) for binding to the cyclin D–Cdk4 complex and, thereby, prevents its phosphorylation and activation. Consequently, the phosphorylation and derepression of Rb is prevented. Activation of growth factor receptor normally leads to suppression of the resting level of p27$^{Kip1}$ expression, but this is counteracted by increases in cAMP. CAK is comprised of cyclin H and Cdk7, the synthesis of which is also growth factor dependent.

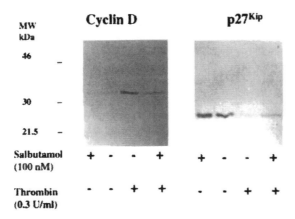

**FIGURE 5** Western blotting for the cell cycle regulatory proteins, cyclin D and p27$^{Kip1}$, following polyacrylamide gel electrophoresis of extracts of airway smooth muscle incubated for 20 h. Cyclin D levels were low or undetectable in the absence of the mitogen thrombin. Thrombin stimulation of cyclin D synthesis was inhibited by salbutamol (added 30 min before thrombin and left in the medium for the remainder of the incubation period). The resting level of p27$^{Kip1}$ was decreased by thrombin and increased by the addition of salbutamol. The suppression of p27$^{Kip1}$ levels by thrombin was partially counteracted by the presence of salbutamol.

cyclin–Cdk complexes is a key event prior to the G1 restriction point, resulting in the dissociation of Rb from E2F, allowing the transcription of genes required for progression through S phase and DNA synthesis. A number of inhibitors of mitogenesis appear to act by interfering with the signalling step(s) that precede the dissociation of inhibitory proteins from the E2F complex.

### b. G1 Cyclins and Cdks

The cyclins are a family of proteins which are synthesised at different rates according to the stage in the cell cycle. The key G1 cyclins are cyclins D and E.[151] Cyclin D1 was first identified as a product expressed in G1 by mouse macrophage cell line (BAC1.2F5A).[152] Cyclins D2 and D3 were identified by using cyclin D1 cDNA as a probe to screen cDNA libraries.[152,153] After mitogenic stimulation, cyclin D1 expression is apparent during the G0/G1 transition and reaches maximal levels prior to G1/S transition.[152] The oscillation of the levels of expression of cyclin D during the cell cycle is moderate in comparison with other cyclins,[151] but its elevation late in G1 is compatible with a role in the passage of cells through the restriction point. A decrease in cyclin D1 accumulation and/or its extrusion from the nucleus may be a prerequisite for the entry of cells into S phase.[154]

Cyclin E mRNA reaches maximal levels in late G1 near the G1/S phase transition, later than the peak of cyclin D levels,[153] and antibodies against cyclin E immunoprecipitate a histone H1 kinase.[155] These observations suggest that cyclin E plays a role in G1/S phase transition or S phase progression rather than at the G1 restriction point.

In cell lines that have been constructed to overexpress cyclin D[156] or cyclin E,[157] the duration of G1 is reduced, the cells are smaller, and there is a diminished requirement for mitogens, indicating the importance of these two cyclins. Microinjection of antibodies against cyclin D1 into fibroblasts overexpressing cyclin D prevented these cells from entering S phase, but these antibodies had no effect when injected near G1/S phase transition.[156,158] Cyclin D localises to the nucleus during G1 and disappears from the nucleus as cells proceed into S phase.[158] Paradoxically, the acute overexpression of cyclin D1 caused by the microinjection of an expression plasmid into fibroblasts has been shown to prevent entry into S phase.[159] This effect may be due to the inhibition of DNA repair in the presence of high levels of cyclin D, which provides an explanation of the difficulty in establishing cell lines with high levels of expression of cyclin D.[156]

Cyclins have no intrinsic protein kinase activity, but function as regulatory elements of protein kinases known as Cdks.[154] Cyclin D associates with Cdk4 or Cdk6.[160-162] Cyclin E associates with Cdk2.[163,164]

### c. Activation of Cyclin–Cdk Complexes

Cyclin–Cdk complexes require phosphorylation by CAK on a conserved threonine residue.[165] CAK is itself a cyclin–Cdk complex comprising cyclin H and Cdk 7. CAK activates Cdk2, Cdk4, and cdc2 complexes.[166,167] Depletion of CAK from mammalian cell lysates by immunoprecipation prevents the activation of these cyclin–Cdk complexes, indicating that CAK is essential for the activation of cyclin–Cdk complexes.[166]

Cyclin D–Cdk4 activity, measured by phosphorylation of Rb fragment, appears first in mid G1 and peaks at G1/S transition.[160,161] In contrast, cyclin E–Cdk2 activity appears 1 to 2 h before entry into S phase and is active during S phase.[163,164] The inhibition of Cdk2 activity prevents mammalian cells from entering S phase.[168-170] The later expression of cyclin E and its complexes with Cdk2, in comparison with cyclin D and the activity of its associated kinase, suggests that cyclin E is essential for the G1/S transition by initiation of DNA replication.[151]

### d. Substrates of Cyclin–Cdk Complexes

Cyclin D, but not cyclin E, directly binds Rb,[171,172] targetting Rb as a substrate for Cdk4 activity.[173] The inducible overexpression of cyclin D1 and E have been shown to hasten the appearance of the hyperphosphorylated form of Rb.[174] The binding of Rb to cyclin D is mediated by the pocket domain of Rb and a Leu-X-Cys-X-Glu amino acid sequence near the amino terminus of the cyclin D1, D2, and D3 proteins. This domain is similar to the sequence used by the adenovirus E1A, SV40 T antigen, and human papilloma E7 oncoproteins to bind the pocket region of Rb.[171]

### Retinoblastoma

The hypophosphorylated form of Rb binds to and inhibits the activity of the transcriptional factor E2F.[175-179] Phosphorylation of Rb by cyclin D-Cdk4 reduces its ability to form inhibitory complexes with E2F.[173] In cells lacking functional Rb, the microinjection of antibodies or antisense plasmids to cyclin D1 does not prevent entry into S phase,[154,180,181] whereas the microinjection of cyclin E antibody prevents cell cycle progression.[154] These observations further support the contention that cyclin E plays a role in the signalling of cell cycle progression downstream of the point at which cyclin D has its regulatory effect.

### E2F

The transcription factor E2F is a sequence-specific, DNA-binding protein complex that was identified independently as a requirement for E1A-dependent transcription of the adenovirus gene[182] and as a differentiation-regulated factor in embryonal carcinoma cells.[183] It was established in HeLa cells that E2F is a heterodimer of DP and E2F proteins. There is a family of five distinct E2F proteins (E2F-1, E2F-2, E2F-3, E2F-4, E2F-5) and a family of three distinct DP proteins (DP-1, DP-2, DP-3), although E2F-1 and DP-1 are the most thoroughly characterised to date.[184] The interaction of DP-1 and E2F-1 results in greater DNA-binding and transcriptional activity and increased affinity for Rb.[185-187] The carboxyl terminal of the DP-1 protein appears to influence the binding of Rb to the DP-1/E2F-1 heterodimer.[188] The level of phosphorylation of DP-1 increases during S phase and correlates with a decreased DNA-binding activity of the heterodimer.[183,188]

E2F transcriptional activity appears to mediate the transition from G1 to S, as the introduction of E2F releases cells from arrest of the cell cycle induced by Rb.[189] Furthermore, E2F microinjection also induces DNA synthesis in quiescent fibroblasts.[190] However, E2F does not induce malignant transformation of rat embryo fibroblasts in cooperation with activated Ras, a common assay for characterisation of proto-oncogenic properties of genes.[191,192] This lack of proto-oncogenic property may be explained by the ability of E2F to induce apoptosis.[193] Several genes have been confirmed to have E2F sites within their promoter regions: p34cdc2, cyclin A, c-Myc, B-Myb, Rb, E2F and DHFR.[183,184]

In addition to phosphorylating Rb, cyclin D–Cdk4 phosphorylates E2F-1, which also inhibits the interaction of E2F with Rb.[194] Interestingly, a majority of hyperphosphorylated Rb exists in E2F complexes at the end of G1 and through S phase.[195] Increased levels of Rb-free E2F complexes may be the result of release of E2F from other pocket-binding proteins (p107 or p130) or the *de novo* synthesis of E2F-1 protein.[196,197] Thus, the phosphorylation of noncomplexed Rb and the synthesis of E2F would produce E2F complexes with transcriptional activity.[184]

### e. *Inhibition of Cyclin-Cdk Complexes*

Inhibitors of mitogenesis can arrest cell cycle progression by the inhibition of formation of cyclin-Cdk complexes or by influencing the association of cyclin–Cdk complexes and protein inhibitors of activation of these complexes. The progression through the cell cycle under mitogenic stimulation is also influenced by a combination of factors that includes the levels of cyclins, Cdks, and Cdk inhibitors. Cdk inhibitors are classed under two groups, the Cip/Kip family and INK family.[151,198]

Transforming growth factor β (TGFβ) inhibits mitogenesis in mink lung epithelial cells and decreases Cdk4 protein levels in these cells.[199] Stimuli that elevate the level of cAMP decrease cyclin D mRNA levels in mouse macrophage cell lines,[200] whereas rapamycin decreases cyclin D levels in osteosarcoma cell lines.[201] The antimitogenic actions of these compounds may be explained by a reduction in cyclin D levels. Cyclin A has also been reported to be downregulated in response to antimitogens,[202-204] although this may be a consequence of cell cycle arrest in G1.[198]

Biochemical analysis of extracts from quiescent cells identified a 27-kDa protein that bound cyclin E–Cdk2, inhibited CAK activation of the Cdk, and reduced the activity of pre-activated cyclin E–Cdk2 complexes.[204,205] Sequencing of p27[Kip1] revealed a domain similar to that found in p21,[206] a cyclin kinase inhibitor that is elevated by the tumor suppressor gene product p53.[207,208] The region of homology between p21 and p27[Kip1] was the domain responsible for binding and inhibiting Cdks.[206] p21 and p27[Kip1] are members of the Cip/Kip family of Cdk inhibitors.[198]

The INK family of Cdk inhibitors consists of p15 and p16, which have multiple ankyrin repeats and no sequence similarity to p21 or p27[Kip1].[209,210] The INK Cdk inhibitors differ functionally from the Cip/Kip inhibitors in targetting isolated Cdk subunits.[198] p16 associates with Cdk4 at the expense of cyclin D.[211,212]

The importance of the balance between cyclin–Cdk complexes and Cdk inhibitors in determining progression through the cell cycle has been demonstrated in at least four different cell lines. (1) In quiescent mink lung epithelial cells high levels of p27[Kip1] are present in association with the cyclin E–Cdk2 complex that is expressed at low levels. The addition of mitogen increases Cdk4 levels and, consequently, cyclin D–Cdk4 complexes which bind p27[Kip1], allowing the appearance of free cyclin D–Cdk4 and cyclin E–Cdk2. The inhibitor of mitogenesis TGFβ prevents an increase in Cdk4 in these cells.[199] (2) In human keratinocytes TGFβ inhibits an increase of Cdk levels on addition of mitogen[202] and elicits a 30-fold increase in p15 mRNA.[209] (3) In mouse macrophages, CSF-1 increases cyclin D levels while reducing p27[Kip1] expression. cAMP causes G1 arrest in these cells via the activation of PKA, which prevents CSF-1-mediated decreases in the levels of p27[Kip1].[213] (4) In human and mouse T-lymphocytes, IL-2 decreases the high levels of p27[Kip1] present in unstimulated cells. Rapamycin acts as an inhibitor of mitogenesis in these cells by inhibiting the IL-2-elicited decrease in p27[Kip1].[214,215]

### f. Termination of E2F Transcriptional Activity

In late G1, E2F associates with cyclin E–Cdk2; however, as cells progress through S phase, cyclin E is replaced with cyclin A.[216] The association of cyclin A with E2F in late S phase allows phosphorylation of DP-1, which decreases the DNA-binding affinity and transcriptional activity of the E2F complex.[217]

### g. Turning off Cyclin–Cdks Complexes

To date, little is known of the mechanism(s) involved in the degradation of cyclin D or cyclin E after G1, when their functions have been completed. Mitotic cyclin complexes are inactivated by ubiquitin-dependent proteolysis of the cyclin subunit,[218] but this mechanism has not been demonstrated for D-type or E-type cyclins.[154] Cyclin E contains PEST sequences (single letter code for amino acids).[153,155] In yeast, the removal of PEST sequences from G1 cyclins prolongs the half-life of these cyclins.[219] Cyclin D–Cdk4 complexes may be inactivated by association with p16. The levels of p16 increase as cells enter S phase,[181] while inactivation of Rb leads to an increase in the expression of p16.[210] Therefore, as cells approach S phase, the release of Rb from E2F may cause an increase in transcription of p16, which then acts to lower the activity of Cdk4 as cells progress through S phase.[151,154]

### 4. Cell-Cycle Regulation in Airway Smooth Muscle

Detailed analyses of cell cycle regulation in airway smooth muscle have yet to be carried out. Thus, the extent to which the foregoing discussion of cyclins, Cdks, CAK, Cdk inhibitors and Rb is relevant to airway smooth muscle is of considerable interest both in the understanding of interactions of currently used anti-asthma agents with biochemical pathways subserving cell proliferation and in the potential for the development of new agents with antiproliferative activity. Our investigations of the effects of salbutamol in human cultured airway smooth muscle suggest that inhibition of thrombin-stimulated cyclin D synthesis and maintenance of $p27^{Kip1}$ levels (see Figure 5) contribute to the antiproliferative effect (Stewart, Schachte, Tomlinson, Harris and Wilson, unpublished observations). It is not yet clear whether the maintenance of $p27^{Kip1}$ levels is more or less important than the inhibition by cAMP of cyclin D synthesis (see Figure 5) or the potential inhibition of the transcriptional activity of c-jun complexes by CREB through competition for limited amounts of CBP (see Section VII.B.2).

# VIII. CONCLUSIONS

The evidence indicating a rise in asthma incidence, morbidity, and mortality has led to a reevaluation of the place of $\beta$-agonists in the treatment of this disease. The recognition of the importance of airway wall remodelling in AHR has also stimulated intense interest in the factors that initiate and modulate growth responses of airway smooth muscle. Fundamental advances in understanding of cell cycle regulation, primarily derived from cancer research, have provided a framework for investigations of these mechanisms in airway smooth muscle which may lead to the development of novel anti-asthma agents which specifically target this important aspect of the pathogenesis of asthma.

# ACKNOWLEDGMENTS

The authors work cited in this review has been supported by grants from the NH&MRC (Australia) and Glaxo-Wellcome R & D (U.K.).

# REFERENCES

1. Barrett, T. E. and Strom, B. L., Inhaled beta-adrenoceptor agonists in asthma: more harm than good? *Am. J. Resp. Crit. Care Med.*, 151, 574, 1995.
2. van Schayck, C. P., Dompeling, E., van Herwaarden, C. L., Folgering, H., Verbeek, A. L., van der Hoogen, H. J., and van Weel, C., How detrimental is chronic use of bronchodilators in asthma and chronic obstructive pulmonary disease, *Am. J. Resp. Crit. Care Med.*, 151, 1995.
3. Devoy, M. A. B., Fuller, R. W., and Palmer, J. B. D., Are there any detrimental effects of the use of long-acting $\beta_2$-agonists in the treatment of asthma? *Chest*, 107, 1116, 1995.
4. Szentivanyi, A., The beta adrenergic theory of the atopic abnormality in bronchial asthma, *J. Allergy*, 42, 203, 1968.

5. Turki, J., Pak, J., Green, S. A., Martin, R. J., and Liggett, S. B., Genetic polymorphisms of the β adrenergic receptor in nocturnal and non-nocturnal asthma: evidence that Gly16 correlates with the nocturnal phenotype, *J. Clin. Invest.*, 95, 1635, 1995.

6. Cockcroft, D. W., Ruffin, R. E., Dolovich, J., and Hargreave, F. E., Allergen-induced increases in non-allergic bronchial reactivity, *Clin. Allergy*, 7, 513, 1977.

7. Juniper, E. F., Kline, P. A., Vanzieleghem, M. A., Ramsdale, H., O'Byrne, P. M., and Hargreave, F. E., Effect of long-term treatment with an inhaled corticosteroid (Budesonide) on airway hyperresponsiveness and clinical asthma in nonsteroid-dependent asthmatics, *Am. Rev. Respir. Dis.*, 142, 832, 1990.

8. James, A. L., Pare, P. D., and Hogg, J. C., The mechanics of airway narrowing in asthma, *Am. Rev. Respir. Dis.*, 139, 242, 1989.

9. Kuwano, K., Bosken, C. H., Pare, P. D., Bai, T. R., Wiggs, B. R., and Hogg, J. C., Small airways dimensions in asthma and chronic airway obstructive pulmonary disease, *Am. Rev. Respir. Dis.*, 148, 1220, 1993.

10. Hossain, S., Quantitative measurement of bronchial muscle in men with asthma, *Am. Rev. Respir. Dis.*, 107, 99, 1973.

11. Dunnill, M. S., Massarella, G. R., and Anderson, J. A., A comparison of the quantitative anatomy of the bronchi in normal subjects, in status asthmaticus, in chronic bronchitis, and in emphysema, *Thorax*, 24, 176, 1969.

12. Lundgren, R., Soderberg, M., Horstedt, P., and Stenling, R., Morphological studies of bronchial mucosal biopsies from asthmatics before and after ten years of treatment with inhaled steroids, *Eur. J. Resp. Dis.*, 1, 883, 1988.

13. Stewart, A. G., Tomlinson, P. R., and Wilson, J. W. *Regulation of airway wall remodelling: prospects for the development of novel antiasthma drugs*, in *Advances in Pharmacology* Vol. 33, Hollinger, M. A., Academic Press, New York, 1995, 209.

14. Townley, R. G., Trapani, I. L., and Szentivanyi, A., Sensitization to anaphylaxis and to some of its pharmacological mediators by blockade of the beta adrenergic receptors, *J. Allergy*, 39, 177, 1967.

15. McCulloch, M. W., Proctor, C., and Rand, M. J., Evidence for an adrenergic homeostatic bronchodilator reflex mechanism, *Eur. J. Pharmacol.*, 2, 214, 1967.

16. Diamond, L., Potentiation of bronchomotor responses by beta adrenergic antagonists, *J. Pharmacol. Exp. Ther.*, 181, 433, 1972.

17. McNeill, R. S., Effect of a β-adrenergic-blocking agent, propranolol, on asthmatics, *Lancet*, 2, 1101, 1964.

18. Zaid, G. and Beall, G. N., Bronchial response to beta-adrenergic blockade, *N. Engl. J. Med.*, 275, 580, 1966.

19. Ouellette, J. J. and Reed, C. E., The effect of partial beta adrenergic blockade on the bronchial response of hay fever subjects to ragweed aerosol, *J. Allergy*, 39, 160, 1967.

20. McReady, S., Conboy, K., and Townley, R., The effect of beta-adrenergic blockade on bronchial sensitivity to methacholine in normal and allergic rhinitis subjects, *J. Allergy*, 41, 108, 1968.

21. McNeill, R. S. and Ingram, C. G., Effect of propranolol on ventilatory function, *Am. J. Cardiol.*, 18, 473, 1966.

22. Parker, C. W. and Smith, J. W., Alterations in cyclic adenosine monophosphate metabolism in human bronchial asthma, *J. Clin. Invest.*, 52, 48, 1973.

23. Shelhamer, J. H., Metcalfe, D. D., Smith, L. J., and Kaliner, M., Abnormal beta adrenergic responsiveness in allergic subjects: analysis of isoproterenol-induced cardiovascular and plasma cyclic adenosine monophosphate responses, *J. Allergy Clin. Immunol.*, 66, 52, 1980.

24. Brooks, S. M., McGowan, K., Bernstein, I. L., Altenau, P., and Peagler, J., Relationship between numbers of beta adrenergic receptors in lymphocytes and disease severity in asthma, *J. Allergy Clin. Immunol.*, 63, 401, 1979.

25. Connolly, M. J., Crowley, J. J., Nielson, C. P., Charan, N. B., and Vestal, R. E., Methacholine reactivity and lymphocyte beta-receptor density and affinity in drug-naive asthmatics and normals, *Am. Rev. Respir. Dis.*, 143, A420, 1991.

26. Nielson, C. P., Crowley, J. J., Vestal, R. E., and Connolly, M. J., Impaired beta-adrenoceptor function, increased leukocyte respiratory burst, and bronchial hyperresponsiveness, *J. Allergy Clin. Immunol.*, 90, 825, 1992.

27. Galant, S. P., Duriseti, L., Underwood, S., and Insel, P. A., Decreased beta-adrenergic receptors on polymorphonuclear leukocytes after adrenergic therapy, *N. Engl. J. Med.*, 299, 933, 1978.

28. Galant, S. P., Duriseti, L., Underwood, S., Allred, S., and Insel, P. A., Beta adrenergic receptors on polymorphonuclear particulates in bronchial asthma, *J. Clin. Invest.*, 65, 577, 1980.

29. Emala, C. W., Arayana, A., Levine, M. A., and Hirshman, C. A., Impaired stimulation of adenylyl cyclase by isoproterenol in leukocyte membranes of BG dogs is similar to reduced stimulation in airway smooth muscle of the same dogs, *Am. J. Respir. Crit. Care Med.*, 149, A332, 1994.

30. Meurs, H., Koeter, G. H., de Vries, K., and Kauffman, H. F., The beta-adrenergic system and allergic bronchial asthma: changes in lymphocyte beta-adrenergic receptor number and adenylate cyclase activity after an allergen-induced asthmatic attack, *J. Allergy Clin. Immunol.*, 70, 272, 1982.

31. Bachelet, M., Vincent, D., Havet, N., Marrash-Chahla, R., Pradalier, A., Dry, J., and Vargaftig, B. B., Reduced responsiveness of adenylate cyclase in alveolar macrophages from patients with asthma, *J. Allergy Clin. Immunol.*, 88, 322, 1991.

32. Barnes, P. J., Dollery, C. T., and MacDermot, J., Increased pulmanory α-adrenergic and reduced β-adrenergic receptors in experimental asthma, *Nature*, 285, 569, 1980.

33. Cheng, J. B. and Townley, R. G., Effects of chronic histamine and ovalbumin aerosols on pulmonary beta adrenergic receptors in sensitized guinea pigs, *Res. Commun. Chem. Pathol. Pharmacol.*, 36, 507, 1982.

34. Shindoh, J., Sugiyama, S., Hayashi, K., Takagi, K., Satake, T., and Ozawa, T., Time course of recovery of beta- and alpha 1-adrenoceptors in experimental asthma, *Clin. Exp. Pharmacol. Physiol.*, 17, 485, 1990.

35. Motojima, S., Yukawa, T., Fukuda, T., and Makino, S., Changes in airway responsiveness and beta- and alpha-1-adrenergic receptors in the lungs of guinea pigs with experimental asthma, *Allergy*, 44, 66, 1989.

36. Gatto, C., Green, T. P., Johnson, M. G., Marchessault, R. P., Seybold, V., and Johnson, D. E., Localization of quantitative changes in pulmonary beta-receptors in ovalbumin-sensitized guinea pigs, *Am. Rev. Respir. Dis.*, 136, 150, 1987.

37. Taki, F., Takagi, K., Satake, T., Sugiyama, S., and Ozawa, T., The role of phospholipase in reduced beta-adrenergic responsiveness in experimental asthma, *Am. Rev. Respir. Dis.*, 133, 362, 1986.

38. Scarpace, P. J. and Bender, B. S., Viral pneumonia attenuates adenylate cyclase but not beta-adrenergic receptors in murine lung, *Am. Rev. Respir. Dis.*, 140, 1602, 1989.

39. Henry, P. J., Rigby, P. J., Mackenzie, J. S., and Goldie, R. G., Effect of respiratory tract viral infection on murine airway beta-adrenoceptor function, distribution and density, *Br. J. Pharmacol.*, 104, 914, 1991.

40. Engels, F., Carstairs, J. R., Barnes, P. J., and Nijkamp, F. P., Autoradiographic localization of changes in pulmonary beta-adrenoceptors in an animal model of atopy, *Eur. J. Pharmacol.*, 164, 139, 164.

41. Lee, J. Y., Uchida, Y., Sakamoto, T., Hirata, A., Hasegawa, S., and Hirata, F., Alteration of G protein levels in antigen-challenged guinea pigs, *J. Pharmacol. Exp. Ther.*, 271, 1713, 1994.

42. Tobias, J. D., Sauder, R. A., and Hirshman, C. A., Reduced sensitivity to β-adrenergic agonists in basenji-greyhound dogs, *J. Appl. Physiol.*, 69, 1212, 1990.

43. Emala, C., Black, C., Curry, C., Levine, M. A., and Hirshman, C. A., Impaired β-adrenergic receptor activation of adenylyl cyclase in airway smooth muscle in the basenji-greyhound dog model of airway hyperresponsiveness, *Am. J. Respir. Cell Mol. Biol.*, 8, 668, 1993.

44. Hungerford, C. L., Emala, C. W., and Hirshman, C. A., Does impaired β-adrenergic stimulation of adenylyl cyclase in trachealis smooth muscle of the BG dog persist in cultured muscle cells? *Am. J. Respir. Crit. Care Med.*, 149, A1083, 1994.

45. Santing, R. E., Schraa, E. O., Vos, B. G., Gores, R. J., Olymulder, C. G., Meurs, H., and Zaagsma, J., Dissociation between bronchial hyperreactivity *in vivo* and reduced beta-adrenoceptor sensitivity *in vitro* in allergen-challenged guinea pigs., *Eur. J. Pharmacol.*, 257, 145, 1994.

46. Wills-Karp, M., Uchida, Y., Lee, J. Y., Jinot, J., Hirata, A., and Hirata, F., Organ culture with proinflammatory cytokines reproduces impairment of the β-adrenoceptor-mediated relaxation in tracheas of a guinea pig antigen model, *Am. J. Respir. Cell Mol. Biol.*, 8, 153, 1993.

47. Raaijmakers, J. A., Beneker, C., van Geffen, E. C., Meisters, T. M., and Pover, P., Inflammatory mediators and beta-adrenoceptor function, *Agents Actions*, 26, 45, 1989.

48. Carstairs, J. R., Nimmo, A. J., and Barnes, P. J., Autoradiographic visualization of beta-adrenoceptor subtypes in human lung, *Am. Rev. Respir. Dis.*, 132, 541, 1985.

49. Spina, D., Rigby, P. J., Paterson, J. W., and Goldie, R. G., Autoradiographic localization of beta-adrenoceptors in asthmatic human lung, *Am. Rev. Respir. Dis.*, 140, 1410, 1989.

50. Spina, D., Rigby, P. J., Paterson, J. W., and Goldie, R. G., Alpha 1-adrenoceptor function and autoradiographic distribution in human asthmatic lung, *Br. J. Pharmacol.*, 97, 701, 1989.

51. Goldie, R. G., Paterson, J. W., Spina, D., and Wale, J. L., Classification of beta-adrenoceptors in human isolated bronchus, *Br. J. Pharmacol.*, 81, 611, 1984.

52. Martin, C. A., Naline, E., Bakdach, H., and Advenier, C., Beta 3-adrenoceptor agonists, BRL 37344 and SR 58611A, do not induce relaxation of human, sheep and guinea-pig airway smooth muscle *in vitro*, *Eur. Respir. J.*, 7, 1610, 1994.

53. Tamaoki, J., Yamauchi, F., Chiyotani, A., Yamawaki, I., Takeuchi, S., and Konno, K., Atypical beta-adrenoceptor-(beta 3-adrenoceptor) mediated relaxation of canine isolated bronchial smooth muscle, *J. Appl. Physiol.*, 74, 297, 1993.

54. Sharma, R. K. and Jeffery, P. K., Airway β-adrenoceptor number in cystic fibrosis and asthma, *Clin. Sci.*, 78, 409, 1990.

55. van Koppen, C. J., Rodrigues de Miranda, J. F., Beld, A. J., van Herwaarden, C. L. A., Lammers, J.-W. J., and Ginneken, C. A. M., Beta adrenoceptor binding and induced relaxation in airway smooth muscle from patients with chronic airflow obstruction, *Thorax*, 44, 28, 1989.

56. Bai, T. R., Mak, J. C. W., and Barnes, P. J., A comparison of β-adrenergic receptors and *in vitro* relaxant responses to isoproterenol in asthmatic airway smooth muscle, *Am. J. Respir. Cell Mol. Biol.*, 6, 647, 1992.

57. Kaliner, M., Shelhamer, J. H., Davis, P. B., Smith, L. J., and Venter, J. C., Autonomic nervous system abnormalities and allergy, *Ann. Intern. Med.*, 96, 349, 1982.

58. Middleton, E., Jr. and Finke, S. R., Metabolic response to epinephrine in bronchial asthma, *J. Allergy*, 42, 288, 1968.

59. Snashall, P. D., Boother, F. A., and Sterling, G. M., The effect of α-adrenoreceptor stimulation on the airways of normal and asthmatic man, *Clin. Sci. Mol. Med.*, 54, 283, 1978.

60. Svedmyr, N. L. V., Larsson, S. A., and Thiringer, G. K., Development of resistance in beta-adrenergic receptors of asthmatic patients, *Chest*, 69, 479, 1976.

61. Goldie, R. G., Spina, D., Henry, P. J., Lulich, K. M., and Paterson, J. W., *In vitro* responsiveness of human asthmatic bronchus to carbachol, histamine, β-adrenoceptor agonists and theophylline, *Br. J. Clin. Pharmacol.*, 22, 669, 1986.

62. Bai, T. R., Abnormalities in airway smooth muscle in fatal asthma, *Am. Rev. Respir. Dis.*, 141, 552, 1990.

63. Bai, T. R., Abnormalities in airway smooth muscle in fatal asthma. A comparison between trachea and bronchus, *Am. Rev. Respir. Dis.*, 143, 441, 1991.

64. Cerrina, J., Ladivric, M. L. R., Labat, C., Raffestin, B., Bayol, A., and Brink, C., Comparison of human bronchial muscle response to histamine *in vivo* with histamine and isoproternol agonists *in vitro*, *Am. Rev. Respir. Dis.*, 123, 156, 1986.

65. Blecher, M., Lewis, S., Hicks, J. M., and Josephs, S., Beta-blocking autoantibodies in pediatric bronchial asthma, *J. Allergy Clin. Immunol.*, 74, 246, 1984.
66. Potter, P. C., Van Wyk, L., White, D., Dakers, B. S., Chung, F. Z., and Dowdle, E. B., Absence of functional inhibition of cloned human beta 2-adrenergic receptors by autoantibodies in asthmatic subjects, *Clin. Exp. Allergy*, 23, 219, 1993.
67. Sears, M. R., Taylor, D. R., Print, C. G., Lake, D. C., Li, Q., Flannery, E. M., Yates, D. M., Lucas, M. K., and Herbison, G. P., Regular inhaled beta-agonist treatment in bronchial asthma, *Lancet*, 336, 1391, 1990.
68. van Shayck, C. P., Dompeling, E., van Herwaarden, C. L., Folgering, H., Verbeek, A. L., van der Hoogen, H. J., and van Weel, C., Bronchodilator treatment in moderate asthma or chronic bronchitis: continuous or on demand? A randomised controlled study, *Br. Med. J.*, 303, 1426, 1991.
69. Haahtela, T., Jarvinen, M., Kava, T., Kirivanta, K., Koskinen, S., Lehtonen, K., Nikander, K., Persson, T., Selroos, O., Sovijarvi, A., Stenius-Aarniala, B., Svahn, T., Tammivara, R., and Laitinen, L., Effects of reducing or discontinuing inhaled budesonide in patients with mild asthma, *N. Engl. J. Med.*, 331, 700, 1994.
70. Grainger, J., Woodman, K., Pearce, N., Crane, J., Burgress, C., Keane, A., and Beasley, R., Prescribed fenoterol and death from asthma in New Zealand 1981–7: a further case-control study, *Thorax*, 46, 105, 1991.
71. Spitzer, W. O., Suissa, S., Ernst, P., Horwitz, R. I., Habbick, B., Cockcroft, D., Boivin, J.-F., McNutt, M., Buist, A. S., and Rebuck, A. S., The use of β-agonists and the risk of death and near death from asthma, *N. Engl. J. Med.*, 326, 501, 1992.
72. Ernst, P., Habbick, B., Suissa, S., Hemmelgarn, B., Cockcroft, D., Buist, A. S., Horwitz, R. I., McNutt, M., and Spitzer, W. O., Is the association between inhaled beta-agonist use and life-threatening asthma because of confounding by severity? *Am. Rev. Respir. Dis.*, 148, 75, 1993.
73. Suissa, S., Ernst, P., Boivin, J.-F., Horwitz, R. I., Habbick, B., Cockcroft, D., Blais, L., McNutt, M., Buist, A. S., and Spitzer, W. O., A cohort analysis of excess mortality in asthma and the use of inhaled β-agonists, *Am. J. Crit. Care Med.*, 149, 604, 1994.
74. Ullman, A. and Svedmyr, N., Salmeterol, a new long-acting inhaled $\beta_2$-adrenoceptor agonist: comparison with salbutamol in adult asthmatic patients, *Thorax*, 43, 674, 1988.
75. Cheung, D., Timmers, M. C., Zwinderman, A. H., Bel, E. H., Dijkman, J. H., and Sterk, P. J., Long-term effects of a long-lasting $\beta_2$-adrenergic agonist, salmeterol, on airway hyperresponsiveness in patients with mild asthma., *N. Engl. J. Med.*, 327, 1198, 1992.
76. Grove, A. and Lipworth, B. J., Bronchodilator subsensitivity to salbutamol after twice daily salmeterol in asthmatic patients, *Lancet*, 346, 201, 1995.
77. Tomlinson, P. R., Wilson, J. W., and Stewart, A. G., Inhibition by salbutamol of the proliferation of human airway smooth muscle cells grown in culture, *Br. J. Pharmacol.*, 111, 641, 1994.
78. Tomlinson, P. R., Wilson, J. W., and Stewart, A. G., The influence of treatment duration on $\beta_2$-adrenoceptor agonist-mediated inhibition of human airway smooth muscle cell proliferation, *Am. J. Respir. Crit. Care Med.*, 151, A48, 1995.
79. Wang, Z.-L., Bramley, A. M., McNamara, A., Pare, P. D., and Bai, T. R., Chronic fenoterol exposure increases *in vivo* and *in vitro* airway responses in guinea pigs, *Am. J. Respir. Crit. Care Med.*, 149, 960, 1994.
80. Kobilka, B. K., Dixon, R. A. F., Frielle, T., Dohlman, H. G., Bolanowski, M. A., Sigal, I. S., Yang-Feng, T. L., Francke, U., Caron, M. G., and Lefkowitz, R. J., cDNA for the human $\beta_2$-adrenergic receptor: a protein with multiple membrane-spanning domains and encoded by a gene whose chromosomal location is shared with that of the receptor for platelet-derived growth factor, *Proc. Natl. Acad. Sci. U.S.A.*, 84, 46, 1987.
81. Frielle, T., Daniel, K. W., Caron, M. G., and Lefkowitz, R. J., Structural basis of β-adrenergic receptor subtype specificity studied with chimeric $\beta_1/\beta_2$-adrenergic receptors, *Proc. Natl. Acad. Sci. U.S.A.*, 85, 9494, 1988.

82. Kobilka, B. K., Kobilka, T. S., Daniel, K., Regan, J. W., Caron, M. G., and Lefkowitz, R. J., Chimeric $\alpha_2$-, $\beta_2$-adrenergic receptors: delineation of domains involved in effector coupling and ligand binding specifity, *Science*, 240, 1310, 1988.
83. O'Dowd, B. F., Hnatowich, M., Regan, J. W., Leader, W. M., Caron, M. G., and Lefkowitz, R. J., Site-directed mutagenesis of the cytoplasmic domains of the human $\beta_2$-adrenergic receptor. Localization of regions involved in G protein-receptor coupling, *J. Biol. Chem.*, 263, 15985, 1988.
84. Liggett, S. B., Bouvier, M., Hausdorff, W. P., O'Dowd, B., Caron, M. G., and Lefkowitz, R. J., Alered patterns of agonist-stimulated cAMP accumulation in cells expressing mutant $\beta_2$-adrenergic receptors lacking phosphorylation sites, *Mol. Pharmacol.*, 36, 641, 1989.
85. Hall, I. P., Daykin, K., and Widdop, S., $\beta_2$-adrenoceptor desensitization in cultured airway smooth muscle, *Clin. Sci.*, 84, 151, 1993.
86. Campbell, P. T., Hnatowich, M., O'Dowd, B. F., Caron, M. G., Lefkowitz, R. J., and Hausdorff, W. P., Mutations of the human $\beta_2$-adrenegic receptor that impair coupling to $G_s$ interfere with receptor down-regulation but not sequestration, *Mol. Pharmacol.*, 39, 192, 1991.
87. Liggett, S. B., Freedman, N. J., Schwinn, D. A., and Lefkowitz, R. J., Structural basis for receptor subtype-specific regulation revealed by a chimeric $\beta_3/\beta_2$-adrenergic receptor, *Proc. Natl. Acad. Sci. U.S.A.*, 90, 3665, 1993.
88. Liggett, S. B., Bouvier, M., O'Dowd, B. F., Caron, M. G., Lefkowitz, R. J., and DeBlasi, A., Substitution of an extracellular cysteine in the $\beta_2$-adrenergic receptor enhances agonist-promoted phosphorylation and receptor desensitization, *Biochem. Biophys. Res. Commun.*, 165, 257, 1989.
89. Hausdorff, W. P., Campbell, P. T., Ostrowski, J., Yu, S. S., Caron, M. G., and Lefkowitz, R. J., A small region of $\beta$-adrenergic receptor is selectively involved in its rapid regulation, *Proc. Natl. Acad. Sci. U.S.A.*, 88, 2979, 1991.
90. Pippig, S., Andexinger, S., and Lohse, M. J., Sequestration and recycling of $\beta_2$-adrenergic receptors permit receptor resensitization, *J. Pharmacol. Exp. Ther.*, 47, 666, 1995.
91. Barnes, P. J., Beta-adrenergic receptors and their regulation, *Am. J. Respir. Crit. Care Med.*, 152, 838, 1995.
92. Bouvier, M., Collins, S., O'Dowd, B. F., Campbell, P. T., de Blasi, A., Kobilka, B. K., MacGregor, C., Irons, G. P., Caron, M. G., and Lefkowitz, R. J., Two distinct pathways for cAMP-mediated down-regulation of the $\beta_2$-adrenergic receptor. Phosphorylation of the receptor and regulation of its mRNA level, *J. Biochem.*, 264, 16786, 1989.
93. Bouvier, M., Hnatowich, M., Collins, S., Kobilka, B. K., Deblasi, A., Lefkowitz, R. J., and Caron, M. G., Expression of a human cDNA encoding the β2-adrenergic receptor in Chinese hamster fibroblasts (CHW): functionality and regulation of the expressed receptors, *Mol. Pharmacol.*, 33, 133, 1988.
94. George, S. T., Berrios, M., Hadcock, J. R., Wang, H., and Malbon, C. C., Receptor density and cAMP accumulation: analysis in CHO cells exhibiting stable expression of a cDNA that encodes the beta$_2$-adrenergic receptor, *Biochem. Biophys. Res. Commun.*, 150, 665, 1988.
95. Reihsaus, E., Innis, M., MacIntyre, N., and Liggett, S. B., Mutations in the gene encoding for the $\beta_2$-adrenergic receptor in normal and asthmatic subjects, *Am. J. Respir. Cell Mol. Biol.*, 8, 334, 1993.
96. Green, S. A., Turki, J., Bejarano, P., Hall, I. P., and Liggett, S. B., Influence of $\beta_2$-adrenergic receptor genotypes on signal transduction in human airway smooth muscle cells, *Am. J. Respir. Cell Mol. Biol.*, 13, 25, 1995.
97. Postma, D. S., Bleecker, E. R., Amelung, P. J., Holroyd, K. J., Xu, J., Panhuysen, C. I. M., Meyers, D. A., and Levitt, R. C., Genetic susceptibility to asthma — bronchial hyperresponsiveness coinherited with a major gene for atopy, *N. Engl. J. Med.*, 333, 894, 1995.
98. Knox, A. J. and Tattersfield, A. E., Airway smooth muscle relaxation, *Thorax*, 50, 894, 1995.

99. McCann, J. D. and Welsh, M. J., Calcium-activated potassium channels in canine airway smooth muscle, *J. Physiol.*, 372, 113, 1986.

100. Kotlikoff, M. I., Potassium currents in canine airway smooth muscle cells, *Am. J. Physiol.*, 259, L384, 1990.

101. Nelson, M. T., Huang, Y., Brayden, J. E., Hescheler, J., and Standen, N. B., Arterial dilations in response to calcitonin gene-related peptide involve activation of K⁺, *Nature*, 344, 771, 1990.

102. Murray, M. A., Boyle, J. P., and Small, R. C., Cromakalim-induced relaxation of guinea-pig isolated trachealis: antagonism by glibenclamide and by phentolamine, *Br. J. Pharmacol.*, 98, 865, 1989.

103. Arch, J. R. S., Buckle, D. R., Bumstead, J., Clarke, G. D., Taylor, J. F., and Taylor, S. G., Evaluation of the potassium channel activator cromakalim (BRL 34915) as a bronchodilator in the guinea-pig: comparison with nifedipine, *Br. J. Pharmacol.*, 95, 763, 1988.

104. Black, J. L., Armour, C. L., Johnson, P. R. A., Alouan, L. A., and Barnes, P. J., The action of potassium channel activator, BRL 38227 (lemakalim), on human airway smooth muscle, *Am. Rev. Respir. Dis.*, 142, 1384, 1990.

105. Kume, H., Takai, A., Tokuno, H., and Tomita, T., Regulation of Ca²⁺-dependent K⁺-channel activity in tracheal myocytes by phosphorylation, *Nature*, 341, 152, 1989.

106. Jones, T. R., Charette, L., Garcia, M. L., and Kaczorowski, G. J., Selective inhibition of relaxation of guinea-pig trachea by charybdotoxin, a potent Ca⁺⁺-activated K⁺ channel inhibitor, *J. Pharmacol. Exp. Ther.*, 255, 697, 1990.

107. Miura, M., Belvisi, M. G., Stretton, C. D., Yacoub, M. H., and Barnes, P. J., Role of potassium channels in bronchodilator responses in human airways, *Am. Rev. Respir. Dis.*, 146, 132, 1992.

108. Kume, H., Grazizno, M. P., and Kotlikoff, M. I., Stimulatory and inhibitory regulation of calcium-activated potassium channels by guanine nucleotide-binding proteins, *Proc. Natl. Acad. Sci. U.S.A.*, 89, 11051, 1992.

109. Snetkov, V. A., Hirst, S. J., Twort, C. H. C., and Ward, J. P. T., Potassium currents in human freshly isolated bronchial smooth muscle cells, *Br. J. Pharmacol.*, 115, 1117-1125, 1995.

110. Boyle, J. P., Tomasic, M., and Kotlikoff, M. I., Delayed rectifier potassium channels in canine and porcine airway smooth muscle cells, *J. Physiol.*, 447, 329, 1992.

111. Murray, M. A., Berry, J. L., Cook, S. J., Foster, R. W., Green, K. A., and Small, R. C., Guinea-pig isolated trachealis: the effects of charybdotoxin on mechanical activity, membrane potential changes and the activity of plasmalemmal K⁺-channels, *Br. J. Pharmacol.*, 103, 1814, 1991.

112. Gimenez-Gallego, G., Navia, M. A., Reuben, J. P., Katz, G. M., Kaczorowski, G. J., and Garcia, M. L., Purification, sequence and model structure of charybdotoxin, a potent selective inhibitor of calcium-activated potassium channels, *Proc. Natl. Acad. Sci. U.S.A.*, 85, 3329, 1988.

113. Anderson, C. S., MacKinnon, R., Smith, C., and Miller, C., Charybdotoxin block of single Ca⁺⁺-activated K⁺ channels. Effects of channel gating, voltage and ionic strength, *J. Gen. Physiol.*, 91, 317, 1988.

114. Sadoshima, J.-I., Akaike, N., Kanide, H., and Nakamura, M., Cyclic AMP modulates Ca-activated K channel in cultured smooth muscle cells of rat aortas, *Am. J. Physiol.*, 255, H754, 1988.

115. Yatani, A., Codina, J., Imoto, Y., Reeves, J. P., Birnbaumer, L., and Brown, A. M., A G protein directly regulates mammalian cardiac calcium channels, *Science*, 238, 1288, 1987.

116. Yatani, A., Imoto, Y., Codina, J., Hamilton, S. L., Brown, A. M., and Birnbaumer, L., The stimulatory G protein of adenylyl cyclase, Gₛ, also stimulates dihydropyridine-sensitive Ca²⁺ channels. Evidence for direct regulation independent of phosphorylation by cAMP-dependent protein kinase or stimulation by a dihydropyridine agonist, *J. Biol. Chem.*, 263, 9887, 1988.

117. Kume, H., Hall, I. P., Washabau, R. J., Takagi, K., and Kotlikoff, M. I., β-Adrenergic agonists regulate $K_{Ca}$ channels in airway smooth muscle by cAMP-dependent and -independent mechanisms, *J. Clin. Invest.*, 93, 371, 1994.

118. Cook, S. J., Small, R. C., Berry, J. L., Chiu, P., Downing, S. J., and Foster, R. W., β-Adrenoceptor subtypes and the opening of plasmalemmal K⁺-channels in trachealis muscle: electrophysiological and mechanical studies in guinea-pig tissue, *Br. J. Pharmacol.*, 109, 1140, 1993.

119. Chiu, P., Cook, S. J., Small, R. C., Berry, J. L., Carpenter, J. R., Downing, S. J., Foster, R. W., Miller, A. J., and Small, A. M., β-Adrenoceptor subtypes and the opening of plasmalemmal K⁺-channels in bovine trachealis muscle: studies of mechanical activity and ion fluxes, *Br. J. Pharmacol.*, 109, 1149, 1993.

120. Cieslinski, L. B., Reeves, M. L., and Torphy, T. J., Cyclic nucleotide phosphodiesterases (PDEs) in canine and human tracheal smooth muscle, *FASEB J.*, 2, A1065, 1988.

121. Giembycz, M. A., Belvisi, M. G., Miura, M., Peters, M. J., Yacoub, M., and Barnes, P. J., Cyclic nucleotide phosphodiesterases in human trachealis and the mechanical effect of isoenzyme-selective inhibitors, *Am. Rev. Respir. Dis.*, 145, A378, 1992.

122. Shahid, M., Philpott, A. J., de Boer, J., Zaagsma, J., and Nicholson, C. D., Cyclic nucleotide phosphodiesterase (PDE) isozyme activities in human peripheral bronchi, *Br. J. Pharmacol.*, 105 (Suppl.), 129P, 1991.

123. Torphy, T. J., Undem, B. J., Cieslinski, L. B., Luttmann, M. A., Reeves, M. L., and Hay, D. W. P., Identification, characterization and functional role of phosphodiesterase isozymes in human airway smooth muscle, *J. Pharmacol. Exp. Ther.*, 265, 1213, 1993.

124. Beavo, J. A., Conti, M., and Heaslip, R. J., Multiple cyclic nucleotide phosphodiesterases, *Mol. Pharmacol.*, 46, 399, 1994.

125. Reeves, M. L., Leigh, B. K., and England, P. K., The identification of a new cyclic phosphodiesterase activity in human and guinea-pig cardiac ventricle, *Biochem. J.*, 241, 535, 1987.

126. Giembycz, M. A. and Barnes, P. J., Selective inhibition of a high affinity type IV cyclic AMP phosphodiesterase in bovine trachealis by AH 21-132. Relevance to the spasmolytic and anti-spasmogenic actions of an AH 21-132 in the intact tissue, *Biochem. Pharmacol.*, 42, 663, 1991.

127. Shahid, M., van Amsterdam, R. G. M., de Boer, J., ten Berge, R. E., Nicholson, C. D., and Zaagsma, J., The presence of five cyclic nucleotide phosphodiesterase isoenzyme activities in bovine tracheal smooth muscle and the functional effects of selective inhibitors, *Br. J. Pharmacol.*, 104, 471, 1991.

128. Tomlinson, P. R., Wilson, J. W., and Stewart, A. G., Salbutamol inhibits the proliferation of human airway smooth muscle cells grown in culture: relationship to elevated cAMP levels, *Biochem. Pharmacol.*, 49, 1809, 1995.

129. Panettieri, R. A., Yadvish, P. A., Kelly, A. M., Rubinstein, N. A., and Kotlikoff, M. I., Histamine stimulates proliferation of airway smooth muscle and induces *c-fos* expression, *Am. J. Physiol.*, 259, L365, 1990.

130. Young, P. G., Skinner, S. J. M., and Black, P. N., Effects of glucocorticoids and b-adrenoceptor agonists on the proliferation of airway smooth muscle, *Eur. J. Pharmacol.*, 273, 137, 1995.

131. Stewart, A. G., Grigoriadis, G., Yeoh, S.-M., and Harris, T. Control of airways smooth muscle proliferation — novel targets for anti-asthma drugs, in *Airway Hyperresponsiveness and Asthma: An Update.* IBC Technical Services Ltd., London, 1992.

132. Noveral, J. P. and Grunstein, M. M., Adrenergic receptor-mediated regulation of cultured rabbit airway smooth muscle cell proliferation, *Am. J. Physiol.*, 267, L291, 1994.

133. Lew, D. B., Nebigil, C., and Malik, K. U., Dual regulation by cAMP of β-hexosaminidase-induced mitogenesis in bovine tracheal myocytes, *Am. J. Respir. Cell Mol. Biol.*, 7, 614, 1992.

134. Dumont, J. E., Jauniaux, J.-C., and Roger, P. P., The cyclic AMP-mediated stimulation of cell proliferation, *Trends Biochem. Sci.*, 14, 67, 1989.

135. Ghosh, T. K., Bian, J., Short, A. D., Rybak, S. L., and Gill, D. L., Persistent intracellular calcium pool depletion by thapsigargin and its influence on cell growth, *J. Biol. Chem.*, 266, 24690, 1991.

136. Mueller, E. and van Breeman, C., Role of intracellular $Ca^{2+}$ sequestration in β-adrenergic relaxation of a smooth muscle, *Nature*, 281, 682, 1979.

137. Assender, J. W., Southgate, K. M., Hallett, M. B., and Newby, A. C., Inhibition of proliferation, but not of $Ca^{2+}$ mobilization, by cyclic AMP and GMP in rabbit aortic smooth-muscle cells, *Biochem. J.*, 288, 527, 1992.

138. Hall, I. P., Donaldson, J., and Hill, S. J., Inhibition of histamine-stimulated inositol phospholipid hydrolysis by agents which increase cyclic AMP levels in bovine tracheal smooth muscle, *Br. J. Pharmacol.*, 97, 603, 1989.

139. Stewart, A. G., Grigoriadis, G., and Harris, T., Mitogenic actions of endothelin-1 and epidermal growth factor in cultured airway smooth muscle, *Clin. Exp. Pharmacol. Physiol.*, 21, 277, 1994.

140. Johnson, P. R. A., Armour, C. L., Carey, D., and Black, J. L., Heparin and $PGE_2$ inhibit DNA synthesis in human airway smooth muscle cells in culture, *Am. J. Phsyiol.*, 269, L514, 1995.

141. Maruno, K., Absood, A., and Said, S. I., VIP inhibits basal and histamine-stimulated proliferation of human airway smooth muscle cells, *Am. J. Phsyiol.*, 268, L1047, 1995.

142. Panettieri, R. A., Cohen, M. D., and Bilgen, G., Airway smooth muscle cell proliferation is inhibited by microinjection of the catalytic subunit of cAMP dependent protein kinase, *Am. Rev. Respir. Dis.*, 147, A252, 1993.

143. Krontiris, T. G., Oncogenes, *N. Engl. J. Med.*, 333, 303, 1995.

144. Roussel, M. F., Theodoras, A. M., Pagano, M., and Sherr, C. J., Rescue of defective mitogenic signalling by D-type cyclins, *Proc. Natl. Acad. Sci. U.S.A.*, 92, 6837, 1995.

145. Cook, S. J. and McCormick, F., Inhibition by cAMP of Ras-dependent activation of Raf, *Science*, 262, 1069, 1993.

146. Wu, J., Dent, P., Jelinek, T., Wolfman, A., Weber, M. J., and Sturgill, T. W., Inhibition of the EGF-activated MAP kinase signaling pathway by adenosine 3′,5′-monophosphate, *Science*, 262, 1065, 1993.

147. Nordheim, A., CREB takes CBP to tango, *Nature*, 370, 177, 1994.

148. Chrivia, J. C., Kwok, R. P. S., Lamb, N., Hagiwara, M., Montminy, M. R., and Goodman, R. H., Phosphorylated CREB binds specifically to the nuclear protein CBP, *Nature*, 365, 855, 1993.

149. Arias, J., Alberts, A. S., Brindle, P., Claret, F. X., Smeal, T., Karin, M., Feramisco, J., and Montminy, M., Activation of cAMP responsive genes relies on a common nuclear factor, *Nature*, 370, 226, 1994.

150. Stewart, A. G., Fernandes, D., and Tomlinson, P. R., The effect of glucocorticoids on proliferation of human cultured airway smooth muscle, *Br. J. Pharmacol.*, 116, 3219, 1995.

151. Sherr, C. J., G1 phase progression: cycling on cue, *Cell*, 79, 551, 1994.

152. Matsushime, H., Roussel, M. F., Ashmun, R. A., and Sherr, C. J., Colony-stimulating factor 1 regulates novel cyclins during the G1 phase of the cell cycle, *Cell*, 65, 701, 1991.

153. Lew, D. J., Dulic, V., and Reed, S. I., Isolation of three novel human cyclins by rescue of G1 cyclin (Cln) function in yeast, *Cell*, 66, 1197, 1991.

154. Draetta, G. F., Mammalian G1 cyclins, *Curr. Opin. Cell Biol.*, 6, 842, 1994.

155. Koff, A., Cross, F., Fisher, A., Schumacher, J., Leguellec, K., Phillippe, M., and Roberts, J. M., Human cyclin E, a new cyclin that interacts with two members of the *CDC2* gene family, *Cell*, 66, 1217, 1991.

156. Quelle, D. E., Ashmun, R. A., Shurtleff, S. A., Kato, J.-Y., Bar-Sagi, D., Roussel, M. F., and Sherr, C. J., Overexpression of mouse D-type cyclins accelerates G1 phase in rodent fibroblasts, *Genes Dev.*, 7, 1559, 1993.

157. Ohtsubo, M. and Roberts, J. M., Cyclin-dependent regulation of G1 in mammalian fibroblasts, *Science*, 259, 1908, 1993.

158. Baldin, V., Lukas, J., Marcote, M. J., Pagano, M., and Draetta, G., Cyclin D1 is a nuclear protein required for cell cycle progression in G1, *Genes Dev.*, 7, 812, 1993.
159. Pagano, M., Theodoras, A. M., Tam, S. W., and Draetta, G., Cyclin D1-mediated inhibition of repair and replicative DNA synthesis in human fibroblasts, *Genes Dev.*, 8, 1627, 1994.
160. Matsushime, H., Quelle, D. E., Shurtleff, S. A., Shibuya, M., Sherr, C. J., and Kato, J.-Y., D-type cyclin-dependent kinase activity in mammalian cells, *Mol. Cell. Biol.*, 14, 2066, 1994.
161. Meyerson, M. and Harlow, E., Identification of G1 kinase activity for cdk6, a novel cyclin D partner, *Mol. Cell. Biol.*, 14, 2077, 1994.
162. Bates, S., Bonetta, L., MacAllan, D., Parry, D., Holder, A., Dickson, C., and Peters, G., Cdk6 (PLSTIRE) and cdk4 (PSK-J3) are distinct subsets of the cyclin-dependent kinases that associate with cyclin D1, *Oncogene*, 9, 71, 1994.
163. Dulic, V., Lees, E., and Reed, S. I., Association of human cyclin E with a periodic G1–S phase protein kinase, *Science*, 257, 1959, 1992.
164. Koff, A., Giordano, A., Desai, D., Yamashita, K., Harper, J. W., Elledge, S., Nishimoto, T., Morgan, D. O., Franza, B. R., and Roberts, J. M., Formation and activation of a cyclin E–cdk2 complex during the G1 phase of the human cell cycle, *Science*, 257, 1689, 1992.
165. Morgan, D. O., Principles of CDK regulation, *Nature*, 374, 131, 1995.
166. Matsuoka, M., Kato, J.-Y., Fisher, R. P., Morgan, D. O., and Sherr, C. J., Activation of cyclin-dependent kinase 4 (cdk4) by mouse MO15-associated kinase, *Mol. Cell. Biol.*, 14, 7265, 1994.
167. Fisher, R. P. and Morgan, D. O., A novel cyclin associates with MO15/CDK7 to form the CDK-activating kinase, *Cell*, 78, 713, 1994.
168. Pagano, M., Pepperkok, R., Lukas, J., Baldin, V., Ansorge, W., Bartek, J., and Draetta, G., Regulation of the cell cycle by the cdk2 protein kinase in cultured human fibroblasts, *J. Cell Biol.*, 121, 101, 1993.
169. Tsai, L.-H., Lees, E., Faha, B., Harlow, E., and Riabowol, K., The cdk2 kinase is required for G1-to-S transition in mammalian cells, *Oncogene*, 8, 1593, 1993.
170. van der Heuvel, S. and Harlow, E., Distinct roles for cyclin-dependent kinases in cell cycle control, *Science*, 262, 2050, 1993.
171. Dowdy, S. F., Hinds, P. W., Louie, K., Reed, S. I., Arnold, A., and Weinberg, R. A., Physical interaction of the retinoblastoma protein with human D cyclins, *Cell*, 73, 499, 1993.
172. Ewen, M. E., Sluss, H. K., Sherr, C. J., Matsushime, H., Kato, J.-Y., and Livingston, D. M., Functional interactions of the retinoblastoma protein with mammalian D-type cyclins, *Cell*, 73, 487, 1993.
173. Kato, J.-Y., Matsushime, H., Hiebert, S. W., Ewen, M. E., and Sherr, C. J., Direct binding of cyclin D to the retinoblastoma gene product (pRb) and pRb phosphorylation by the cyclin D-dependent kinase CDK4, *Genes Dev.*, 7, 331, 1993.
174. Resnitzky, D., Gossen, M., Bujard, H., and Reed, S. I., Acceleration of the G1/S phase transition by expression of cyclins D1 and E with an inducible system, *Mol. Cell. Biol.*, 14, 1669, 1994.
175. Hiebert, S. W., Chellappan, S. P., Horowitz, J. M., and Nevins, J. R., The interaction of RB with E2F coincides with an inhibition of the transcriptional activity of E2F, *Genes Dev.*, 6, 177, 1992.
176. Chellappan, S. P., Hiebert, S., Mudryi, M., Horowitz, J. M., and Nevins, J. R., The E2F transcription factor is a cellular target for the RB protein, *Cell*, 65, 1053, 1991.
177. Helin, K., Lees, J. A., Vidal, M., Dyson, N., Harlow, E., and Fattaey, A., A cDNA encoding a pRB-binding protein with properties of the transcription factor E2F, *Cell*, 70, 337, 1992.
178. Kaelin, W. G., Krek, W., Sellers, W. R., DeCaprio, J. A., Ajchenbaum, F., Fuchs, C. S., Chittenden, T., Li, Y., Farnham, P. J., Blanar, M. A., Livingston, D. M., and Flemington, E. K., Expression cloning of a cDNA encoding a retinoblastoma-binding protein with E2F-like properties, *Cell*, 70, 351, 1992.

179. Shirodkar, S., Ewen, M., DeCaprio, J. A., Morgan, J., Livingston, D. M., and Chittenden, T., The transcription factor E2F interacts with the retinoblastoma product and a p107–cyclin A complex in a cell cycle-regulated manner, *Cell*, 68, 157, 1992.

180. Lukas, J., Muller, H., Bartkova, J., Spitkovsky, D., Kjerulff, A. A., Jansen-Durr, P., Strauss, M., and Bartek, J., DNA tumor virus oncoproteins and retinoblastoma gene mutations share the ability to relieve the cell's requirement for cyclin D1 function in G1, *J. Cell Biol.*, 125, 625, 1994.

181. Tam, S. W., Theodoras, A. M., Shay, J. W., Draetta, G. F., and Pagano, M., Differential expression and regulation of cyclin D1 protein in normal and tumor human cells: association with Cdk4 is required for cyclin D1 function in G1 progression, *Oncogene*, 9, 2663, 1994.

182. Kovesdi, I., Reichel, R., and Nevins, J. R., Identification of a cellular transcription factor involved in E1A *trans*-activation, *Cell*, 45, 219, 1986.

183. La Thangue, N. B. and Rigby, P. W. J., An adenovirus E1A-like transcription factor is regulated during the differentiation of murine embryonal carcinoma stem cells, *Cell*, 49, 507, 1987.

184. Muller, R., Transcriptional regulation during the mammalian cell cycle, *Trends Genet.*, 11, 173, 1995.

185. Bandara, L. R., Buck, V. M., Zamanian, M., Johnston, L. H., and La Thangue, N. B., Functional synergy between DP-1 and E2F-1 in the cell cycle-regulating transcription factor DRTF1/E2F, *EMBO J.*, 12, 4317, 1993.

186. Helin, K., Wu, C.-L., Fattaey, A. R., Lees, J. A., Dynlacht, B. D., Ngwu, C., and Harlow, E., Heterodimerization of the transcription factors E2F-1 and DP-1 leads to cooperative *trans*-activation, *Genes Dev.*, 7, 1850, 1993.

187. Krek, W., Livingston, D. M., and Shirodkar, S., Binding to DNA and the retinoblastoma gene product promoted by complex formation of different E2F family members, *Science*, 262, 1557, 1993.

188. Bandara, L. R., Lam, E. W.-F., Sorensen, T. S., Zamanian, M., Girling, R., and La Thangue, N. B., DP-1: a cell cycle-regulated and phosphorylated component of transcription factor DRTF1/E2F which is functionally important for recognition by pRb and the adenovirus E4 orf 6/7 protein, *EMBO J.*, 13, 3104, 1994.

189. Zhu, L., van der Heuvel, S., Helin, K., Fattaey, A., Ewen, M., Livingston, D., Dyson, N., and Harlow, E., Inhibition of cell proliferation by p107, a relative of the retinoblastoma protein, *Genes Dev.*, 7, 1111, 1993.

190. Johnson, D. G., Schwarz, J. K., Cress, W. D., and Nevins, J. R., Expression of transcription factor E2F1 induces quiescent cells to enter S phase, *Nature*, 365, 349, 1993.

191. Beijersbergen, R. L., Kerkhoven, R. M., Zhu, L., Carlee, L., Voorhoeve, P. M., and Bernards, R., E2F-4, a new member of the E2F gene family, has oncogenic activity and associates with p107 *in vivo*, *Genes Dev.*, 8, 2680, 1994.

192. Jooss, K., Lam, E. W.-F., Bybee, A., Girling, R., Muller, R., and La Thangue, N. B., Proto-oncogenic properties of the DP family of proteins, *Oncogene*, 10, 1529, 1995.

193. Chen, L. I., Nishinaka, T., Kwan, K., Kitabayashi, I., Yokoyama, K., Fu, Y.-H. F., Grunwald, S., and Chiu, R., The retinoblastoma gene product RB stimulates Sp1-mediated transcription by liberating Sp1 from a negative regulator, *Mol. Cell Biol.*, 14, 4380, 1994.

194. Fagan, R., Flint, K. J., and Jones, N., Phosphorylation of E2F-1 modulates its interaction with the retinoblastoma gene product and the adenoviral E4 19 kDa protein, *Cell*, 78, 799, 1994.

195. Schwarz, J. K., Devoto, S. H., Smith, E. J., Chellappan, S. P., Jakoi, L., and Nevins, J. R., Interactions of the p107 and Rb proteins with E2F during the cell proliferation response, *EMBO J.*, 12, 1013, 1993.

196. Johnson, D. G., Ohtani, K., and Nevins, J. R., Autoregulatory control of *E2F1* expression in response to positive and negative regulators of cell cycle progression, *Genes Dev.*, 8, 1514, 1994.

197. Hsiao, K.-M., McMahon, S. L., and Farnham, P. J., Multiple DNA elements are required for the growth regulation of the mouse *E2F1* promoter, *Genes Dev.*, 8, 1526, 1994.

198. Massague, J. and Polyak, K., Mammalian antiproliferative signals and their targets, *Curr. Opin. Genet. Dev.*, 5, 91, 1995.

199. Ewen, M. E., Sluss, H. K., Whitehouse, L. L., and Livingston, D. M., TGFβ inhibition of cdk4 synthesis is linked to cell cycle arrest, *Cell*, 74, 1009, 1993.

200. Cocks, B. G., Vairo, G., Bodrug, S. E., and Hamilton, J. A., Suppression of growth factor-induced CYL1 cyclin gene expression by antiproliferative agents, *J. Biol. Chem.*, 267, 12307, 1992.

201. Albers, M. W., Williams, R. T., Brown, E. J., Tanaka, A., Halt, F. L., and Schreiber, S. L., FKBP-rapamycin inhibits a cyclin-dependent kinase activity and a cyclin D1–cdk association in early G1 of osteosarcoma cell line, *J. Biol. Chem.*, 268, 22825, 1993.

202. Geng, Y. and Weinberg, R. A., Transforming growth factor β effects on expression of G1 cyclins and cyclin-dependent protein kinases, *Proc. Natl. Acad. Sci. U.S.A.*, 90, 10315, 1993.

203. Morice, W. G., Wiederrecht, G., Brunn, G. J., Siekierka, J. J., and Abraham, R. T., Rapamycin inhibition of interleukin-2-dependent p33$^{cdk2}$ and p34$^{cdk2}$ kinase activation in T lymphocytes, *J. Biol. Chem.*, 268, 22737, 1993.

204. Slingerland, J. M., Hengst, L., Pan, C.-H., Alexander, D., Stampfer, M. R., and Reed, S. I., A novel inhibitor of cyclin–cdk activity detected in transforming growth factor β-arrested epithelial cells, *Mol. Cell. Biol.*, 14, 3683, 1994.

205. Polyak, K., Kato, J.-Y., Solomon, M. J., Sherr, C. J., Massague, J., Roberts, J. M., and Koff, A., p27$^{Kip1}$, a cyclin–Cdk inhibitor, links transforming growth factor-β and contact inhibition to cell cycle arrest, *Genes Dev.*, 8, 9, 1994.

206. Polyak, K., Lee, M.-H., Erdjument-Bromage, H., Koff, A., Roberts, J. M., Tempst, P., and Massague, J., Cloning of p27$^{Kip1}$, a cyclin-dependent kinase inhibitor and a potential mediator of extracellular antimitogen signals, *Cell*, 78, 59, 1994.

207. Harper, J. W., Adam, G. R., Wei, N., Keyomars, K., and Elledge, S. J., The p21 cdk-interacting protein Cip1 is a potent inhibitor of G1 cyclin-dependent kinases, *Cell*, 75, 805, 1993.

208. El-Deiry, W. S., Tokino, T., Velculescu, V. E., Levy, D. B., Parsons, R., Trent, J. M., Lin, D., Mercer, W. E., Kinzler, K. W., and Vogelstein, B., *WAF1*, a potential mediator of p53 tumor suppression, *Cell*, 75, 817, 1993.

209. Hannon, G. J. and Beach, D., p15$^{INK4B}$ is a potential effector of TGF-β-induced cell cycle arrest, *Nature*, 371, 257, 1994.

210. Serrano, M., Hannon, G. J., and Beach, D., A new regulatory motif in cell-cycle control causing specific inhibition of cyclin D/cdk4, *Nature*, 366, 704, 1993.

211. Xiong, Y., Hannon, G. J., Zhang, H., Casso, D., Kobayashi, R., and Beach, D., p21 is a universal inhibitor of cyclin kinases, *Nature*, 366, 701, 1993.

212. Bates, S., Parry, D., Bonetta, L., Vousden, K., Dickson, C., and Peters, G., Absence of cyclin D/cdk complexes in cells lacking functional retinoblastoma protein, *Oncogene*, 9, 1633, 1994.

213. Kato, J.-Y., Matsuoka, M., Polyak, K., Massague, J., and Sherr, C. J., Cyclic AMP-induced G1 phase arrest mediated by an inhibitor (p27$^{Kip1}$) of cyclin-dependent kinase 4 activation, *Cell*, 79, 487, 1994.

214. Fripo, E. J., Koff, A., Solomon, M. J., and Roberts, J. M., Inactivation of a cdk2 inhibitor during interleukin 2-induced proliferation of human T lymphocytes, *Mol. Cell. Biol.*, 14, 4889, 1994.

215. Nourse, J., Fripo, E., Flanagan, W. M., Coats, S., Polyak, K., Lee, M.-H., Massague, J., Crabtree, G. R., and Roberts, J. M., Interleukin-2-mediated elimination of the p27$^{Kip1}$ cyclin-dependent kinase inhibitor prevented by rapamycin, *Nature*, 372, 570, 1994.

216. Lees, E., Faha, B., Dulic, V., Reed, S. I., and Harlow, E., Cyclin E/cdk2 and cyclin A/cdk2 kinases associate with p107 and E2F in a temporally distinct manner, *Genes Dev.*, 6, 1874, 1992.

217. Krek, W., Ewen, M. E., Shirodkar, S., Arany, Z., Kaelin, W. G., and Livingston, D. M., Negative regulation of the growth-promoting transcription factor E2F-1 by a stably bound cyclin A-dependent protein kinase, *Cell*, 78, 161, 1994.
218. Schwob, E., Bohm, T., Mendenhall, M. D., and Nasmyth, K., The B-type cyclin kinase inhibitor p40$^{SIC1}$ controls the G1 to S transition in S. cerevisiae, *Cell*, 79, 233, 1994.
219. Nash, R., Tokiwa, G., Anand, S., Erickson, K., and Futcher, A. B., The *WHI1+* gene of *Saccharomyces cerevisiae* tethers cell division to cell size and is a cyclin homolog, *EMBO J.*, 7, 4335, 1988.
220. Strader, C. D., Sigal, I. S., Register, R. B., Candelore, M. R., Rands, E., and Dixon, R. A. F., Identification of residues required for ligand binding to the β-adrenergic receptor, *Proc. Natl. Acad. Sci. U.S.A.*, 84, 4384, 1987.
221. Strader, C. D., Candelore, M. R., Hill, W. S., Sigal, I. S., and Dixon, R. A. F., Identification of two serine residues involved in agonist activation of the β-adrenergic receptor, *J. Biol. Chem.*, 264, 13572, 1989.
222. Fraser, C. M., Chung, F.-Z., Wang, C.-D., and Venter, J. C., Site-directed mutagenesis of human β-adrenergic receptors: substitution of aspartic acid-130 by asparagine produces a receptor with high-affinity agonist binding that is uncoupled from adenylate cyclase, *Proc. Natl. Acad. Sci. U.S.A.*, 85, 5478, 1988.
223. Strader, C. D., Dixon, R. A. F., Cheung, A. H., Canderlore, M. R., Blake, A. D., and Sigal, I. S., Mutations that uncouple the β-adrenergic receptor from G$_s$ and increase agonist affinity, *J. Biol. Chem.*, 262, 16439, 1987.
224. Liggett, S. B., Caron, M. G., Lefkowitz, R. J., and Hnatowich, M., Coupling of a mutated form of the human β$_2$-adrenergic receptor to G$_i$ and G$_s$. Requirement for multiple cytoplasmic domains in the coupling process, *J. Biol. Chem.*, 266, 4816, 1991.

# INDEX

## A

Printed and bound by CPI Group (UK) Ltd, Croydon, CR0 4YY

17/10/2024

01775690-0015